De-Medicalizing Misery

Psychiatry, Psychology and the Human Condition

Edited by

Mark Rapley
University of East London, UK

Joanna Moncrieff
University College London, UK

Jacqui Dillon
Hearing Voices Network, Sheffield, UK

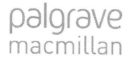

First published 2011 by
PALGRAVE MACMILLAN

Palgrave Macmillan in the UK is an imprint of Macmillan Publishers Limited, registered in England, company number 785998, of Houndmills, Basingstoke, Hampshire RG21 6XS.

Palgrave Macmillan in the US is a division of St Martin's Press LLC, 175 Fifth Avenue, New York, NY 10010.

Palgrave Macmillan is the global academic imprint of the above companies and has companies and representatives throughout the world.

Palgrave® and Macmillan® are registered trademarks in the United States, the United Kingdom, Europe and other countries.

ISBN 978–0–230–24271–5   hardback
ISBN 978–0–230–30791–9   paperback

This book is printed on paper suitable for recycling and made from fully managed and sustained forest sources. Logging, pulping and manufacturing processes are expected to conform to the environmental regulations of the country of origin.

A catalogue record for this book is available from the British Library.

A catalog record for this book is available from the Library of Congress.

Printed and bound in Great Britain by
CPI Antony Rowe, Chippenham and Eastbourne

Contents

v

Preface

Rudi Dallos

Occasionally I come across a book that is both inspiring and discomfiting. This book reveals that, in fact, both feelings are necessary. I have recently written about how, with the much lauded contemporary emphasis on reflective practice, we need to include a 'complacency monitor' to help us think about our clinical practice. This book is a valuable addition to what we might usefully keep at our desk, bedside or even in our holiday reading, in a pile called 'Books to Monitor Complacency'.

De-Medicalizing Misery offers a rich array of ideas. It offers an historical, political and philosophical summary, analysis and critique of the assumptions and practices of the psy professions, including clinical psychology. Historical accounts can be fascinating but they can also be dismissed with the comforting statement that 'yes but it isn't like that now ... we live in more enlightened times'. Alongside this runs the common wish to kill the messenger. But the messengers in this book deserve to live and to write another day. A major contribution of the book is that the historical is linked to the contemporary, and in fact it is argued forcefully that it is mistaken to assume that we have simply transcended some of the more clearly barbaric practices of psychiatry, such as electro-convulsive shock therapy, lobotomy and drug treatment in modern approaches to clinical psychology, psychotherapy and psychiatry. We are reminded that most of the psycho-therapies and their implementation in the NHS, especially in the form of time-limited, 'quick fix' applications, are fundamentally based in the medical model, for example in the use of DSM-based diagnosis in driving the selection of evidence-based models of therapy.

To reiterate, this book is not a comfortable read. My personal wish would be to avoid some uncomfortable ideas about how we may, by our presence and participation in multi-disciplinary teams, be implicitly condoning compulsory treatment, medication and confinement. Though ideologically we may claim to disagree with such practice it is argued we are made culpable by association. As I felt myself writhing at this realization I became all the more uncomfortable as I read Jacqui Dillon's account of her experience of childhood sexual abuse and the subsequent medicalization of her experience by the 'caring' professions. As well as feeling moved by the quiet dignity of her account, I was also shaken to think again about the many people who even more quietly put up with being labelled and medicated. I have experience in my own family with my two half-brothers – even now in my high status position as a Professor of Clinical Psychology I have witnessed my suggestion that their so-called schizophrenia may be related to experiences of abuse and emotional damage in their childhoods being politely tolerated but then ignored. I can understand why it so easy to slip into medicalizing because, to be honest, I have found my brothers at times to be incredibly difficult, a strain and even infuriating. I too have sometimes wanted a quick answer and a quick fix to their troubled and troublesome states. But deep down, like many family members, I wanted professionals to understand our lives and traumas and help them and us to find support, and work – to help build a life for them, not just offer a slow death through medication.

As someone who has both experienced significant problems in my own family and also worked with families in the practice of 'family therapy', I was delighted to see the extensive discussion of the family's role in the causation of mental illness. In their chapter, Carlton Coulter and Mark Rapley get to the heart of some of the core issues regarding 'mental illness': in a succinct passage they state that 'being in some way responsible for an outcome does not, inevitably and necessarily, imply the intent to cause'. In my experience with families many do indeed hold themselves responsible but struggle with exactly this dilemma, that the distress experienced by their child was not what they had intended. What I often find is that their intentions had been to do things 'better' than had been the often miserable, painful and shameful experience of their own childhoods. They/we had so much wanted things to be different. As this book makes clear, helping parents to 'do it better' is not simply, or even predominantly, about clinical intervention, parent education or training. It is also about helping to reveal and to resist the madness-making paradoxes and practices of the mental health professions, and in turn to show how these are shaped and maintained by wider regimes of societally based inequality and oppression.

Like the authors of the chapters in this book I am very sympathetic to the constraints of professionals working in the NHS and social care systems. But even if well intentioned, we also need to feel uncomfortable and, hopefully, provoked to make changes in how we see people such as Jacqui. Her account, and the other chapters in this book, clarify that the transformation required is so much more than well-meaning attempts at the empowerment of families. If professionals like me can so easily be ignored by the medical professions what hope for many who are less privileged?

Acknowledgements

This book arose from a series of conferences co-convened by the School of Psychology at the University of East London, the Critical Psychiatry Network and the Hearing Voices Network. We are grateful to all of these organizations for their support, and particularly to Sue Meade at UEL for all her hard work as conference organiser.

Some chapters are reworks and updates of previously published work. Joanna Moncrieff's chapter is based on a paper entitled 'The creation of the concept of an antidepressant: An historical analysis' (Moncrieff, J. (2008), *Social Science and Medicine*, 66, 2346–55); Lucy Johnstone's chapter is based on her paper 'Can trauma cause "psychosis"? Revisiting another taboo subject. A critical overview of the recent literature' (Johnstone, L. (2007) *Journal of Critical Psychology, Counselling and Psychotherapy*, 7, 4, 211–20). David Smail's chapter is based on a talk originally given at Balliol College, Oxford, in May 1996. The second part of Sami Timimi's chapter is based on Timimi, S. (2009) 'The Use of Psycho-pharmaceuticals to Control Boys' Behaviour: A Tale of Badly Behaving Drug Companies and Doctors', *Arab Journal of Psychiatry*, 20, 2, 147–60. Jacqui Dillon's chapter is a revised version of a piece originally published as part of *Telling Stories? Attachment based approaches to the treatment of psychosis*, edited by Sarah Benamer, Karnac Books (2010). Irving Kirsch's chapter is an updating of Kirsch, I. (2009) 'Antidepressants and the placebo response', *Epidemiologia e Psichiatria Sociale*, 18, 318–22. We are also grateful to PCCS Books for permission to reproduce material from Romme, M., Escher, S., Dillon, J., Corstens, D. & Morris, M. (2009) *Living with Voices: 50 stories of recovery* (p. 119) in her chapter.

Other thanks are also due: Mark Rapley would like to thank Mary Boyle, John Clements, Craig Newnes and Alec McHoul for their enduring friendship and inspiration. For him, this book is for Ella. Joanna Moncrieff would like to thank the Wellcome Trust for funding her historical research on antidepressants, and Professor Virginia Berridge for supervising this work. Jacqui Dillon would like to thank Marius Romme and Sandra Escher for having the integrity to listen to, and learn from, those deemed to be 'lacking in insight' and Orit Badouk Epstein, a gifted therapist and exceptional human being, for everything. David Harper would like to thank Mary Boyle and Ian Parker for comments on an earlier version of his chapter. He also acknowledges Miles Mandelson and the Psychology Service at Whiston Hospital. Mersey Regional Health Authority provided funding (Small Grant No. 670) for part of the research informing his chapter.

Notes on Contributors

James Bourne is a recently qualified clinical psychologist. His chapter is based on genealogical research that he carried out while training on the UEL doctoral program in clinical psychology. He is currently working with children and families in London.

Mary Boyle is Professor Emeritus of Clinical Psychology at the University of East London, UK, where she was director of the doctoral programme in clinical psychology until 2006. She has published widely in the areas of critical and feminist psychology. Her work includes *Schizophrenia: A scientific delusion?* and *Rethinking Abortion: Psychology, gender, power and the law.*

Patrick Bracken is a consultant psychiatrist and Clinical Director of Mental Health Services in West Cork, Eire. He was formerly Professor of Philosophy, Diversity and Mental Health at the University of Central Lancashire and is now an International Fellow of the University. He coedited *Rethinking the Trauma of War* with Dr Celia Petty in 1998. His own book *Trauma: Culture, meaning and philosophy* was published in 2002. With his colleague, Professor Phil Thomas, he published *Postpsychiatry: Mental health in a postmodern world* in 2005.

Carlton Coulter is a clinical psychologist who lives and works in east London. He is particularly interested in commonsense understandings of distress, and the issues of power and ethics in therapy.

Rudi Dallos is Professor of Clinical Psychology and Programme Director of the Doctor of Clinical Psychology Training Programme, University of Plymouth, UK. Aside from his love of rock and blues guitar he is an associate editor of *Psychology and Psychotherapy*, coeditor of *Clinical Child Psychology and Psychiatry* and book reviews editor for the *Journal of Family Therapy*. In addition to numerous journal papers he is the author of *Attachment Narrative Therapy*; co-author with Arlene Vetere of *Research Methods in Psychotherapy* and, with Lucy Johnstone, of *Formulation in Psychotherapy*.

Jacqui Dillon is the Chair of the National Hearing Voices Network, England, a user led charity which works to promote acceptance and understanding of the experiences of hearing voices, seeing visions, tactile sensations and other sensory experiences. She is an international speaker and trainer specializing in hearing voices, 'psychosis' and trauma. Jacqui is also a member of the campaign coordinating committee for CASL – the Campaign to Abolish the Schizophrenia Label. With Professor Marius Romme and Dr Sandra Escher she is coeditor of *Recovered Voices: An Anthology of 50 Voice Hearers Stories of Recovery.*

Duncan Double is a consultant psychiatrist in Norfolk & Waveney Mental Health NHS Foundation Trust and Honorary Senior Lecturer at the University of East Anglia. He is a foundation member and the website editor of the Critical Psychiatry Network (www.criticalpsychiatry.co.uk). He is also editor of *Critical psychiatry: The limits of madness* (Palgrave Macmillan).

Suman Fernando was a consultant psychiatrist in Enfield for over 20 years and then an academic at the Tizard Centre, University of Kent at Canterbury, UK. He is involved in voluntary organisations serving black and minority ethnic (BME) communities in London and Sri Lanka and lectures on issues of race and culture in mental health in UK and Canada. He is Honorary Senior Lecturer in the European Centre for Migration and Social Care (MASC) at the University of Kent and Honorary Professor in the Department of Applied Social Studies, London Metropolitan University. His books include *Mental Health, Race and Culture* (2nd edition, 2002; *Cultural Diversity, Mental Health and Psychiatry: The struggle against racism,* (2003) and *Mental Health in a Multi-ethnic Society* (1995). His website is at http://www.sumanfernando.com/

David J. Harper is Reader in Clinical Psychology at the University of East London, UK. His research interests are in critical psychology and social constructionist approaches in mental health, particularly in relation to psychosis. He works one session a week as a consultant clinical psychologist for East London NHS Foundation Trust.

Lucy Johnstone is a clinical psychologist and counselling psychologist, and formerly Programme Director of the Bristol Clinical Psychology Doctorate, UK. She has worked in adult mental health settings for a number of years, and has a particular interest in the more severe forms of mental distress. She is the author of *Users and Abusers of Psychiatry,* and with Rudi Dallos coeditor of *Formulation in Psychology and Psychotherapy: Making sense of people's problems,* as well as a number of other articles and chapters taking a critical perspective on traditional psychiatric practice.

Irving Kirsch is Professor of Psychology at the University of Hull, UK. His meta-analyses of antidepressant medication efficacy studies have been covered widely in the media. His research is focused on suggestion, with particular attention to placebo effects and hypnosis.

Joanna Moncrieff is Senior Lecturer in the Department of Mental Health Sciences at University College London and a practising consultant psychiatrist at the North East London Foundation Trust, UK. She has spent her academic career reevaluating the nature and efficacy of psychiatric drugs and exploring the history and politics of psychiatry. She is the co-chair of the Critical Psychiatry Network, and has campaigned against the dominance of the biomedical approach to psychiatry, the extension of psychiatric coercion and the influence of the pharmaceutical industry, in alliance with service user groups. She is the author of *The Myth of the Chemical Cure* (Palgrave Macmillan), *A Straight Talking Introduction to Psychiatric Drugs*, and numerous papers and book chapters.

Craig Newnes is a dad, gardener, an ex-Director of Psychological Therapies and a past-Chair of the BPS Psychotherapy Section, UK. He is editor of the *Journal of Critical Psychology, Counselling and Psychotherapy* and commissioning editor for the Critical Division of PCCS Books. His latest book is *Making and Breaking Children's Lives*. In 2005 received the CCHR Human Rights Award for speaking out about the Psy-complex. Nowadays he tires easily.

Nimisha Patel is Reader in Clinical Psychology on the Doctoral Degree Programme in Clinical Psychology, University of East London, UK and Lead Consultant Clinical Psychologist and Head of Audit, Evaluation and Research at the Medical Foundation for the Care of Victims of Torture.

Mark Rapley is Professor of Clinical Psychology at the University of East London, UK. He is the author of *The Social Construction of Intellectual Disability, Quality of Life Research* and, with Susan Hansen and Alec McHoul, *Beyond Help*. He lives in London, but wishes he didn't.

David Smail has written a number of books on psychotherapy and psychology, most recently *Power, Interest and Psychology*. Now retired, he was for many years, head of clinical psychology services in Nottingham and Special Professor of Clinical Psychology at Nottingham University, UK. He has a website at www.davidsmail.info/

Ewen Speed is Lecturer in Medical Sociology in the Department of Health and Human Sciences at the University of Essex, UK. He has written about discourses of mental health (and mental illness) drawing particular attention to the potential for passive acceptance or active resistance that different discourses of mental health and illness can offer the service user.

Philip Thomas is a writer and Honorary Visiting Professor in the Department of Social Sciences and Humanities in the University of Bradford, UK. He worked as a consultant psychiatrist in the NHS for over 20 years, and left clinical practice in 2004 to focus on writing and academic work.

Sami Timimi is a consultant child-and-adolescent-psychiatrist in the National Health Service, UK and Visiting Professor of Child and Adolescent Psychiatry at the University of Lincoln, UK. He is the author or editor of several books including *Naughty Boys* (Palgrave Macmillan) and *Liberatory Psychiatry*.

Arlene Vetere is Professor of Clinical Psychology at Surrey University, UK and a UKCP registered systemic psychotherapist. She is current president of the European Family Therapy Association. Her latest book, with Rudi Dallos, is called *Systemic Therapy and Attachment Narratives: Applications across a range of diverse settings*.

1

Carving Nature at its Joints? DSM and the Medicalization of Everyday Life

Mark Rapley, Joanna Moncrieff and Jacqui Dillon

> There's a place in Freud where he says, 'with regard to matters of chemistry or physics or things like that, laymen would not venture an opinion. With regard to psychology it's quite different; anybody feels free to make psychological remarks'. And part of the business he thought he was engaged in was changing that around; that is, cojointly to develop psychology and educate laymen, so that laymen would know that they don't know anything about it and that there are people who do, so that they would eventually stop making psychological remarks.
>
> (Sacks, 1992: 217)

It is surely now apparent that after nearly 130 years of recognizably modern psychiatry and psychology (the 'disease' *Dementia Praecox* first appeared as a recognizable diagnosis in the fourth German edition of Emil Kraepelin's *Lehrbuch der Psychiatrie* in 1893 and William James published his *Principles of Psychology* in 1890), the enterprise is, to put it mildly, problematic. The architects of modern biological psychiatry have constructed a system that does little justice to the myriad problems it claims to address, while creating multiple iatrogenic problems for those to whom it is applied. Mainstream psychology likewise, while sometimes appearing to offer alternative approaches, essentially supports the positivist psychiatric project of codifying human suffering into disease-like categories. Yet, it would seem, more than a century of intensive psychiatric research has yet to find *any* form of organic grounding for the overwhelming majority of the 'mental disorders' listed in the DSM and psychology likewise has failed to provide any coherent alternative justification for this attempt to catalogue the 'problems of living' (Szasz, 1960: 115). As such we – along with many others, including parts of the popular media (Carey, 2010; Laurance, 2010) – are compelled to conclude that the effort to codify various forms of misery and disturbing conduct *as if* they were physical diseases, far from being another triumph of modern science – carving nature at its joints *a la* Linnæus or the periodic table (Mendeleev, 1901) – is, rather, best regarded as fiction or, more kindly, in Barthes' sense, as mythology.

But that mythology defines our present. It would seem that Sigmund's project (ably assisted by the pharmaceutical industry and the professions of psychiatry, clinical psychology and their associated partners in the psy-complex (Rose, 1996)) has been a spectacular success. Not in the way that he imagined, for sure, but resoundingly to the benefit of his professional heirs and successors: that is to say we inhabit a culture positively drowning in a cacophony of American Psychiatric Association-authorized 'psychological remarks' (Hansen, McHoul & Rapley, 2003).

In this book we draw together a range of contributors who, like us, take the view that the human costs of the medicalization of misery and madness outweigh any benefit that the metaphoric transformation of suffering into 'disease' may once have offered. With the impending arrival of DSM 5 (the future reach of which may be presaged by a presence on Twitter and Facebook – with 10,227 Facebook 'fans' as of 17 February 2011!) it is timely to ask whether there may be better ways to make sense of the range of human experiences we have come to know as 'mental disorders'.[1] The timeliness of this questioning is only enhanced by the ever-widening net of 'mental disorder' that the DSM seeks to cast over unhappiness, personal misfortune and troubling conduct. For example, the devoted website DSM5.org alerts us to the fact that the appropriate expert committee has now set out revised criteria for 'Reactive Attachment Disorder of Infancy and Early Childhood' (see Box 1.1).

As the criteria illustrate, the APA (advised by 'more than 600 global experts in the field of mental health' and 'representing 38,000 physician leaders in mental health', DSM5.org, 2010) seriously suggests that children being miserable (having 'limited positive affect') and distressed (showing 'irritability, sadness, or fearfulness') – is best described as the child having a 'mental disorder' afflicting *them*. That this is not an inexplicable or 'inappropriate' 'condition', but the well-documented, entirely understandable and absolutely sensible consequence of long-standing child abuse is, actually, apparent from

Box 1.1 Proposed DSM-V Criteria for Reactive Attachment Disorder of Infancy or Early Childhood

A   A pattern of markedly disturbed and developmentally inappropriate attachment behaviors, evident before 5 years of age, in which the child rarely or minimally turns preferentially to a discriminated attachment figure for comfort, support, protection and nurturance. The *disorder* appears as a consistent pattern of inhibited, emotionally withdrawn behavior in which the child rarely or minimally directs attachment behaviors towards any adult caregivers, as manifest by both of the following:

(1)   Rarely or minimally seeks comfort when distressed.
(2)   Rarely or minimally responds to comfort offered when distressed.

B   A persistent *social and emotional disturbance* characterized by at least 2 of the following:

(1)   Relative lack of social and emotional responsiveness to others.
(2)   Limited positive affect.
(3)   Episodes of *unexplained* irritability, sadness, or fearfulness which are evident during nonthreatening interactions with adult caregivers.

C   Does not meet the criteria for Autistic Spectrum Disorder.

D   *Pathogenic care* as evidenced by at least one of the following:

(1)   *Persistent disregard of the child's basic emotional needs* for comfort, stimulation, and affection (i.e., neglect).
(2)   *Persistent disregard of the child's basic physical needs.*
(3)   *Repeated changes of primary caregiver* that prevent formation of stable attachments (e.g., frequent changes in foster care).
(4)   *Rearing in unusual settings* such as institutions with high child/caregiver ratios that limit opportunities to form selective attachments.

E   There is a presumption that the care in Criterion D is responsible for the disturbed behavior in Criterion A (e.g., the disturbances in Criterion A began following the pathogenic care in Criterion D).

F   The child has a developmental age of at least 9 months. (DSM5. org, 2010, our emphases).

the criteria. However, instead of stating the obvious fact that abusive childrearing practices produce distressed children who have learnt to be fearful of adults, highly convoluted language is used to concede, in Criterion E, that children's conduct which has *already been claimed* as a 'mental disorder' is 'presumed' to be the outcome of 'pathogenic care'.[2]

As others have pointed out, to describe what are actually, and essentially, morally troubling issues – in this case children behaving in ways which make manifest their adult-created misery – (misery consequent upon 'persistent disregard of ... basic emotional needs (i.e., neglect) ... persistent disregard of ... basic physical needs') or straightforwardly matters of material circumstance (being brought up in 'unusual settings such as institutions with high child/caregiver ratios' or being subject to 'pathogenic care') as *medical conditions* is to make a moral – not a 'scientific' – choice in and of itself (cf. Bentall, 1992), and moreover, strains the medical metaphor past breaking.

Although Reactive Adjustment Disorder may seem an extreme example, the more familiar 'mental disorders' share the same dynamics, with more or less understandable reactions to life's challenges de-contextualized and transformed into internal individual pathology – whether labelled as depression, psychosis or some other diagnosis. In other words, the relentless widening of the mythical net of 'mental disorder' is seriously corrosive of the sense that we can have, and make, of our selves and our circumstances.

Quite aside from serving the sorts of professional and commercial interests documented by Irving Kirsch, Sami Timimi, David Smail, Duncan Double, Joanna Moncrieff and Craig Newnes among others in this volume, this corrosion of the dignity of 'lay' human selfhood perpetuated by the medicalization of suffering and difference thrives because it sanitizes and simplifies. The moral complexity and ambiguity that is inherent in the enterprise of policing human conduct is neatly reduced to the morally neutral and more predictable activity of managing a bodily disease. In Szasz's words, the myth that is 'mental illness' functions to 'render more palatable the bitter pill of moral conflict in human relations' (Szasz, 1960). Medicalization enables those who work in the mental health professions to manage the human suffering that they are daily confronted with, and also the nagging concern that there is little that they can do to help. In the process, as Mary Boyle and David Smail point out in their contributions, the people behind the 'disorders' may be overlooked, and the social circumstances that cause or contribute to their suffering often go unexamined and unchallenged.

Much of this volume is dedicated to exposing the linguistic contortions by which the transposition of social, moral and political issues into disease is achieved. In keeping with our position, and following Schütz (1962), here then we deliberately employ the vernacular. That is to say, we *can* (and here *do*) talk, sensibly, in everyday terms, about madness, grief, misery, distress, confusion, hopelessness, craziness, despair and so on through the rich and perfectly well-fitted lexicon of human suffering that the English language provides. In doing so we hope to foreground a contrast to Freud, Kraepelin, the APA et al. and the other weavers of the mythic language by which contemporary psy has rendered laymen unable to make 'psychological remarks' uninflected by its nostrums. That is we do not take the view that 'psychological remarks' should be the exclusive preserve of the professions: rather we take the view that ordinary people, using ordinary language, 'have perfectly good and sufficient descriptions of themselves' (McHoul, 2008: 4).

Taking seriously Wittgenstein's remark that 'our talk gets its meaning from the rest of our proceedings' (1975: 229), what we seek to do in this collection is, then, to return the capacity to make meaningful psychological remarks to its proper place in 'our proceedings', to restore to quotidian discourse a way of 'inventing ourselves' (*pace* Rose, 1996) that, unlike contemporary psy, recognizes and respects the essential *humanness* of the human condition.

De-Medicalizing Misery is, simply, a shorthand term for this project. Resisting the psychiatrization and psychologization of almost every aspect of human experience, and finding a way to place what are, frequently, essentially *moral and political* – not *medical* – matters back at the centre of our understanding of human suffering is a massive and multifaceted task. In consequence our contributors address a range of aspects of this project.

At this point we feel it important to gratefully acknowledge the observation of an anonymous reviewer that our contributors take various different approaches. Whereas some of the contributions are recognizably standard academic pieces, others are personal viewpoints and hence – while perhaps not best judged according to conventional academic standards – offer a complementarity to 'academic' material. Equally, the volume is not intended as a comprehensive critique of psychiatry and psychology: we acknowledge that many other writers, from diverse disciplinary fields, have made cogent and powerful critiques of this area. In particular we are conscious that much of the debate in sociology is perhaps under-represented. Of course, since Goffman's (1961) *Asylums* and Garfinkel's earlier observations on degradation ceremonies (1956a, b) sociologists have elaborated on these foundations and made penetrating critiques of the psy professions, and a debt to their work is owed not only by us as editors but also by many of our contributors. More recently, the sociological work of academics such as Pilgrim and Rogers (2003; 2005; 2010) and McCabe and colleagues (2002; 2004), while clearly congruent with our project, makes an important and distinctive contribution. This perspective is not omitted by design, but rather the selection of contributors to this volume reflects many factors, including prosaic practical considerations as well as issues of topicality at the time of writing. We hope, however, that this does not unduly detract from the relevance of the collection presented here.

In opening, Phil Thomas and Pat Bracken straightforwardly ask 'what does it mean to "demedicalize misery"?' and examine how the persistence of dualist thought in Western philosophy and culture helps in sustaining the idea of 'mental' illness as the ghostly partner in crime of 'physical' illness. Maintaining the focus on the 'macro' – the epistemological, the political and the discursive – Mary Boyle examines the strategies that psychology and psychiatry deploy in their relentless efforts to 'make the world go away', and how they benefit from these endeavours, at whatever cost to theoretical coherence and practical utility. Some of the upshots of this Cartesian legacy, and professional efforts to discount the materiality of the world in the production of distress, are examined by Suman Fernando. He notes that the disciplines that inform mental health services (mainly psychiatry and Western psychology) have grown out of a particular culturally determined understanding of the human condition, ideologies about life and so on, generally termed 'Western culture', and are at variance with – sometimes in conflict with – understandings and ideologies in 'other' cultures: such a reality disjuncture, he suggests, plays a crucial role in the disproportionate pathologization of non-white citizens in the UK.

Developing the concentration on the incoherence of medicalized understandings of forms of conduct, Dave Harper critically interrogates the notion that being wary, mistrustful and suspicious of others is best understood as a specific form of psychiatric disturbance, a 'symptom' of 'mental disorder' known as 'paranoia'. In passing, paranoia is a particularly interesting inversion of what is now commonplace psychiatric practice in that – etymologically at least – it appears since the early 1800s to have suffered relegation from being a generalized descriptor of insanity *tout court* to being merely a 'symptom' of other forms of madness (from Gk. paranoia 'mental derangement, madness', from *paranoos* 'mentally ill, insane' from *para* – 'beside, beyond' + *noos* 'mind': Online Etymology Dictionary, 2010). In an examination of the more 'traditional' trajectory of psychiatric disease creation, James Bourne examines how everyday, but socially problematic, ways of being-in-the-world which may once have been described as resulting from a 'flawed character' or a 'lack of breeding' mutated into the psychiatric 'condition' called 'Borderline Personality Disorder'.

Our focus on the use of language to cast the mythical net of 'mental disorder' continues in chapters by Arlene Vetere, Lucy Johnston and Sami Timimi. Here – picking up on some of Mary Boyle's arguments about the essentially *social* nature of distress – the focus is on the way in which psy actively seeks to divorce persons from their social worlds in making sense of madness and misery, and to delete from our thinking of ourselves notions such as Sartre's (1944/1989) insight that '*l'enfer: c'est les autres*'. Sami Timimi explores how psychiatric discourse about children's emotions and behaviour, centred as they are around the notion that inconvenient behaviour can be helpfully curbed by the use of drugs, have contributed to a dramatic change in our views about, and practices towards, childhood and child-rearing. Both Arlene Vetere and Lucy Johnstone examine the relationship between terrifying childhood experiences ('trauma') and later difficulties in living, sometimes described as 'psychosis'.

Contra DSM5.org, Vetere makes it abundantly clear that children who grow up exposed to chronic fear, sadness, shame, worry, the threat of – and actual – violence in their lives are – unsurprisingly – often likely to learn to find the world frightening, and people in it a doubtful source of kindness and love. That some of the ways that the grown-ups these children become deal with the lasting lessons of their childhood are described as 'symptomatic' of 'mental disorder' obliterates their suffering and invalidates their experience and sense of self; one of the ways such children may come to be described is as 'having' a 'psychosis'.

The term 'psychosis', Johnstone argues, is presented as more user-friendly and less stigmatizing than a diagnosis of 'schizophrenia'. However, she shows clearly that it is equally, if not more, problematic in terms of reliability, validity and so on, while its woolliness serves to disguise and defuse fundamental critiques about the nature, purpose and consequences of psychiatric diagnosis. While Vetere's and Johnstone's chapters are based on a review of academic literature and empirical social research, Jacqui Dillon describes, from first-hand experience, exactly what this life course means. The wider social consequences of the psychiatric endeavour are outlined in chapters by Ewen Speed, Jacqui Dillon and Carlton Coulter and Mark Rapley. We have noted that one of the effects of the widespread acceptance of the medicalized mythology of the present is that it obliterates suffering and invalidates experience. Countering this silencing, and providing a platform for voices of the mad and their families, is an essential part of our project. As such, Ewen's chapter discusses the politics of self-identification among recipients of mental health services. Picking up from Sami Timimi's chapter on the medicalization of childhood, Carlton Coulter and Mark Rapley examine the anguish and uncertainty expressed by the parents of children diagnosed as 'psychotic' occasioned by the conflicting stories that psychiatry tells about parental responsibility, 'mental-illness-as-biological-derangement' and 'mental health literacy' in trying to make sense of their moral accountability for their child's distress.[3]

Quite aside from the adverse effects on persons and families of their acceptance – in good faith – of the contemporary mythology of interiorized, individualized mental pathology, psychiatry's claims about its scientificity demand further scrutiny. In chapters by Joanna Moncrieff, Irving Kirsch and Duncan Double the idea, the evidence and the means by which we have come to be persuaded of the contemporary cultural commonsense that 'depression' is a 'chemical imbalance in the brain' are explored. Joanna Moncrieff lays bare how the very idea that there could be such a thing as an 'antidepressant' was constructed to present psychiatry as a modern medical enterprise with proper medical treatments and not, as we are so often assured, a consequence of sophisticated research on brain biochemistry. Irving Kirsch subsequently – and comprehensively – debunks the hypothesis that the *soi-disant* 'antidepressants' have a specific biochemical effect on a 'mental disorder' called 'depression'. The ill effects of such cultural commonsense are explored by Duncan Double, who asks why doctors were so slow to recognize antidepressant-discontinuation problems. While Moncrieff and Kirsch demonstrate that the scientific status of what WHO claims is the world's leading cause of disability is lacking, Duncan Double shows very clearly what is at stake, and how this stake is managed.

If Moncrieff, Double and Kirsch are sceptical about the efficacy of the pharmacological 'magic bullet', Nimisha Patel, David Smail and

Craig Newnes are similarly sceptical about the much vaunted efficacy of psychological – as opposed to medical – understandings of misery and the much vaunted solution to it, the 'talking cure' – psychotherapy. The workings of the world, of material reality, are central to Craig Newnes' analysis of the harms done as part of the political game clinical psychology has played to ensure the profession's survival. Smail continues this line of analysis and suggests that therapeutic psychology, 'the great red herring of the twentieth century', is not – as proponents of NICE guidelines would have it – the pinnacle of 'evidence-based practice', but rather an ideological masterstroke which obscures the significance for emotional suffering of the social structure of material reality. Nimisha Patel takes the issue of torture as a worked example of the pitfalls of neglecting to acknowledge and to theorize the socio-political context in making sense of distress.

To return to where we started, it would seem that a rethink of the ways we currently comprehend – and respond to – madness and misery is long overdue. However much psy might wish it, the world will not 'go away'. It is time to call time on Sigmund's project. We close this collection, then, with some very brief concluding remarks by Jacqui Dillon, Joanna Moncrieff and Mark Rapley offering some observations on what such a reconfigured understanding may look like, and some – tentative – pointers towards that goal.

2
Dualisms and the Myth of Mental Illness

Philip Thomas and Patrick Bracken

What does it mean to 'de-medicalize misery'? Does it mean that we should no longer think of states of despair, sadness and madness in medical terms? Does it mean that there is no proper role for doctors in trying to work with and help those so afflicted? And if that is so, then what is to be done about the systems that Western societies have set up to help, such as mental health and primary care services, all of which are predicated on the assumption that misery and madness are, among other things, medical conditions? Are all these to be dismantled? If so, what should take their place? These are not rhetorical questions; they serve the point of drawing attention to the fact that words have important consequence, if we mean what we say.

The idea that we should de-medicalize misery has a mixed pedigree. The arguments that have made it possible for us to say such a thing originate in vastly different ideologies and forms of knowledge. Sociology, history, philosophy, Marxism, right-wing libertarianism, and more recently some survivors and service users, as well as academics in anthropology, feminism, post-colonial and cultural studies have all made contributions of one sort or another to the argument that the profession of medicine has no legitimate role to play in misery and madness. They have all, to varying degrees, raised serious questions about the role of medical knowledge and doctors in this field.

One of the most pungent and enduring critics of the role of medicine in misery is the American psychiatrist and academic, Thomas Szasz. It is exactly 50 years since the publication of his paper the *Myth of Mental Illness* (Szasz, 1960), in which he argued that hysteria is better understood as a problem of personal behaviour aimed at seeking help. A year later in the book of the same name, he extended his argument to the full range of psychiatric conditions, including schizophrenia. His ideas have been enormously influential, paradoxically nowhere more so than in the profession of psychiatry itself. Wilson (1993) has described how the onslaught of Szasz and other anti psychiatrists[1] led to a hardening of the profession's positivistic tendencies, and the emergence of DSM 3 and neo-Kraepelinism.

In this chapter we extend our analysis of Szasz's ideas that we started elsewhere (Bracken & Thomas, 2010). Here we focus on some aspects of the philosophical assumptions that underpin Szasz's arguments, specifically in so far as these are relevant to the idea that we should, or could, de-medicalize misery and madness We begin with a detailed examination of Part One of the *Myth of Mental Illness*, drawing attention to the philosophical ideas about the nature of subjectivity that lie at the heart of his arguments – Cartesian dualism. Although Cartesianism has been immensely influential in Western philosophy over the last 350 years, key strands of thought in Continental philosophy in the twentieth century have exposed the failure of Cartesianism to provide anything like a realistic account of human subjectivity. For this reason we turn to the philosophy of Maurice Merleau-Ponty, particularly his view that we are embodied beings, to examine the implications of Szasz's ideas for our understandings of ourselves. We also draw on recent work in anthropology that reveals the complex relationship between neurological disease, psychosis and culture. We conclude that, rather than de-medicalizing misery, we really require a completely different form of medicine, one that unlike Szasz, avoids the pitfalls of dualisms.

Our distaste for dualistic approaches to human reality stems ultimately, not from philosophy, but from our experiences as doctors, and in particular, from our work with individuals and families from non-Western communities. Through this work we have become sensitized to the different ways in which human beings experience their bodies in relation to disease, distress and states of madness. While Szasz might be right that certain pathological processes can be identified in human bodies cross-culturally, the reality is that the human experience of disease varies greatly and cannot be disentangled from the cultural context in which the individual exists. Likewise, all forms of medical understanding and practice are laden with cultural assumptions, values and operate according to different priorities. Szasz rightly sees psychiatry in this light but fails to see that psychiatry is not alone in this.

Body or mind in the *Myth of Mental Illness*

In the introduction to the *Myth of Mental Illness*, Szasz declares that the methods and subject matter of psychiatry have more in common with studies in linguistics and philosophy. Despite this, psychiatry's contemporary conceptual framework remains firmly within the tradition of medicine, and is thus rooted in the natural sciences. He sees this as an anomaly, and he highlights the confusion that exists in psychiatry over the relationship between the physical and mental worlds, through a logical analysis of language use influenced by the ideas of the Vienna Circle.[2] Later Szasz turns to American pragmatism, particularly the ideas of George Herbert Mead, to develop a model of the doctor-patient relationship based in game playing. He also draws on Popper's critique of historicism,[3] arguing that the key principles of natural science, causality and determinism cannot be carried over into the human sciences. This is because he is concerned about the negative implications such a move would have for the possibility of free will. Here, however, we are primarily concerned with Szasz's views about the relationships between the physical and mental worlds, and his reliance on the philosophy of the Vienna Circle.

His analysis begins with an examination of the philosophical assumptions that are to be found in the work of the founders of psychoanalysis, focussing particularly on Charcot and Freud's writing on hysteria and conversion syndromes. Szasz points out that hysteria developed in the reverse order from that which usually characterizes the way in which medicine identifies new diseases. Charcot effectively created a new criterion for what constitutes a disease: 'paresis was proved to be a disease; hysteria was declared to be one' (Szasz, 1974: 12). He points out that Charcot was in a position to make such a declaration,[4] but beneath this he identifies a deep-seated confusion about the body-mind relationship. This persists in contemporary psychiatry. Szasz may have a point here, but we will argue that his position is dualistic. He denies that those conditions identified as psychiatric disorders have any bodily basis, and, furthermore, that they are all to be accounted for in moral terms, or in terms of problem behaviours:

> This dichotomy is reflected in the two basic contemporary psychiatric methods, namely the physicochemical and the psychosocial. In the days of Charcot and Freud, however, only the former was recognized as belonging to science and medicine. Interest in the latter was synonymous with charlatanry and quackery.[5]
>
> (Szasz, 1974: 27–8)

Szasz insists that there are clear limits to what we can legitimately describe as illness. Disturbances in bodily functions are correctly to be understood in terms of pathology, but difficulties in our beliefs, emotions, relationships and behaviour are primarily moral problems, and it is not appropriate to talk of these in terms of illness. This view has been a firm and consistent feature of Szasz's writings throughout his illustrious career extending over 50 years. In a recent work he writes as follows: 'I maintain that mental illness is a metaphorical disease: that bodily illness stands in the same relation to mental illness as a defective television set stands to a bad program' (Szasz, 2007: 6).

He proposes that we require two distinct discourses, one to describe the functioning of the television set, another to describe the quality of the programme. By extension, we cannot 'cure' psychological problems by interfering with the body of the person who experiences these problems, just as tinkering around with the internal components of a television set will not provide a better programme. We should not use the language and logic of pathology to frame psychological problems.

This confusion between mental worlds and physical worlds lies at the heart of the problem of psychiatry, as Szasz sees it. It is a stumbling block (to use his expression) that underpins the differential diagnosis between hysteria and neurological disorders. It also stands in the way of a 'systematic theory of personal conduct free of brain-mythological components' (Szasz, 1974: 28). This is important in understanding Szasz's position. One of his objectives in disposing of a neurobiological account of human action is to clear the way for a moral basis for personal conduct in the second part of his book. But in trying to dispose of what might be seen as psychiatry's confused monism he substitutes instead body-mind dualism.

This emerges most clearly in his account of Freud and Breuer's early description of hysteria in Chapters 4 and 5. Szasz argues that Freud's theory of conversion helped to deal with the dualistic question of how an emotional problem can present as a physical symptom. He acknowledges that such a question presupposes Cartesian dualism (although he does not specify what sort of dualism arising from Descartes' philosophy he is referring to), and then argues that the concept of conversion is misleading because, as we have seen, it involves confusion between two different languages or modes of representation, the psychological and physical. However, Szasz's solution to the problem of the body-mind relationship as far as psychiatry and medicine are concerned is to abandon one wing of it altogether:

> The only viable alternative to this familiar but false perspective is to abandon the entire medical approach to mental illness and to

substitute new approaches for it appropriate to the ethical, political, psychological and social problems from which psychiatric patients suffer and which psychiatrists ostensibly seek to remedy.

(Szasz, 1974: 79)

Szasz insists that we see everything in black or white. It makes no sense, he argues, to use the language of pathology to talk about distress or madness, because these are fundamentally moral problems of one sort or another. The language of pathology is only relevant to physical diseases affecting the body. In terms of how we think and act as doctors, the two worlds, mental and physical, must be kept apart.

It is his argument about the confusion in psychiatry when dealing with the mental and physical worlds that reveals most clearly the influence of the philosophy of the Vienna Circle. He draws on the work of Moritz Schlick (one of the founder members of the Circle), citing his warning against the confused use of words from 'different languages'. He points out that this is precisely what happens when we talk about 'psychosomatic' medicine, and he goes on to attack psychiatry's use of words such as 'organic', 'psychogenic', and 'mental illness' as further instances of 'linguistic misuse'. He is particularly critical of the work of Franz Alexander who, in the emerging field of psychosomatic medicine, made the distinction between conversion hysteria and organ neurosis. Alexander saw no distinction between mental and physical worlds as far as illness was concerned. Szasz accuses him of

> ignor[ing] the linguistic and legal, epistemological and social, and all the other distinctions between psychological and physiological events and pursuits, and simply assert[ing] that 'psychic and somatic phenomena take place in the same biological system and are probably two aspects of the same process'.
>
> (Szasz, 1974: 87)

Szasz argues that if we make no distinction between medicine and psychology, then why should we bother to distinguish between medicine and religion, or medicine and the law, or medicine and politics. By implication this is an absurd position. At the same time he asserts his own opposition to any form of holism (as opposed to dualism):

> In any case, we cannot have it both ways: we must choose between the psychophysical symmetry of modern psychosomatic medicine, fashionable in medicine and psychiatry today, and the psychophysical

hierarchy of modern philosophy, opposing contemporary efforts to medicalize moral problems.

(Szasz, 1974:87)[6]

We broadly agree with Szasz's analysis of the problem of the body in relation to psychiatry, at least as far as there is no clear evidence that the different categories of 'mental illnesses' as currently defined have readily identifiable pathological causes. Elsewhere we have written about the limitations and failings of the biomedical model in psychiatry (Bracken & Thomas, 2005; see Chapter 6). However, we part company with him when he starts to prescribe what sort of suffering is legitimate from a medical point of view. We believe that his imposition of a strictly dualistic solution to the mind-body relationship in medicine and psychiatry is seriously misguided. His insistence that bodily and mental worlds are distinct domains to be spoken about only in their own terms overlooks the symbolic meaning of the body and biology in our lives. Although he correctly, in our view, points out that the concept of mental illness is a metaphor, he fails to acknowledge that diseases, physical illnesses and the body all possess metaphorical significance and meaning in our lives.[7]

Elsewhere, we have contrasted Szasz's analysis of the problems of psychiatry with the work of Michel Foucault. Szasz's approach is predicated on a number of simple binary distinctions (Bracken & Thomas, 2010). In this chapter we are focussing in detail on one aspect of this, his understanding of the body-mind relationship and the role it plays in relation to physical illness, distress and madness. An important consequence of this is his claim in Chapter 3 of the *Myth of Mental Illness*, that in physical medicine culture has no role to play. He asserts that the manifestations of physical diseases are largely independent of culture or socio-political conditions in general: '[A] diphtheritic membrane was the same and looked the same whether it occurred in a patient in Czarist Russia or Victorian England' (Szasz, 1974: 48). He maximizes the polarization between mental and physical illness by asserting that although the 'phenomenology' (his word) of bodily illness such as tuberculosis is not influenced by socio-cultural factors, this is most certainly the case as far as mental illness is concerned:

[t]he phenomenology of so-called mental illness ... depend[s] upon and var[ies] with the educational, economic, religious, social and political character of the individual and the society in which it occurs.

(Szasz, 1974: 48–9)[8]

It may be the case that when people from different cultural or religious backgrounds become ill, their bodies display the same physical derangements. But the danger here is that we overlook the relationship between culture and the personal meaning and significance of bodily disease. Szasz engineers a radical disconnection between the world of culture and medicine, which in his analysis can only be spoken about in terms given to us by natural science. At a stroke he dismisses the work of medical anthropologists and writers in the field of medical humanities, who have shown that diseases have meanings for us, and that the interaction between meaning and pathology is a complex and vital factor in understanding the outcome of disease and treatment.

Before we move on to a philosophical critique of dualisms in the *Myth of Mental Illness* we will briefly summarize what we have gleaned so far.

Szasz sets out three main propositions. First is the idea that mental diseases are metaphorical, and thus not real; second is the idea that physical diseases are 'real' in the literal sense; third, that the 'phenomenology' of physical disease is the same across cultures. Although we agree with his first and second propositions, we disagree with his third proposition. Our position is that while physical diseases are 'real' in the sense that they can be identified through material changes in the physical body, they are at the same time saturated with significance and meanings for us. And in just the same way, our subjectivity is such that we struggle to search for meaning and significance in our states of madness and distress. We will show that the difficulty with Szasz's third proposition is that the nature of human subjectivity is such that it is simply not possible to make polarized distinctions between a physically based medicine and the world of culture and meaning. To do this we will first examine the origins of Szasz's ideas about the relation between body and mind, through the work of the French Enlightenment philosopher René Descartes.

Descartes and dualism

We are primarily concerned here with the implications of different forms of dualism for the way in which we experience physical disease, madness and distress. Our analysis is influenced by the work of Hubert Dreyfus (1991). Different types of dualism have figured prominently in Western philosophy for thousands of years, but it is through the Enlightenment and the philosophy of Descartes that we can begin to understand the impact of dualism in contemporary thought. Dreyfus (1991) points out that Descartes' philosophy reinvigorated a tradition that can be traced back to Plato. In common with many Enlightenment thinkers, Descartes was preoccupied with the problem of knowledge and certainty. He was heavily influenced by Galileo's work in mathematics and astronomy, and he wanted to put philosophy on a similarly secure footing. Could we be as certain of the accuracy and truthfulness of our thoughts about the world as we could be about the solution to a mathematical problem, or the prediction of the positions of the planets? He argued that it was possible to achieve this through reflexive clarity, a systematic reflection on the contents of the mind to distinguish between that which was obviously correct from that which was not, and mapping the ways in which our internal representations of the external world were ordered and related. This principle formed the basis for what subsequently became scientific explorations of subjectivity, for example Husserlian phenomenology, psychoanalysis (as originally conceived by Freud), the origins of the project of modern psychology, especially cognitivism (Bracken & Thomas, 2008), and theories of artificial intelligence.[9]

A central plank in Descartes' philosophy is a belief in the possibility of reflexive clarity, and the importance of defining and mapping the ways in which internal (or mental) representations of the external world are ordered and related. However, a consequence of this is different forms of dualism. These arise as follows: Cartesianism operates on a fundamental distinction between the 'inner' world of the mind and the 'outer' physical world with which it is in contact. This separation of the inner and the outer is predicated upon Descartes' metaphysical (or ontological) separation of the world into two kinds of substance, the soul from the material body in which it resided. The body is characterized by the fact that it possesses 'extension'; it occupies space. It is thus *res extensa* (or a thing that is extended in space). In contrast to this the soul is characterized by thought, and is thus 'a thing which thinks', a *res cogitans*. This view of the self as a thing or substance has had major implications, and two in particular are relevant to understanding the shortcomings of Szasz's arguments. The first of these is the metaphysical notion of two separate substances existing in the world, body and mind. This has given rise to an extensive and on-going debate about the relationship between the two. In addition, there is also the separation of the mind from the outside world that follows in the wake of Descartes' metaphysical dualism. We might call this his 'epistemological dualism',[10] in which the subject is in contact with an outside world and has knowledge of it through sensations that are synthesized and built up into mental representations of the world.[11] The point is that in this Cartesian view the mind becomes 'self-contained'. It stands outside the world and has a relationship to it. Mind ('subjectivity', or our experience of ourselves and the world) becomes something conceivable apart from and separate from this relation. It knows the world from the outside. Thus, there is an epistemological separation of mind from world. It is this epistemological separation, based ultimately, as we have seen, on Descartes' metaphysical dualism, which provides the basis for what is known as the representational theory of mind and thought, concerned as it is with the relationship between inner states of mind and outer states of the world. It is this view of subjectivity that Szasz draws on when he insists that the mental world (metaphysical) cannot be spoken with the language that we use to talk about the natural world (physical), or for that matter that culture and disease are separate worlds.

Embodiment and the philosophy of Merleau-Ponty

Cartesianism has been immensely influential in Western thought. It provides the basis for the scientific view of the world, the idea that it is possible for us to have a detached and objective perspective on the natural world, one that gives us a 'truthful' account of reality.[12] Psychology and medicine have extended this perspective to subjectivity, our bodies and our 'selves'. The mind has become a 'thing' to be studied according to the principles of scientific enquiry, as has the body. This approach has yielded great benefits as far as the treatment of (bodily) disease is concerned, but it has its limitations. Elsewhere, we have used the philosophy of Martin Heidegger to draw attention to these, especially the way in which they fail to account for the way in which our subjectivity is bound to social contexts, is embodied and tied to temporality in a unique way (Bracken & Thomas, 2005). Here, we turn to the philosophy of Maurice Merleau-Ponty to examine in detail the implication of Szasz's ideas about the relationships between body, mind and culture for our understanding of disease and illness. We will use his philosophy to argue that it is simply not possible to separate out physical and mental domains as far as subjectivity is concerned in the way that Szasz suggests. The physical body (biology included) is inextricably bound up with the way we experience ourselves, and the world in which we live. This is especially so when it comes to understanding what happens to us in states of disease, illness and madness. Culture and history play a central role in making this possible.

In *Phenomenology of Perception*, Merleau-Ponty (1962) begins by examining neurological and psychological theories of perception. He is critical of the idea that scientific theories can provide anything like a complete account of our experience of the world. This is because these approaches to subjectivity fragment it, analyse it and then break it down into different components (mental, physical and so on). Such an approach is partial and incomplete; as Langer (1989: 7) puts it , it is simply not possible to undo the bond between the human subject and the world, and then re-forge it. Merleau-Ponty is not in principle opposed to scientific accounts of experience, but he argues that science itself is derivative and secondary to what he calls pre-objective experience (i.e. our experience of the world as it already presents itself to us).

Merleau-Ponty argues that the starting point for any account of experience must be experience itself. This is because the world of experience is present to us before anything else. For Matthews (2002) this view of phenomenology is part of a tradition that means abandoning a scientific conception of phenomenology in favour of a description of being-in-the-world. Like Heidegger, Merleau-Ponty was concerned not with scientific explanations of experience, but with descriptions of it, so the phenomenological reduction also meant setting to one side scientific explanations and theories.[13] This aspect of his work has given rise to the view that Merleau-Ponty was anti-scientific, a view that Matthews strongly contests.[14] The human activity of scientific enquiry is itself a product of human experience and history; it involves a very particular way of encountering the world. To achieve this scientific encounter, we systematically strip values from the way in which we 'see' the natural and human worlds. We do this through all the techniques we use to rid science of 'bias'. For example, the language of science does not involve value descriptions such as 'nice, friendly, pleasant, helpful'. But our value orientation to the world is primary and foundational. It is from this context that we have developed the scientific way of understanding. In spite of this, the scientific way of understanding the world is often presented as something that gives us a view of the world 'as it really is'. The irony of biological reductionism in psychology and psychiatry is that it is essentially an attempt to move in the other direction: to use the 'de-valued' language of the physical sciences to explain the value-laden (and 'messy') world of human psychology from whence they sprang in the first place. Scientific accounts of human experience do not stand outside that experience; they are created by it.

Merleau-Ponty points out that phenomenological philosophy means looking at the world afresh. This is because we are so accustomed to a scientific view of the world, our bodies, and ourselves that we take it for granted. This is where we begin to understand why Szasz is mistaken in claiming that it is only possible to talk about disease through the language of natural science. The scientific view is taken for granted as a foundational and truthful account of reality. This is an objective view, one that sees the world and everything in it, other people and our own bodies included, as objects existing in the world apart from ourselves. The philosopher Thomas Nagel has described this as the 'view from nowhere' (Nagel, 1986). Its objectivity is seen to be free of values. Merleau-Ponty is not opposed to this perspective, but he objects to the idea that it is capable of offering us a complete view of reality. This is because it obscures the fundamental fact that our view of reality is already given through our existence, our being-in-the-world.

An important consequence of this is that our relationship to the world is not one that can be captured through 'inner' representations of external reality such as cognitive schema or information processing, built up through operations on individual sensations or sense data.[15] We cannot grasp human experience as if it were simply a matter of having 'true' thoughts about the world. The world as we experience it does not consist of myriad discrete sensations as the objectivism of science would have us believe, but it is presented to us as a coherent, meaningful (usually) whole. In addition to this, we are physically present in the world through our bodies, so we stand in a closer relationship to it than if we were disembodied pure consciousness. Our bodies place us in a specific place and time, so our experience of the world and our relationship to it cannot be a view from nowhere; it is situated in a specific culture and history. For this reason, Merleau-Ponty's view of phenomenology means that we must accept the cultural and historical realities of human experience. Matthews puts it this way:

> If what I am cannot be understood except in terms of my manifold relationships, practical and emotional as well as purely intellectual, with the world that I inhabit, then the phenomenological description of my experience cannot be achieved without reference to my social and historical situation.
>
> (Matthews, 2002: 39)

For this reason we may regard Merleau-Ponty's phenomenology as a hermeneutic phenomenology. It is not possible for us to see the world around us as free of value and meaning.

We have seen that Merleau-Ponty uses the word perception to refer to the nature of pre-reflective experience. In this sense, perception is primary, because the world as we perceive it, as it reveals itself to us through being as Heidegger might say, provides the basis for all aspects of our experience. The body is vital in making this possible, and for this reason he develops the idea of the body-subject in order to see that the body is so much more than a physiological mechanism, an object reduced to the deterministic rules of physiology and causality. It is the means through which being-in-the-world becomes possible.

The significance of the body-subject

We can begin to understand the importance of the body in Merleau-Ponty's thought through the following extended quote from Matthews:

> The world as experienced by a particular subject cannot be a mere collection of independent and merely externally related objects, but must be conceived of as unified by its relations to that subject and his or her projects in it: as a system of meanings. That is the sense in which, for each of us, the world is 'my world'. Thus the subject can be conceived of only in relation to a world, and the world can be conceived of only in relation to a subject. The subject must be 'in the world' both in the way that objects are and in a way that transcends the mode of being of objects.
>
> (Matthews, 2002: 57)

It is through the body that I, as a subject, am 'in the world', and it is through the body that the world becomes open to me. This moves us away from the Cartesian view of the subject as a disembodied mind or brain, something cut off from the world and capable only of a remote relationship with it. Being-in-the-world is only possible because human beings are very special objects in the world. They are living organisms conscious of their environments, and capable of interacting meaningfully with their environments. It is through the body that we act in and on the world in ways that are meaningful for us. We are dependent on our physical senses, given to us by our bodies, for our awareness of our environments.

Burkitt (1999: 75) points out that Cartesianism privileges vision in terms of how we experience the world. He argues that we are more than spectators; our bodies mean that the world is apparent to us through all our senses. We depend on our bodies to move through the environment in order to interact meaningfully with it. This means that any state or condition of the body that impairs our ability to act meaningfully in the world has to be laden with significance.[16] Our brains play a central role in enabling these activities, and thus having the brains that we have is vital to us being conscious beings in the way in which we are conscious beings.[17] It also means that the body, like other objects in the world, has symbolic meaning. Merleau-Ponty uses the expression body-subject to emphasize the unity of experience with the physical basis of the body.[18] This is not to say that we cannot study the body scientifically, and regard it as an object in the world subject to cause and effect like other objects, but the normal way in which we encounter other people is as body-subjects like ourselves, or as Matthews puts it, as an expression of other people's way of being-in-the-world. We can no more separate them from their embodiment than we can separate ourselves from our own bodies: 'in this way, the world as we perceive it is again a world of meanings, which include our own bodies and other embodied persons as having particular sorts of meaning for us' (Matthews, 2002: 60).

Body and meaning in disease

Merleau-Ponty's philosophy of embodiment has its limitations. Burkitt (1999) argues that although it sets out a convincing set of arguments for the importance of the body in meaning, it falls short of linking the body properly to the symbolic. Neither does it really engage with the different types of power relationships that have, at different times in history, influenced the body and its role in subjectivity (for example, through the suppression or encouragement of different forms of sexuality). However, while this is beyond the scope of our chapter, we do need to pay attention to the link between the body and the symbolic, because this is central to our arguments about the limitations of Szasz's ideas. At this point we turn to empirical work from medical anthropology that deals specifically with the symbolic meaning of disease and disturbances in bodily function linked to this.

Anthropologists have turned to the concept of embodiment as a methodology that has helped to reformulate theories of culture, self and experience. It provides a way of charting a middle course between body and culture that recognizes the importance of both, and at the same time avoids the pitfalls of dualisms. The anthropologist Thomas Csordas (1994) points out, that embodiment problematizes the distinctions between body and mind, culture and biology, gender and sex. His work (Csordas, 1994a) shows that cultural meaning is an intrinsic feature of embodied experience. He defines embodiment as follows:

> Embodiment, in the sense I am using it, is a methodological standpoint in which bodily experience is understood to be the existential

ground of culture and self, and therefore a valuable starting point for their analysis.

(Csordas, 1994a: 269)

There are two issues that require clarification here. The first is the relationship between embodiment and biology; the second is the identification of embodiment as a starting point in preobjective experience, or being-in-the-world. In response to the first, he argues that both biology and culture are forms of objectification (or representation), so it is essential that we move away from our dependence on both, preferably by describing experience in terms of an experiential understanding of being-in-the-world. We can see how he does this through his account of the case of a thirty-year-old Navajo man, Dan, who was a participant in a large-scale study of the illness experiences of Navajo cancer patients. He had been diagnosed as suffering from an astrocytoma affecting the left temporal-parietal lobe. After the tumour was removed he received chemo- and radiotherapy, and developed seizures and a wide variety of neurological and psychiatric symptoms, including headaches and olfactory auras, poor sleep, difficulty expressing his thoughts, blunted affect, disorganized thinking and rambling speech. After surgery he also lost his limited ability to understand Navajo. His attempts to rehabilitate his language skills using word puzzles in magazines were only partially successful.

One evening at an early stage in the post-operative period, Dan had an encounter with the Holy People,[19] which 'comprised a lengthy auditory experience, followed by a compulsion to talk that relieved his intense headache pain and left him with a "happy and good feeling"' (Csordas, 1994a: 273). At the time he had this experience his cognitive abilities were still seriously impaired, but his understanding of the event was that this encounter had resulted from a new way of praying, one that was different from the mode of prayer he had learnt as a child. His family agreed. His father (himself a ritual leader) confirmed that, within the cultural tradition, this change in Dan indicated that he would become a healer or medicine man.

Csordas points out that Dan's problems with verbal fluency made it very difficult for others to understand him, but it was clear that his family and community saw the utterances that arose within the neurological context of his aphasic difficulties as being inspired by the Holy People, but only when Dan stopped trying to fight the aphasia. In other words, his family and community regarded his aphasic utterances as significant and meaningful within the context of their culture. Subsequently Dan participated in four peyote rituals with the elders. These lasted all night, and involved singing, prayer, peyote ingestion and quiet conversation.

In his account of the ritual six months later, he claimed that he had won the support of the elders. Csordas gives three points in support of this. First, Dan claimed that the divine inspiration he had experienced was a consequence of his healing, and that the peyotists should therefore pay attention to what he had to say. Even though part of his 'brain was cut out' (Csordas, 1994a: 275) he had been inspired by the Holy People to speak Holy words. Second, the other participants at the rituals agreed that Dan's prayers must have been correct, because if they had not been so he would have become ill during the rituals, which he hadn't. This indicated within the tradition that his words had incurred divine approval.[20] Finally, Dan argued that the reason his words were difficult to understand, especially by the elders in the ritual, was because they reflected in part the concerns of a younger generation of Navajo people, who, like Dan, had moved away and attended college, and had had life experiences that the older generation had not had. According to Dan's account, the elders agreed with this view, and could see that his words were aimed at a younger generation. Indeed, his words helped the elders to understand some of the problems facing their grandchildren. Some were moved to tears by his words. Csordas points out that anthropologists who have worked closely with Navajo peyote rituals see this as an accepted reaction indicating that the participants are deeply moved by a speaker's sincerity.

Dan attached deep significance to the loss of his ability to communicate in Navajo while still being able to speak in English. He concluded that this was because the Holy People wanted him to address young people in English. Most spoke little or no Navajo, and were therefore unable to engage with traditional prayers and rituals, which were part of their heritage. This frustrated them because they were unable to gain benefit from prayer and ritual, but Dan was now in a position to be able to help them with this. Although he had lost what Navajo he had, within his culture and community his illness brought a new meaning and significance into Dan's life, and with it a positive new identity. It formed the basis of his recovery.

Conclusions

Csordas' work, based in the philosophies of Merleau-Ponty and Heidegger, draws out the richness and complexity of experiences in disease and psychosis. We can begin to see how Dan understood and made sense of his experiences, meaning that is suspended between his bodily (neurological) disturbances, his culture and the support and approval of his family and community. We might say that one of his neurological symptoms, his loss of language, was existentially important for Dan because it also symbolized a wider concern in the Navajo community of the loss of culture and tradition experienced by the younger people. We can see how culture and community carry and validate the meaning of Dan's experiences, which otherwise would simply be seen in terms of neurological or cognitive deficits. More than that, we can see how, as a result of placing Dan's experiences within a spiritual framework shared with his community, he emerges with a positive identity, one that gives him a unique and significant role in helping a younger generation of Navajo. In other words we can begin to see how culture and meaning interact with biology and identity to bring about the conditions that are necessary for the emergence of recovery.

Seen in this light, the dualism that characterizes Szasz's ideas is not only theoretically problematic, but it just does not make clinical sense. David Pilgrim (2007) points out that grounds for questioning the scientific basis of psychiatric conditions are also applicable to many physical disorders. Many chronic physical conditions, especially those encountered in primary care, such as arthritis, psoriasis, irritable bowel syndrome and asthma have no clearly established aetiology and low treatment specificity. Szasz pays no heed to this.[21] All these conditions have psychological and cultural dimensions as well as a physical basis; if doctors fail to engage with all three of these then they are failing to engage properly with patients. The importance of this emerges in the work of Daniel Moerman, an anthropologist who has devoted his academic life to studying what he calls the meaning effect in medicine. Much of his work deals with the placebo response, which he prefers to call the meaning response. He draws attention to many studies that show how the formal properties of placebos, such as their colour, and whether they are in tablet, capsule or injection form, influence their potency. He also cites studies that show that sham surgery is effective in relieving symptoms, such as operations for angina (sham internal mammary ligation), pacemaker implantation, laser treatment for severe angina, as well as surgery for prolapsed intervertebral discs and Meniere's disease. In summarizing these studies, Moerman makes the following point:

> Much of the meaning of medicine, of the meaning response (and in the narrowest sense, the placebo response), is a cultural phenomenon engaged in a complex interplay of the meanings of disease and illness. The modern triumph of a universalist biology tends to blind us

to the dramatic variation in the ways that people experience their own physiology based on who they are and what they know.

(Moerman, 2002: 70)

The key issue, we suggest, is that medicine has struggled with dualism since Descartes. We are so deeply accustomed to thinking about ourselves as human beings in terms of either the body or the mind, and at the same time locking culture outside in the cold, that as doctors we have to resort to philosophically suspect and clinically awkward concepts such as 'psychosomatic' medicine to bridge the gulf. It follows from our analysis that misery is not in need of de-medicalizing; instead it requires a different type of medicine, one informed by insights to be gleaned from existential phenomenology. For a brief period there was a tradition in European psychiatry and philosophy that showed that this was possible. Sadly, the work of Ludwig Binswanger, Eugene Minkowski and others, which was brought to the attention of the English-speaking world by May et al. (1958), lies buried beneath the fallout from the polarized arguments of Szasz and his followers, crushed by the evidence-based Behemoth that psychiatry has become. We should not de-medicalize misery, but instead try to answer the question that Rollo May (1958a: 3) poses: 'can we be sure ... that we are seeing the patient as he really is, knowing him in his own reality; or are we seeing merely a projection of our own theories about him'?

3
Making the World Go Away, and How Psychology and Psychiatry Benefit

Mary Boyle

This chapter is based on two propositions. The first is that if we are ever to de-medicalize misery, then both the impact of people's environments and their life experiences, as major causes of emotional distress, *and* the social significance of these connections will have to be made more prominent. The second proposition is that both psychiatry and clinical psychology so avoid giving prominence to people's contexts in their theory, research and practice that we might reasonably ask why. Are they acting in accordance with evidence, has research demonstrated that life experience is not very important or, given what we know of the links between avoidance and fear, are psychiatry and clinical psychology actually rather fearful of context? This matter can be settled quickly. The evidence that what has happened and is happening to people in their lives plays a major role in creating various forms of emotional distress and behavioural problems – including psychosis – is very strong (Bentall, 2003; Read et al., 2005; Stoppard, 2000; Tew, 2005; Wilkinson & Pickett, 2009). As Bentall (2003) and Falloon (2000) have pointed out, this evidence is stronger than any we have for genetic or biological causes. So, if context is not at the forefront of psychiatric and clinical psychological theory and practice, then the avoidance is likely to be associated with something other than neutral presentation of evidence.

In this chapter, I want to examine this avoidance of context in three ways. First, I'll discuss some of the strategies which psychiatry and clinical psychology use to avoid confronting the importance of people's social situations and life experiences not only in causing distress, but also in accounting for the particular forms it takes and how it might be alleviated and prevented. Second, when we observe avoidance of something on this scale, then we might reasonably ask, 'What is the threat?'

I will therefore make some suggestions about the nature of the threats to clinical psychology and psychiatry from acknowledging the importance of context. Finally, can anything be done? Are there ways of addressing these threats, decreasing avoidance and making people's environments and experiences more central in theory and practice?

The avoidance strategies

For clarity, these will be divided into what might be called 'pure avoidance', where context is entirely avoided, and 'safety behaviours', a term referring to behaviour adopted to neutralize threat when a feared object or situation cannot be completely avoided, for example sitting near the exit in the cinema in case of a panic attack, or only using a lift if accompanied by a friend. But when, as in this case, the feared 'object', the possible role of social context of causing distress, is less specific, then safety behaviours too are likely to be less immediately obvious.

It is important to emphasize that I am not suggesting that these strategies are consciously or deliberately devised and deployed to serve a particular purpose. They are, rather, part of everyday discursive, theoretical, empirical and clinical practice, whose origins and effects are rarely questioned. Indeed, within the mainstream it is not assumed that these practices *have* origins and effects apart from reflecting reality and furthering scientific progress.

Pure avoidance strategies

In psychiatry, the most obvious pure avoidance strategy is simply to convert distress and problem behaviour to 'symptoms' and 'disorders' and to focus entirely on these and their associated diagnostic categories. It is possible to talk extensively about people, and to produce vast amounts of research, using this strategy without once mentioning any life experience as in, for example, the study of symptom clusters, the development of symptom checklists, computations of diagnostic reliability or of the relationships between symptoms and diagnoses, and diagnoses and outcomes.

In clinical psychology, the counterpart of this is to focus on intrapsychic attributes. Psychology has invented a great many of them, usually expressed as abnormalities and deficits, to characterize people who use psychiatric services. Kenneth Gergen (1997) has called this a 'discourse of deficit' and its popularity can be gauged by the length of the list of psychological 'abnormalities' suggested as causal factors in the case of just two 'symptoms' – hearing voices and expressing very unusual beliefs. People who have these experiences have been variously described as having: defective judgement; abnormal perceptual biases; defective speech processing mechanisms; defective reality testing; parasitic memories; pathologically stored linguistic information; deficits in internal monitoring systems and an abnormal self-serving bias; and described as being hasty, over confident and suggestible, as well as making excessively external attributions and jumping to conclusions.

As with the strategy of converting experience to symptoms or disorders, a great deal of research can be and is carried out using intrapsychic attributes without ever mentioning context and life experience, including developing scales to measure 'deficits', correlating scales with each other, factor-analysing them, comparing groups on them, relating them to performance on experimental tasks and so on, none of which involves moving beyond the person's inner world of psychic 'pathology'. This avoidance strategy complements psychiatry's focus on diagnoses and disorders as these are often used as the starting point for researching 'psychopathology'.

With their exclusive focus on individuals, these discursive and research practices involve and produce a third avoidance strategy: looking for causes in brains and minds and not in people's lives. It is this strategy which regularly shapes lists of research and funding priorities for human misery; the US National Institute of Mental Health, for example, highlighted genetics, neuroimaging post-mortem studies and developmental neurobiology as research priorities for 'schizophrenia' (Hyman, 2000), while Goldberg claimed that 'the greatest changes to our knowledge of mental disorders can be expected from a combination of [brain] imaging with other technologies – for example, electrophysiological data or neuropsychological data' (2000: 649).

Pure avoidance strategies thus work together to produce the overall effect of obscuring the fact that there is even a person behind these symptoms and deficits, far less one with an actual, contextualized, life. And, by rarely or never mentioning context, such strategies have the effect of making it look as if it is simply not relevant in explaining distress.

These are tried and tested strategies but more recently a new example of pure avoidance has appeared in relation to the 2006 Layard initiative to increase access to psychological therapy. The (then) UK Labour government believed (accurately) that there are high levels of depression and anxiety in the UK population but seemed reluctant to become involved in debates about why this should be; the focus instead has been on returning people to work and reducing Incapacity Benefit payments.

So, instead of discussions about the causes of such widespread anxiety and depression, a curious situation has arisen where 'depression' and 'anxiety' are no longer semi-technical names for various forms of misery whose existence still has to be explained. Instead, depression and anxiety have been promoted to being the major causes of a separate problem called 'misery' or, as the LSE's (2006: 1) *Depression Report* puts it: 'crippling depression and chronic anxiety are the biggest causes of misery in Britain today'. Note that depression and anxiety have been given the status of first causes, rather like supernatural deities whose own existence requires no explanation. Should we now ask what causes misery, the official answer is anxiety and depression.

Safety behaviours

As I noted earlier, the evidence causally linking social context to distress and behavioural problems is plentiful and robust so that there is a limit to how far clinical psychology and psychiatry can avoid it without raising questions about their status as evidence based disciplines or professions. Avoidance strategies using safety behaviours – where context does feature in a theoretical account – are therefore crucial in creating an image of professions open to evidence, while ensuring that the evidence never seems to point to the conclusion that social context and life experiences are major causes of distress and therefore ought to be targets for intervention. Because these safety behaviours are so important, they are numerous and come in various guises. The major ones, however, appear to be:

Producing adverse environments as consequence not cause

This strategy involves presenting the kinds of environments so often associated with distress such as poverty, unemployment, poor relationships, social isolation, domestic and sexual violence, as *consequences* rather than *causes* of 'having a mental disorder'. For example, evidence that social class was negatively linked to psychiatric status led speedily to the 'downward drift' hypothesis arguing that psychological problems caused people to slip down the social hierarchy rather than the other way around, in spite of evidence to the contrary (Link et al., 1986; Muntaner et al., 1991). Similarly, links between 'relapse' of those diagnosed as schizophrenic and negative patterns of family interaction have led to claims that this negative behaviour is a response to a relative's 'schizophrenia' (Kavanagh, 1992; Coulter & Rapley, this volume). By contrast, evidence suggesting a causal link between family interaction and psychosis (Doanne et al., 1981; Goldstein, 1987; Tienari, 1991) is rarely mentioned in the mainstream literature.

The consequential strategy has been boosted by ideas about stigma and discrimination (Thornicroft, 2006) as these seem to provide mechanisms whereby service users become socially disadvantaged. I do not think it is farfetched to suggest that one of the reasons the ideas of stigma and discrimination have become such popular topics in psychiatry and clinical psychology is because they fit so well with the consequential strategy, and distract attention from the role of discrimination and other forms of social disadvantage in causing psychological problems in the first place. Of course there is credibility in the idea that emotional distress and behavioural problems have adverse social consequences. In seeing a focus on consequences as an avoidance strategy therefore, it is not a matter of denying any credibility to these claims; what is striking is the speed and enthusiasm with which a consequential argument is made when psychiatric diagnoses are associated with social adversity and the similar speed with which a causal argument is made when diagnoses are (far more weakly) associated with biological variables. The overall message from this strategy is that things only start to go wrong in people's lives *after* they have become 'mentally disordered' for other, probably biological, reasons.

The vulnerability–stress hypothesis

When this hypothesis was introduced in the 1970s by Joseph Zubin, the idea that people became 'mentally ill' through an interaction of pre-existing vulnerabilities and current environmental stressors seemed so reasonable as to be difficult to question. But the hypothesis did not, as Zubin had perhaps hoped, lead to a clear account of the nature of these vulnerabilities, how they had arisen and how the environment interacted with them to produce particular patterns of distress. Instead, the hypothesis (quickly promoted to the status of a 'model') has, with its close relative the biopsychosocial model, become an extraordinarily useful and effective strategy for downplaying the impact of life experiences on emotional distress (see Coulter & Rapley, this volume). One of the advantages of this strategy is that unlike the consequential strategy described above, it actually acknowledges a causal role for the environment (stress) thus averting criticism that this aspect is being ignored. But as soon as context or life experiences are invoked, they are negated by the implication that negative experiences are not inherently stressful but are made so by pre-existing vulnerability so that only 'the vulnerable' are adversely affected – 'normal' people would be able to cope. Part of the power of this strategy lies in the inventiveness of its proponents in generating supposed vulnerabilities (for example, McGlashan and Johannessen, 1996, list around 55, mostly biological, for 'schizophrenia' alone) and in the non-specific nature of these attributes, for example that the faulty brain 'overreacts' to the environment (Tienari et al., 1994; Warner, 2000). Such suggestions cover virtually any eventuality. Indeed, it is difficult not to be struck by the efforts made by proponents of the vulnerability–stress hypothesis to preserve the primacy of biology and to downplay even the most aversive environments such as a lifetime of racial discrimination and social disadvantage or serious sexual abuse, without the slightest theoretical or empirical justification. McGorry (2000) for example suggests that '[low] vitamin D also provides a possible explanation for the increased risk of schizophrenia in second generation dark-skinned migrants who have moved to live in cooler climates (their skin is less efficient at producing vitamin D)' (61; parenthesis in original). In a more oblique argument, Fowler et al., (2006) seem to suggest that childhood sexual abuse may exert some of its harmful effects via a genetic or constitutional inability to contextually integrate information. It is perhaps only a matter of time before it is claimed that some 'vulnerable' people are over-sensitive to sexual abuse.

To digress for a moment, the vulnerability–stress strategy is also now explicitly used by the alcohol and gambling industries to argue against restrictions on their commercial activities. They imply that 'normal' people are not affected by the widespread availability of alcohol or gambling, but that only a small group of 'the vulnerable' needs special protection and that this can be provided by, for example, industry-funded treatment programmes or age-appropriate advertising. This illustrates how quickly these professional strategies can become part of everyday social currency and be used to protect interests well beyond those of professionals.

It's all in the past

A third safety strategy is closely related to the vulnerability–stress hypothesis and underpins much cognitive behaviour therapy. The basic premise of traditional CBT is that dysfunctional assumptions about self and the world develop as a result of negative childhood experiences. These 'schemata' are then reactivated by later critical incidents (such as failing an exam, a relationship breakdown) mediated by negative automatic thoughts of which the person may not be aware. These cognitive patterns are said to produce negative affective states such as depression and anxiety.

Here, the potentially damaging effects of adverse environments are directly acknowledged but placed firmly out of reach and out of sight in the past, in the person's early experience; its main role is to create a person who now thinks dysfunctionally, irrationally or idiosyncratically about a seemingly benign or only averagely difficult present. But it is dangerously easy to 'forget' these past events and focus only on the cognitive present, which CBT explicitly does. Indeed, it is increasingly common to refer to cognitive accounts as theories of problem *maintenance* so that questions about early adverse experiences may no longer even be asked, far less answered.

This safety strategy, most popularly exemplified by cognitive theory and therapy, therefore obscures the potential impact of context in two distinct ways. The first is by theoretically placing experiences acknowledged as being very negative (for example, abuse, neglect or bullying) in the distant past so that their remoteness, and the fact that they cannot now be changed, appear to justify lack of close attention to them. The second is by constructing the present as a series of triggers or critical incidents which by implication are not sufficient in themselves to produce serious emotional distress. This construction is greatly facilitated by the use in textbooks of examples of triggers which are, if not exactly mundane, then relatively common such as being ignored by an acquaintance, failing an exam or being rejected following a job interview rather than, say, being evicted from your home or suffering repeated racial abuse. The theory underlying traditional CBT can thus be seen as a sophisticated version of the vulnerability–stress hypothesis – and this is no doubt part of its popularity as a safety strategy for psychology and psychiatry. The additional element of a vulnerability created by specific negative early life experiences, rather than non-specific genes or biology, is not as threatening as it might be in terms of foregrounding the environment because, as I've noted, the remoteness of these events seems to justify keeping them well in the theoretical and practical background.

Finally, three safety behaviours which often appear as a group – sanitize, quantify but do not theorize. By sanitize, I mean the use of neutral or 'technical' language such as expressed emotion, low social support, stress, life events, and so on to refer to highly negative life experiences which are then further sanitized by being converted to numbers stripped not only of factual description but also of all personal meaning. The result is that what has actually happened to people is rarely spelled out, making it much easier for others to assume that the experiences of those who receive psychiatric diagnoses cannot be that negative or important in causing distress in comparison to putative biological or psychological deficits. This approach also encourages descriptive and rather simplistic research, for example linking 'amounts' of sanitized variables (number of life events; scores on scales of expressed emotion) to 'symptom' ratings, relapse, treatment response and so on. While some of this research has been important in highlighting statistical links between life experience and distress, detailed analytical theorizing about the nature of these links is usually avoided. I will return later to why that might be and why it is so important.

What is the threat?

Before I discuss why confronting the potential importance of the environment in causing distress should be so threatening to psychiatry and clinical psychology, it is worth emphasizing several points. As I said earlier, I am not suggesting that strategies for avoiding context are used in a planned and conscious way. Like any defence mechanism they are a mixture of the conscious and the unconscious, the articulated and the unarticulated. The strategies undoubtedly gain credibility from their partial truth – people *are* discriminated against if they use psychiatric services and their early experiences *do* influence how they react to future events. And no doubt the biological, psychological and social do interact in producing human action and emotion. But strategies which avoid confronting the importance of context in initiating and maintaining distress also gain credibility from the symbiotic relationship between psychological and psychiatric theory and method and Western, particularly North American, cultural assumptions about the primacy of the autonomous individual. Mainstream psychology and psychiatry, without ever acknowledging the fact, have been profoundly influenced by these assumptions in seeing their role as the study of decontextualized individuals whose behaviour, cognitions and emotions are best accounted for by reference to their brains and minds. Thus, the DSM conceptualizes each of the 'mental disorders' listed as: 'a clinically significant behavioural or psychological syndrome or pattern that occurs *in an individual*' (1994: xxi–xxii, emphasis added). As for psychology, Raitt and Zeedyk have summed up the situation well in commenting that 'to "do" psychology is almost necessarily to provide an individualistic account of behaviour' (2000: 56).

The result is that what I have called here avoidance strategies are never seen as such by those who employ them; instead they manifest themselves as taken for granted, routine, ways of speaking, theorizing, researching and practising but their effect is to create an academic and professional context in which the focus on deficiencies of individuals as both the primary source of their distress and the primary target of change, seems beyond question. This not only deflects attention from what the person has experienced but also, and as we shall we see crucially, from who and what else were involved in these experiences. Credible and taken for granted these practices might be, but we are still entitled to look behind them, to call them avoidance strategies linked to fear and threat, because they involve ignoring and manipulating so much evidence about the importance of context. It is also difficult to convey just how extensive and pervasive these avoidance strategies are, the ease and fluency with which they are used. I would suggest that, in one way or another, they feature in well over 90 per cent of mainstream psychiatric and clinical psychology literature. What might motivate this? What is it about acknowledging social context or life experiences as major causes of emotional and psychological problems, as crucial in understanding their meaning, and what is it about theorizing the nature and significance of these links that is so threatening to psychiatry and psychology? Obviously, there is no one answer to this but I want to suggest some fundamental aspects of the threat which may help to explain why so much effort is made to neutralize it. Although there are similarities and overlaps in the nature of the threat to psychiatry and clinical psychology, there are important differences so I will deal with the two groups separately.

For psychiatry, the fundamental threat is *not* that people's behavioural, emotional and psychological problems can be shown to be statistically correlated with their life experiences and social context. As we have seen, these statistical relationships can easily be dealt with – neutralized – by the vulnerability–stress hypothesis or by consequentialist arguments. What is truly threatening to psychiatry is evidence that both the *form and content* of emotional distress and 'disordered' behaviour are *systematically, meaningfully and inseparably related* to social context and life experience. The reason this is so threatening is because the medical model which underlies both the modern DSM and hence psychiatry's authority, is explicitly justified on the basis that those behaviours and experiences said to constitute mental disorders are *not* meaningful and intelligible, that instead they are outward symptoms of an internal pathology and therefore not subject to the same rules as so-called normal behaviour or normal distress – hence the use of a medical framework to explain them.

As Jacobs and Cohen (2010) point out, placing certain instances of distress in a pathology framework involves presenting the person not as feeling or behaving intelligibly given their history and current situation but as having become, 'through no intention or action of his of her own ... the setting for the operation of impersonal, harmful cause-effect processes' – the biochemical imbalances, structural brain abnormalities and gene defects invoked in so much psychiatric theorizing. The problem for psychiatry – and the magnitude of the problem can hardly be overstated – is that it has never been able reliably to identify these 'impersonal, harmful, cause-effect processes' which supposedly justify the medical model, far less show that they are operating in any particular distressed individual. Clearly, a way out of this difficulty must be found. The DSM argues, then, that in order to be considered a mental disorder, a person's 'symptoms' or 'impairments' 'must not be merely an expectable and culturally sanctioned response to a particular event, for example the death of a loved one. Whatever its original cause, it must currently be considered a manifestation of a behavioural, psychological or biological dysfunction in the individual' (1994; xxi–xxii). The first part of this criterion is clearly absurd. It assumes the existence of a 'database', which psychiatrists can consult listing which responses every 'culture' both expects and sanctions in relation to every imaginable set of life circumstances. Not only that, but the criterion conflates the absence of cultural expectation or sanction, assuming this could ever be demonstrated, with the presence of internal pathology and dysfunction (see Boyle, 2002a for a more detailed discussion of this point). The second part is equally absurd. Who is entitled to 'consider' that the person's distress is a 'manifestation of internal dysfunction' and why should mere consideration be taken as evidence?

Psychiatry, then, insofar as it sees itself as a medical specialty, dependent on the DSM, is in an extremely difficult position. By its own definition (although not usually stated quite so bluntly), its subject matter is meaningless distress, distress which is not intelligible in terms of a person's culture, life experiences or current circumstances. Yet psychiatry cannot identify the non-cultural, non-social, non-personal processes supposedly responsible and can only offer criteria for distinguishing meaningful and meaningless distress which, to put it mildly, are not fit for purpose. As Jacobs (2009) and Jacobs and Cohen (2010) have shown, attempting to square this particular circle leads the authors of the DSM into labyrinthine and often contradictory arguments and attempts at justification. It is no wonder that psychiatry is so fearful of context and has to devise so many strategies to avoid it, because context constantly threatens to make emotional and behavioural problems intelligible or, to put it another way, it threatens to abolish psychiatry's self-defined subject matter.

What about clinical psychology? Why do mainstream clinical psychology and its parent discipline psychology, use these avoidance strategies every bit as much as psychiatry to limit our understanding of distress – when on the face of it psychology has nothing to fear from making distress psychologically and socially intelligible, indeed that would seem to be one of its major purposes. Again, there is obviously no one answer to this but I want to suggest two closely related possible answers.

The first concerns psychology's extreme insecurity about its academic and social acceptance as a science. This may be traced to the discipline's roots in philosophy but whatever its origins, psychology deals with this insecurity by identifying with and superficially imitating disciplines such as physics, biology, neuroscience and medicine, whose scientific status is more secure in the public mind and by distancing itself from disciplines such as sociology and anthropology which may be seen, however inaccurately, as less scientific. A second related reason for avoiding context is that psychology is also greatly preoccupied with avoiding accusations of social and political bias, of being influenced by values rather than disinterestedly pursuing truth (Boyle, 1997). It is therefore very concerned to be seen as engaged only in research whose claims to objectivity are accepted by the public and whose results can more easily be presented as fact rather than opinion. It is partly for these reasons that psychology is much more comfortable talking about brains and minds than about poverty, sexual violence and racial oppression, that it has made experimental and quantitative methods so fundamental to the discipline (Danziger, 1985) and that attempts to introduce alternative methods may be met with such hostility (see Morgan, 1998). For similar reasons, mainstream clinical psychology has followed the lead of its parent discipline in avoiding socially and politically sensitive topics and in giving the highest status to experimental and quantitative methods. This, together with the pressing need to be accepted by and coexist with psychiatry in order to function as a profession, has led it to impose on 'abnormal' behaviour and experiences a language and theoretical framework derived from the study of the body and to imply a discontinuity between 'normal' and 'abnormal' behaviour and experiences.

This is not to say that experimental and quantitative methods, or a knowledge of biological processes, have no place in the study of human behaviour. But identifying so strongly with the natural and biological sciences has meant that even when psychology and clinical psychology tentatively engage with social context or the social meaning of behaviour and experience, there are severe limitations on what they can say. This is not because it is intrinsically unscientific to study context and meaning but because they may not be particularly relevant to the disciplines psychology rather cravenly imitates and whose methods – developed for a non-social subject matter – were not designed to answer questions about context or human relationships and whose theoretical frameworks were not designed to generate such questions. Unfortunately, in imitating the style rather than the substance of prestigious disciplines, psychology has paid insufficient attention to the cautions of philosophers of science that there is no one scientific method but rather methods designed to suit particular subject matters and to render particular problems soluble (Chalmers, 1990; Kuhn, 1970).

But there is more going on here than a craving to be recognized as a science and a mistaken idea of what this might mean. Modern psychology not only relies on experimental and quantitative methods but, as I noted earlier, also presents its subject matter as the study of individual minds. In an early and detailed analysis, Sampson (1981) argued that far from being self-evident, this choice of subject matter functions to maintain the social and ideological status quo, not least by cutting people off from an understanding of how mental operations relate to social and historical practice, and from effective action to change their *actual* circumstances rather than their *subjective understanding* of these circumstances. Sampson linked the focus on individual minds to the increasing dominance of cognitivism in modern psychology, a trend which has become even more pronounced since his paper, and is also reflected in clinical psychology's adoption of cognitive behaviour therapy as its major therapeutic approach (House & Lowenthal, 2008). It is notable that the rise of cognitivism since the mid 1970s has paralleled an increasing social and political emphasis on the individual and particularly the individual as consumer, a correlation that is unlikely to be accidental. Context, in the sense that it refers to people's circumstances, to their interactions to the external world, is not, therefore, a neutral term and attending to or ignoring it are not neutral acts to be explained merely through a preference for one or other theoretical models. Just how un-neutral context is, can be gauged by listing those aspects most consistently related to distress and problem behaviour – child abuse and neglect, school and workplace bullying, domestic and sexual violence, discrimination, poverty and unemployment. It is not difficult to work out that these events involve relatively powerful groups – governments, corporations, men, white people, adults – damaging less powerful groups. In the case of emotional distress, then, context seems to include or even equate to the operation of power. This suggests that another way of looking at mainstream psychology's dominant theories and methods, and the strategies I have discussed here for avoiding social context, is to say that they are actually ways of obscuring the operation of power and of protecting relatively powerful groups from scrutiny.

Mainstream psychology and clinical psychology operate routinely to offer this protection but from time to time extraordinary measures are called for. An obvious example is the swift collaboration of parents, researchers and professionals in the invention of 'false memory syndrome' in the face of allegations from women in therapy about child sexual abuse. This medical sounding label went well beyond denying the allegations – mainly against fathers and which may or may not have been true – to the wholesale pathologization and invalidation of the women concerned. The censorship of any suggestion that what happens in families might have causal links to the initiation of psychosis can be seen in a similar light. The less subtle aspects of this censorship range from accusations of blaming the parents, or being old fashioned and out of touch with evidence, to being told bluntly that you cannot say that. And mainstream clinical psychology – and psychiatry – have readily agreed not to say it, relying instead on the safety behaviours of invoking the vulnerability–stress hypothesis and the claim that negative family environments are a consequence of a pre-existing mental disorder.

So by minimizing or denying the importance of life experiences and social context – by choosing not to expose the operation of power – mainstream psychology gains the double advantage of both appearing more 'scientific' and also avoiding the risk of offending the powerful by seeming to implicate them in causing distress to others; here, the powerful actually means any group that might make a public fuss over suggestions that they harm others and be taken seriously; it does not usually include users of mental health services who in fact often find themselves accused of being a major source of harm to others. In following psychology in minimizing context, clinical psychology gains the added advantage of placating psychiatry, which, for the reasons I discussed earlier, is as keen as psychology to avoid making context central. In fact, what we seem to have are three very insecure groups who have implicitly agreed not to expose the operation of power in return for academic and professional privileges.

What can be done?

Can anything be done about this? Is it possible to reduce clinical psychology's and psychiatry's fear and avoidance of people's environment as a potential cause of their distress? Exposure to what you fear is a very effective way of reducing fear and avoidance. In this case, however, the threat to clinical psychology and psychiatry is very real and rational; it is doubtful that either profession, especially psychiatry, could survive in its current form if people's context and life experiences were made central. Mere exposure to evidence about context is therefore unlikely to be the whole answer as it will simply be neutralized in the ways I have described. On the other hand, without exposure – by which I mean that prominence is given to context and life experience at every possible opportunity in practice, theory and research – nothing will change. What is important is to create exposure to context while minimizing the opportunity to use any of the avoidance strategies I've discussed. Full discussion of what this might entail is beyond the scope of this chapter, but I will make some initial suggestions (see also Boyle, 2006).

First, it is imperative to be aware of what is at stake. If psychology's and psychiatry's neglect of social context is simply seen as an oversight to be corrected by the provision of evidence, rather than as a highly strategic and complex defence mechanism, then we may be very unprepared for the strength and, I have to say, at times aggressiveness of resistance to any attempt to insert context as cause into discussions of emotional or behavioural problems. And if what is at stake is borne in mind then we can respond to the underlying fear rather than the overt resistance, which should at least make for some interesting discussions.

More specifically, I would argue that a persistent emphasis on the intelligibility and meaningfulness of emotional distress, 'bizarre' psychological experiences and problem behaviours are essential in challenging strategies for avoiding context. This is because all of the strategies, some blatantly others very subtly, act to undermine these aspects of distress and because it is the apparent absence of intelligibility which makes it so easy and so apparently necessary to apply a medical model or any model based on individual deficits in which context plays only a minor or no role. Emphasizing intelligibility does not simply mean proclaiming the fact although that always helps; it means that every presentation of distress, in theory, research, teaching, case discussions, media presentations and everyday conversations between service users and professionals would have at its centre, unless there is strong evidence to the contrary, the idea that people's feelings and actions are consonant with their past and present experiences. It also means taking great care not to resort to those safety strategies which admit (some) intelligibility with one hand and snatch it away with the other, invoking biological vulnerabilities, cognitive dysfunctions or psychological deficits. Most of all, perhaps, it means being aware that 'abnormal' experience and behaviour often seem unintelligible because we do not know enough about what someone has experienced and because as a society we are reluctant to acknowledge how damaging some 'normal' social practices, such as gender role socialization or consumerism may be.

Closely related to this is the need to acknowledge the importance of language. The avoidance strategies discussed are also powerful linguistic devices which have the effect of making context seem not very important or even irrelevant for understanding or alleviating people's problems. It is not just the almost exclusive use of a vocabulary of symptoms, deficits, disorders and vulnerabilities or sanitized ways of describing life experiences; it is the absence of crucial concepts like inequality, power, subordination and resistance. It is also the extensive use of the passive voice which keeps damaging agents invisible, saying for example, 'women with low social support are vulnerable to depression' rather than something like, 'women who live with oppressive men are made miserable' (Pilgrim & Bentall, 1999). I would argue that these linguistic devices are so powerful that it will be almost impossible to challenge context-avoidance strategies and make context more central, without entirely abandoning medical language, including the term 'mental health', because using this language is the quickest and most effective way of implying lack of intelligibility and suggesting a pathological or deficient individual. At the very least, using this language means that extra work has to be done to reinstate context and meaning which never sit easily with talk of illness, symptoms or disorders. It could be the difference, for example, between saying 'John is a widower with psychotic symptoms' and saying 'the critical voices John hears may be part of a painful debate he is having with himself about whether he cared enough for his wife when she was dying'. The difficulty with this, of course, is that researchers and professionals are all very fluent in context-free or context-'lite' language – it is the first language they are taught – so that talking in ways which make life experiences and their social meanings central, as distinct from absent or secondary, is literally to speak a foreign language and risk sounding rather strange. Like any novel and potentially hazardous undertaking, it is therefore perhaps best done the presence of allies (see Johnstone,

2000; Miller & McLelland, 2006 and Jacobs, 2009 for examples of speaking in this way). Our attempts to speak differently would gain much support from research into how talk and language work in various settings – consultations, ward rounds, case discussions, teaching sessions, media reports and research literature – to make context seem unimportant in explaining distress. What happens when service users talk about their life experiences in consultations? How do professionals frame questions about such experiences or present them in formulations? How do they respond to media questions about the causes of mental distress?

Important though language is, however, if we are going to make social context more prominent, to make distress meaningful and intelligible, we cannot do so without good theory. It is not enough to say, for example, that ethnicity is linked to psychosis or that gender is linked to depression; we have to be able to explicate how particular social structures, power relationships, patterns of family interaction, employment practices, economic and social policies and so on manifest themselves in particular forms and content of distress and behavioural problems. In other words we need theories which explicitly link the social and the behavioural/psychological, exactly the kind of theories which mainstream psychology and psychiatry have been reluctant to develop.

Fortunately, there are many relevant theoretical ideas outside the mainstream, for example in critical and feminist psychology, in other disciplines, notably anthropology, and increasingly in 'popular' writing (for example, Seidenberg & Decrow, 1983; Dryden, 1999; Johnstone, 2000; Smail, 2001; Stoppard, 2000; Littlewood, 2002; Barber, 2007; Malson & Burns, 2009; Wilkinson & Pickett, 2009). Equally there are theories within mainstream psychology such as social learning theory which are very capable of being contextualized (Jukes, 1999). Without theory we end up only with unexplained correlations between the environment and distress which, as we have seen, are all too easily manipulated to make context hazy or invisible.

Finally, I have noted psychology's (and psychiatry's) insecurity about their scientific status. Given this, it is perhaps unsurprising that challenges to the mainstream are often met not with curious questioning but with a recitation of research said to support traditional theory and practice. This means – not unreasonably – that challenging strategies which avoid context must involve close familiarity with the strengths and weaknesses of evidence offered in support of them as well as of evidence for the primary role of context in causing distress.

These suggestions may seem rather abstract, nothing you can go out and do tomorrow. But if we do not address the power and persistence of strategies for avoiding context, and the fear that motivates them, and if we do not with equal persistence make it difficult to use them, then the possibility of de-medicalizing misery seems very remote.

4
Cultural Diversity and Racism: An Historical Perspective

Suman Fernando

Introduction

Cultural diversity is not something new in the United Kingdom (UK) – after all there have been waves of immigration over the centuries. What was new during the 1960s and 1970s, was that diversity became more visible because of the settlement of large numbers of people within the UK, whose cultural roots were from Asia, Africa and the Caribbean, rather than Europe – people who *looked* different mainly because of the colour of their skins. With society being composed of people who were different in 'race', attitudes, which until then had largely been kept safely in the colonies and other foreign parts, were suddenly evident in the UK. Chickens had come home to roost. It is in this context that a variety of problems in the mental health field – sometimes called 'ethnic issues' have emerged during the past 25 or 20 years. What we see, then, is that Black and Minority Ethnic (BME) people are more often diagnosed as schizophrenic; compulsorily detained under Mental Health Act; admitted as 'offender patients'; held by police under Section 136 of Mental Health Act; transferred to locked wards from open wards and not referred for psychotherapy.

Instead of exploring these issues head-on, this paper takes a historical perspective of the problems presented after discussing very briefly the terms culture, 'race', racism and ethnicity. In doing so the paper will discuss the current practice of psychiatry in relation to issues around race and culture.

Culture

At one time culture was seen as a relatively fixed system of traditional beliefs that are passed on from generation to generation – for example by Leighton and Hughes (1961) who defined culture as being composed of 'shared patterns of belief, feeling and adaptation which people carry in their minds'. But, this approach has given way to a view of culture as something that cannot be clearly defined, as something living, dynamic and changing – a flexible system of values and worldviews that people live by and create and re-create continuously, a system by which we define our identities and negotiate our lives (see Fernando, 2003, 2010). And so, understanding culture, training in cultural understanding, or learning about one's own or other people's cultures is about seeking an awareness of group norms being created in the here-and-now in a context of the lived experience of people.

The multicultural society of modern Britain shows evidence of many diverse cultural influences – for example from Asia, Africa and the Caribbean – as well as those geographically closer in Europe. This plurality of cultures involves us all – we are all culturally 'hybrid'; yet there are groups or communities in our society that we can point to as 'cultural groups' distinguished by certain cultural forms – of marriage customs, main language and so on. But unlike in some other countries, notably the United States of America (USA), these British cultural groups are seldom cut off from each other and from the main majority culture. In other words, what is characteristic of most parts of the UK is that there is intermingling of peoples and cultures.

This way of seeing culture as a flexible system is very important in the mental health field not least because we inherit a background of racist ideas about 'culture' and cultural difference – discussed later in this paper. What is also important to grasp is that the disciplines that inform mental health services (mainly psychiatry and Western psychology) have grown out of a particular culturally determined understanding of the human condition, ideologies about life and so on, generally termed 'western culture', and hence they are at variance with – sometimes in conflict with – understandings and ideologies in 'other' cultures. There is a sort of culture clash between psychiatry and Western psychology on the one hand and a multicultural society on the other. In short, society is multicultural but the disciplines are uni-cultural.

Race and racism

The concept of 'race' as we understand it is based on selected aspects of physical appearance such as skin colour and generally assumed to be a biologically determined entity. However this idea of 'race' has been dismissed in scientific circles as a basis for dividing up the human race. As Rose et al. (1984: 127) put it: 'Human "racial" differentiation is indeed only skin deep. Any use of racial categories must take its justification from some other source than biology.' One source of course is the socio-political and so some people refer to it as 'social-race' (Omi & Winant, 1994). But the tendency to think of people in terms of their 'race', 'race thinking' (Barzun, 1965), persists in spite of the unscientific nature of race itself as an entity. And this race thinking, allied to ways of thinking that place different races in a hierarchic scale or ladder, is at the heart of both personal racism, usually called 'race prejudice', as well as more generalized attitudes, behaviours and institutional practices that have racist implications, referred to as just 'racism' (for further discussion see Fernando, 2003, 2010).

The nature of racism is often driven by history and context (Goldberg, 1993); and the ways in which people experience racism varies. Thus racism during American slavery differs from post-slavery segregationism and each from current expressions of racism in the USA. Racism in South Africa during the times of apartheid differs from that expressed through inequalities in the post apartheid era. Nineteenth-century-British racism in the colonies differs from current manifestations of racism in the UK. Racism experienced by a person who *looks* African or Caribbean is different to that experienced by someone who *looks* Chinese or South Asian or wears clothes that indicate a particular religious adherence.

In the mental health field, racism can work through in a variety of ways in systems of control epitomized in forensic psychiatry. Stereotypes of dangerousness play a big part here (see later); risk assessments are strongly permeated by an image of black violence that is evident in Western media and the 'common-sense' of the person-in-the-street. But stereotypes are not static and their effect varies from time to time, often as a result of political concerns or events taken up in the media. Changes in legislation (for e.g. in the Mental Health Act) often promote certain ways of thinking among professionals.

Philomena Essed (1990) talks of the 'everyday racism' experienced in myriads of little ways through ways of behaving and socializing – the way people look at you (or don't look), see you (or don't see), the drip-drip-drip that builds up. People who exhibit racism are not necessarily overtly (racially) prejudiced, although if one examines their attitudes in some depth racist attitudes may be uncovered. In fact racism may be manifested in social and political systems because people – black and white – unwittingly collude in it, usually because they gain in some way from doing so.

Ethnicity

'Ethnicity' is essentially about self-perception – how people see themselves in terms of both 'race' and 'culture' – set in a historical background (of where we come from) experienced as part of family or community (see Hall, 1992; Senior & Bhopal, 1994). So if racism is felt as a powerful force in society now or in the past, people from various backgrounds or cultures may see themselves largely in racial terms (e.g. as 'black people') but also (or alternatively) identify in 'cultural' terms of history, religion or parental birthplace (e.g. as 'Irish', 'Muslim', 'Caribbean' or 'Asian'). The current tendency in the UK is to refer to 'black and minority ethnic communities' or BME communities, leaving open the issues of what exactly an ethnic community comprises. But this means that recent immigrants, especially refugees and asylum seekers, often get left out of the BME category and may be called 'migrants' (as different to BME) – a category of exclusion in many parts of Europe, including of course the UK. This topic is discussed in updated form and greater detail elsewhere (Fernando, 2010).

Psychiatry

Psychiatry as we know it today arose about 200 – 300 years ago from two main sources. First, the need to control and 'put away' lunatics wandering and disturbing the more affluent areas of European cities. Second, a growing medical interest in matters to do with the mind in European medical circles. The two influences came together in medical domination over people considered 'mad' and the definition of lunacy in terms of illnesses. As it developed as a medical discipline, various categories of illness were constructed, so that various problems – problems for individuals, for families, and for society in general – were construed as mental health problems, as 'illness' – with pathology located in different parts of the individual mind – thinking, emotions, intellect and so on. Yet, psychiatry and its counterpart clinical psychology did not develop in a vacuum.

The construction of illness happened in a particular social and political context. By copying the medical approach of defining problems as 'illness', psychiatry and the mental illnesses it constructed achieved a sort of prestige of being 'real' in a biological sense although there is little to justify this. But objective biological tools for detecting or measuring mental illness have *never* been there for psychiatry, mainly because it is concerned with the 'mind' – a concept rather than a 'thing' – associated with subjective emotions, feelings and so on. The result is that psychiatry and its illness models have always been open to permeation by social and political forces and have always reflected these forces in its theory and practice.

The way that psychiatry and (Western) psychology developed as a part of the European 'Enlightenment', when reason took precedence over other forms of understanding and the values of liberty, individual rights and democracy emerged as influences in Western culture, are described in detail elsewhere (Fernando, 2010). But it is noteworthy that, as Toni Morrison (1990) points out, this enlightenment of European thought happened during the heyday of slavery and colonialism when powerful myths of racism were being refined and integrated into European culture. It could be argued that racism is indeed a 'European value' permeating much of post-enlightenment-European thinking, including that which underpins Western psychology and psychiatry.

Racism in psychiatry

In the nineteenth century, there was contentious discussion as to whether there was greater or lesser amount of madness among non-Europeans (usually called primitives or savages) compared to white people. Three theories were rife: (a) the 'noble savage' idea that uncivilized (i.e. non-European) people were free from madness; (b) that savages were mentally degenerate anyway; and (c) that it all depended on context; for instance, statistics in USA allegedly showed that mental illness was more often reported among freed slaves compared to those who were still in slavery (Thomas & Sillen, 1972). It was taken to mean that slavery was conducive to mental health for black people. Significantly, we are still pre-occupied with a question about race and the modern equivalent of madness, namely schizophrenia.

In the mid-nineteenth century, black slaves who persistently escaped were diagnosed as suffering from a disease of the mind called *drapetomania*, named after the Greek words meaning 'run away' and 'mad or crazy' (Cartwright, 1851). When John Langdon Down (1866) surveyed so-called idiots and imbeciles resident in institutions around London, he identified them as 'racial throwbacks' to Ethiopian, Malay and Mongolian racial types – mostly, he said, they were 'Mongols'. He was in fact reflecting an explanation for pathology that was common at the time – the ideology of 'degeneration' (Morel, 1852). The underlying thesis was that social conflict, aggression, insanity and criminality were all signs of individual pathology representing reversal (throwback) to a racially primitive stage of development, either mentally or physically, or both (Pick, 1989) – an explanation that Kraepelin (1904) took on in constructing dementia praecox (which became 'schizophrenia').

When Kraepelin (1913) observed that guilt was not seen in Javanese people who became depressed, his conclusion was that Javanese were 'a psychically underdeveloped population' akin to 'immature European youth' (Kraepelin, 1921: 171). Stanley Hall (1904), founder of the *American Journal of Psychology* and first president of the American Psychological Association (Thomas & Sillen, 1972: 7), described, in a standard text on adolescence, Asians, Chinese, Africans and Indigenous Americans as psychologically 'adolescent races' who 'live a life of feeling emotion and impulse' (1904: 80). Swiss psychologist Carl Jung observed that white Americans were culturally different to (white) Europeans because they were adversely affected by 'racial infection' from living too close to black people. 'The inferior man exercises a tremendous pull upon civilized beings who are forced to live with him because he fascinates the inferior layers of our psyche' (Jung, 1930:196).

The idea that black people are underdeveloped white people (that pervades the so-called knowledge that informs psychiatry and psychology) dies hard and, I think, still underpins much of what emerges today as tests in psychology and more generally as explanations for differences in expression of distress – for example usually as a 'lack' of something among black people.

In the years following World War II, Carothers (1971), hailed by WHO as an expert on the 'African Mind', reported that Africans did not get depressed because they (like African-Americans) lacked 'a sense of responsibility' (1953: 148); and that their thinking resembled that of 'leucotomised Europeans'. More recently, Leff (1973, 1981), after analysing observations across the world, concluded that people from Africa and Asia as well as black Americans (the politically 'Black') have a less developed ability to differentiate emotions when compared with Europeans and white Americans – a finding interpreted by him as representing the 'historical development of emotional differentiation', an 'evolutionary process' (1981: 65–6). These ideas are in line with recurring versions of the racist IQ movement in psychology (e.g. Herrnstein & Murray, 1994) that represent the general 'under-development' thesis implicit in psychiatry and (Western) psychology referred to later in this paper.

Racism in psychiatry today

Twenty first-century Britain, like many other Western societies, has made overt racism unacceptable. So what we are often faced with is institutional racism obscured to a large extent by political correctness in discourse. In this context the main racial issue in psychiatry – as well as in other systems such as education and law enforcement – is identified as institutional racism which has been defined in the Macpherson report (Home Office, 1999) into the way the police mishandled the investigation of the murder in 1993 of Stephen Lawrence, a black teenager:

> The collective failure of an organisation to provide an appropriate and professional service to people because of their colour, culture or ethnic origin. It can be seen or detected in processes, attitudes and behaviour that amount to discrimination through unwitting prejudice, ignorance, thoughtlessness and racist stereotyping that disadvantages minority ethnic people.
>
> (Home Office, 1999: 28)

Various themes – images, stereotypes, ways of thinking, ways of researching, traditions – affect the way psychiatry and psychology function in British society and possibly in all predominantly white societies of Europe and North America. A theme apart from that of 'dangerousness' is the perception of black people and their cultures as underdeveloped in terms of expressing sophisticated emotions (as evident in the studies by Leff referred to earlier), particularly depression, and so seeing black people as being unable to handle emotional problems without suppressive – indeed oppressive – medication or other intrusive interventions to change ways of thinking.

The discourse around psychiatry and psychology often forgets that psychiatry is not just a medical discipline involved in helping people described as 'ill' but, from the very beginning, it has been concerned with social control – and of course still is concerned with control, especially in the field of forensic psychiatry. The new discourses in mental health that we hear so much about – for example, 'recovery', 'spirituality', 'values-based practice' and 'wellbeing' – have no place in forensic services or the 'hard end' of psychiatry where patients are invariably dealt with in the traditional narrow illness model. This aspect of the psychiatric system is one that specially concerns BME communities, especially people who look African or 'black'.

'Subtle racism' was the term used to describe the ideology at Broadmoor Hospital by a team asked to inquire into the death of Orville Blackwood way back in 1993, the year that Stephen Lawrence was murdered. Orville was a black man (inevitably diagnosed as 'schizophrenic') who died in a seclusion room – the third to do so within a short time – hence the inquiry (Special Hospitals Service Authority, 1993). The report was subtitled 'Big, Black and Dangerous' reflecting the racist stereotype that they found to be prevalent in British forensic psychiatry. At places like Broadmoor Hospital (the foremost British Forensic institute) that I used to visit in the 1980s and 1990s, racism is easily hidden under the medical umbrella of psychiatry, with clinical judgement being paramount. Ten years after the Blackwood inquiry (and several more deaths in psychiatric custody) the inquiry report into the death of David Bennett (Norfolk, Suffolk and Cambridgeshire Strategic Health Authority, 2003) draws similar lessons to those given in the Blackwood report. After ambiguous statements by government ministers, at first admitting and later denying that racism existed in mental health systems, none of the recommendations of either report has been acted upon.

The situation today is that Government quotes work being done under the plan *Delivering Race Equality* (Department of Health, 2005) as the answer to what it calls 'racial inequalities' in the mental health system. I do not think anyone on the ground who is actually involved in DRE work thinks it will deliver much to change the mental health system (Fernando, 2007) The only lasting achievement of DRE is to provide us with even more information on racial inequality through its yearly one-day census reports justifying our fears that little has changed since the 1980s.

Conclusions

Psychiatry is a child of Western culture – there is no Ayurvedic psychiatry or psychiatry in Chinese Traditional Medicine (TCM) or a psychiatry of Africa or First Nations of America (also called indigenous peoples or aboriginals of America). So a major problem for British society, which is culturally hybrid, is the unicultural and racist nature of psychiatry and the fact that the psychology it draws on is entirely Western psychology – nothing at all from the many other psychologies of the world. Incidentally, the fact that psychiatry, like Coca-Cola, has been sold or applied – or one might say, imposed – all over the world says something about power and status rather than about usefulness or validity. But it goes on unrelentingly – as a form of imperialism (Fernando, 2010).

Mental health services are underpinned by psychiatry, and I think unlikely to change much unless psychiatry itself changes in some fundamental way. So BME communities generally welcome the critical psychiatry movement and the alternative ways of seeing human problems being put up by (for example) 'Hearing Voices Network'. But in a multicultural society that is not enough. Not just psychiatry, or just the biomedical model that informs it, but the movements critical of psychiatry too, have roots in west-European culture. If we are to reach out for an understanding of human beings that is universal, multicultural and nonracist, we must draw from a plethora of world cultures, and address racism in all its forms.

In searching for alternatives we must look for inspiration to systems of medicine and the psychologies within (for example) Ayurveda (of India), TCM and African systems (pejoratively and unjustly termed 'witchcraft' by Western anthropologists) and I think we need to turn to the great religions of the world; for example Buddhism is much more a psychology than a religion in Western terminology. Yet, this is not simple; these non-European systems have been underdeveloped – often suppressed – for 200 years; some are almost stuck in a time warp. Indeed (for example) the once-highly-advanced systems of North American First Nations were illegal in Canada until the 1960s and only recently been allowed to function at all. Even today, Ayurveda has low priority in terms of government spending even in Asian countries, with governments that still suffer from colonial thinking – and Western money often provided through non-governmental organizations (NGOs) calls the tune.

A historical view shows that psychiatry is racist primarily because it comes from a west-European social context that was itself racist, right from the Enlightenment onwards; so alternatives to psychiatry, as they develop (and I sincerely hope they do), run the risk of being racist because (in a way) racism is the natural – 'normal' – state of affairs, the default position. So to continue the analogy, unless one customizes the alternatives we are trying to build up, unless we make active efforts to be anti-racist, racism is likely to pervade these too.

5
The Social Context of Paranoia

David J. Harper

'Psychiatry', suggests Hornstein (2009a: 6), 'is the most contested field in medicine' and, as Bracken and Thomas (2001: 724) note, '[i]t is hard to imagine the emergence of "antipaediatrics" or "critical anaesthetics" movements'. But why is this so? One of the reasons is that there is often a fundamental disagreement about the meaning attributed to experience and, who has the right to confer that meaning. Experiences like paranoia are often decontextualized and stripped of meaning. For example, psychiatry variously classifies paranoia as a subtype of schizophrenia, a separate delusional disorder or as a type of personality disorder. Yet arcane discussions of the differences between diagnostic subtypes distract from commonalities in the way paranoia is experienced.

In this chapter I investigate the concept of paranoia, paying attention to its contested nature. I take a deliberately broad view, seeing it as an apparently unwarranted fear and belief that others intend to harm one in some way, leading us to respond to others in a fearful, wary and even hostile manner. Deciding on the best way to address such distressing feelings very much depends on what we think paranoia is and so, the chapter begins with an examination of some of the conceptual assumptions embedded in the notion.

Problematizing paranoia

One of the core assumptions made when diagnosing paranoia is that the person is fearful or hostile because their beliefs about the intentions of others are false. In simple terms, their beliefs are delusional. According to the American Psychiatric Association a delusion is:

> A false belief based on incorrect inference about external reality that is firmly sustained despite what almost everyone else believes and despite

what constitutes incontrovertible and obvious proof or evidence to the contrary. The belief is not one ordinarily accepted by other members of the person's culture or subculture (e.g. it s not an article or religious faith). When a false belief involves a value judgement, it is regarded as a delusion only when the judgement is so extreme as to defy credibility. Delusional conviction occurs on a continuum and can sometimes be inferred from an individual's behaviour. It is often difficult to distinguish between a delusion and an overvalued idea.

(APA, 2000: 821)

For a delusion to be considered paranoid (or 'persecutory' in psychiatric terms) the central theme of the belief is that the person (or someone close to them) is being victimized or conspired against in some way and there is an explicit intention to harm them.

Definitions like these have been challenged on conceptual and empirical grounds over the years (e.g. Boyle, 2002a; David, 1999; Freeman & Garety, 2000; Harper, 1996, 2004; Moor & Tucker, 1979; Oltmanns, 1988; Spitzer, 1995). Indeed, one commentator has noted that 'despite the façade created by psychiatric textbooks, there is no acceptable (rather than accepted) definition of a delusion' (David, 1999: 17). There have been attempts to relabel delusions as 'abnormal beliefs' or 'unusual beliefs'. Oltmanns (1988) has argued that rather than trying to settle on a fixed definition of delusion, it might be better to elucidate seven 'defining characteristics' by which delusions might be recognized with none of the characteristics being seen either as essential or sufficient for a diagnosis. This approach clearly provides some flexibility but this can also be problematic in that diagnoses can prove to be too flexible. As the Rosenhan (1973) study showed it can be quite hard to prove that one does not fulfil psychiatric criteria once one has been given a diagnosis, and diagnosers appear to show a great deal of flexibility in which criteria they draw on and how they interpret them (Harper, 1994). For example, if a person does not fit the criteria for delusion, the DSM definition of paranoid personality disorder is very similar: 'distrust and suspiciousness of others such that their motives are interpreted as malevolent ... individuals with this disorder assume that other people will exploit, harm or deceive them, even if no evidence exists to support this expectation' (APA, 2000: 690).

Boyle (2002a: 279) argues that diagnostic debates are so long-lived because researchers have an 'assumptive framework' which remains 'unexamined or even unarticulated'. In this chapter, I examine the assumptive framework of contemporary notions of paranoia and delusion and argue that the Oltmanns approach, like that of the DSM-IV, rests on four fundamental assumptions that obscure more helpful ways of looking at relatively enduring beliefs, fears and ways of relating to others.

Naive realism

One of the most basic problems is the assumption that it is possible to prove that a person's beliefs are false – a naively realist worldview. Yet we know that most people end up with a diagnosis of paranoia without independent empirical investigation – probably the most that will have happened is a psychiatric interview with the person and possibly a family member. Maher has argued that assessment of the plausibility of a person's beliefs is 'typically made by a clinician on the basis of "common sense", and not on the basis of a systematic evaluation of empirical data [and that it is not] customary to present counter evidence to the patient; it is not even common to present vigorous counterargument' (Maher, 1992: 261). These observations have empirical support: based on a study of outpatient psychiatric consultations McCabe et al. reported that '[w]hen patients attempted to present their psychotic symptoms as a topic of conversation, the doctors hesitated and avoided answering the patients' questions, indicating reluctance to engage with these concerns' (2002: 1150). It is ironic that service users are required to provide proof for their claims but the threshold appears to be lower for professionals. Indeed, researchers often report examples of delusions that either turned out to be true or which had a 'kernel of truth' in them (Barrett, 1988).

If the diagnosis of a delusion is based more on a judgment of plausibility than an empirical investigation, then it means that different diagnosers may arrive at different conclusions – posing problems for the reliability of diagnoses of delusions. Of the few studies of diagnostic reliability reported, despite significant methodological weaknesses, quite varied results are found with judgments of the bizarreness of delusions, particularly poor (Bell, Halligan & Ellis, 2006; Harper, 1999). However, how many of us could say that we have objective evidence for any, let alone all, of our beliefs? Is it even possible or desirable to have 'evidence' for political, ethical and spiritual or religious beliefs? So the idea that beliefs are straightforwardly empirically verifiable is problematic. Given this, it is perhaps not unsurprising that judging whether a belief is abnormal in some way is even more of a challenge.

How abnormal are abnormal beliefs?

It is commonly assumed that the kinds of beliefs which are diagnosed as delusional are rare and such beliefs are statistically abnormal. However, when surveys of the general public are conducted, we find that potentially 'delusional' beliefs are not as unusual as might be thought. For example, one UK survey reported that 45 per cent of people believed in telepathy, 45 per cent believed in the ability to predict the future, 42 per cent believed in hypnotism, 39 per cent believed in life after death, 39 per cent believed in faith healing and 31 per cent of people believed in ghosts (Social Surveys/Gallup Poll Ltd, 1995). A more recent American Gallup survey reported slightly lower percentages though belief in ESP was at 41 per cent, but 73 per cent of Americans believed in at least one of 10 paranormal items (Moore, 2005).

It is even harder to evaluate beliefs when it comes to social judgments about others. A 1994 Gallup survey reported that 24 per cent of people admitted lying at least once the previous day and 64 per cent thought they had been lied to at least once the previous day (Social Surveys/ Gallup Poll Ltd, 1994). In a further survey, 60 per cent of people felt that one could not be too careful in dealing with people and only 37 per cent felt most people could be trusted (Social Surveys/Gallup Poll Ltd, 1997). Given these levels of trust in others it seems that some level of paranoia is relatively commonplace.

An objection to this might be that belief in ghosts and so on is a different matter to belief in something 'properly' delusional. However, Emmanuelle Peters and colleagues at the Institute of Psychiatry have conducted some interesting studies using the *Peters Delusions Inventory* or PDI (Peters, Joseph & Garety, 1999a), a short self-report questionnaire containing questions about beliefs drawn from schedules of psychiatric symptoms. It is deliberately phrased using everyday words rather than psychiatric terminology – examples include 'do you ever feel as if people seem to drop hints about you or say things with a double meaning?' and 'do you ever feel as if you are being persecuted in some way?' For each belief three ratings are made: the conviction with which it is held; the amount of distress associated with it; and the extent to which the person is preoccupied with it.

In one study Peters and her colleagues reported that although 'psychotic inpatients' had higher scores on the PDI than the general population (Peters et al., 1999a) there was also considerable overlap between the two groups. In other words, some members of the general public scored *higher* on the delusions survey than those who were psychiatric inpatients. This finding has since been replicated using a much larger general population sample (Peters et al., 2004). Where the two groups in this study appeared to differ was that the general public was less preoccupied with, distressed by and convinced by their beliefs.

In a separate investigation, Peters et al. (1999b) compared members of New Religious Movements (Druids and Hare Krishnas), non-religious people, Christians and 'deluded people' on their scores on the PDI measure. They found no differences between the members of New Religious Movements and 'deluded people' in terms of either the number of beliefs held or the strength with which they were held. The only differences between the groups were in how preoccupied the participants were with their beliefs and how distressed they were about them.

Thus, whereas traditional psychiatric approaches assume that it is the *fact* of holding a belief considered delusional that is the problem, this research indicates that the key issue is the *relationship* people have with their beliefs – in other words, whether your beliefs get in the way of the life you wish to lead.

A number of studies report similar results with the PDI in France, the Netherlands and New Zealand, with anywhere between 3–20 per cent of the population holding beliefs which would, conventionally, be regarded as delusional. In another study, nearly half of a sample of British college students reported an experience of paranoia including a clear statement that they felt there had been a planned intention to harm them – the key criterion for a diagnosis of a paranoid or persecutory delusion (Ellett, Lopes & Chadwick, 2003). Freeman has noted that a 'conservative estimate is that 10–15 per cent of the general population regularly experience paranoid thoughts' (Freeman, 2007: 430). In a community survey of a random sample of 7076 people in the Netherlands, van Os et al. (2000) reported that 8.7 per cent of the sample had delusional beliefs but that 3.3 per cent had 'true' delusions. In other words, 8.7 per cent of the population held beliefs that fulfilled most of the diagnostic criteria for delusions but did not require clinical intervention – they did not appear to be causing the person or those around them clinically significant levels of distress or causing problems in their daily life. This means that although 5.4 per cent of the sample had beliefs which psychiatrists would diagnose as delusions, they were managing to go about their everyday lives apparently without problems. Similarly, a survey of the US general population suggested that 4.41 per cent of the population met the criteria for a diagnosis of paranoid personality disorder (Grant et al., 2004).

What are we to make of surveys like these? They show that 'paranoid' experiences are not nearly as unusual or abnormal as we are led to believe. Since referrals to mental health services in no way match these levels, this either indicates a serious level of under diagnosis or that many people with such experiences do not require help from mental health services. How might some people manage to hold beliefs which might be seen as delusional, and yet manage to avoid being referred to, or seeking help from, mental health services? Weeks and James (1997) have researched the similar topic of 'eccentricity' and identify a number of people who remain happy and engaged with the world despite holding unconventional views. Sun Ra and David Icke are examples of people whose beliefs others might find unusual but who do not appear to have experienced distress because of their beliefs or been in receipt of mental health services.

Sun Ra was a black American avant-garde musician who, from the 1950s until his death in 1993, led a jazz group called the Arkestra. He claimed to be from the planet Saturn, tracing this realization to a religious vision he had in the 1930s (Szwed, 1998). He has been the subject of a number of documentary films including Don Letts' *Brother from Another Planet – The Sun Ra Story*. David Icke was a BBC TV sports presenter who became involved in the Green party in the late 1980s. A week after resigning from the Green Party he held a press conference to announce that he had become a 'channel for the Christ spirit' and predicted that the world would end in 1997 after a series of natural disasters. He has gone on to write a number of books about his ideas, in particular that the world is being run by a race of shape-shifting alien lizards who have interbred with humans and can appear in human form (see www.davidicke.com). According to journalist Jon Ronson his career is 'a global sensation' and 'he lectures to packed houses all over the world' (Ronson, 2001: 151).

Is paranoia meaningless?

The influence of biological and reductionist traditions in psychiatry has meant that mental health professionals have traditionally been little interested in the content of people's experiences. Thus, historically, there has been more interest in *whether* someone heard a voice rather than in *what the voice said*. Similarly, the assumption has generally been that beliefs seen as delusional or paranoid are meaningless – an 'empty speech act' (Berrios, 1991) – and that exploring them will mean that the clinician is 'colluding' with the belief.

However, there is mounting evidence that such beliefs are full of meaning. One study reported that those with a diagnosis of delusions scored as highly on a measure of purpose and meaning in life as those training to be Anglican priests (Roberts, 1991). This suggests that these beliefs may actually give people a meaning in life even though, in the case of those who feel paranoid, the meaning may not be at all pleasant (Harper, 2008). This is, perhaps, not that surprising: if you are unemployed, poor and living alone on a frightening housing estate with little money to spend in occupying yourself, it may be functional to imagine you are Jesus, or are being followed by MI5. Other research has reported finding a correspondence between the themes in a person's 'delusions' and their everyday life or their past (Rhodes & Jakes, 2000).

An important line of research has been the investigation of links between paranoid beliefs, social inequality and victimization. For example, John Mirowsky and Catherine Ross (1983) conducted a survey of the general population in El Paso, Texas and across the border in Juarez, Mexico. They reported that those with the most paranoid beliefs tended to be working class Mexican women – those who were in social positions characterized by powerlessness, the threat of victimization and exploitation. Again, this should not be all that surprising. When you are not fully in control of your life – when, for example, you could be sacked from your poorly paid job at any moment – in a very real sense others *are* in control of your life and it may feel as if they are persecuting you.

Racism also plays a part here, and a range of empirical work indicates that it may be one of the causes of the high rates of psychosis in the black population. For example, black and Asian people in the UK are 50 per cent more likely to be diagnosed with schizophrenia than white people (King et al., 1994). Moreover, the prevalence of schizophrenia diagnoses is higher among black people living in majority white areas (Boydell et al., 2001). A community survey in the Netherlands noted that those meeting diagnostic criteria for delusions were more likely to report having experienced discrimination previously (Janssen et al., 2003). Similarly, Karlsen and Nazroo (2002) have noted that those belonging to minority ethnic groups were much more likely to have psychotic symptoms if they reported experiencing racist victimization in the previous year. Lastly, experiences of victimization and stressful life events were among the correlates of psychotic symptoms in a large UK community survey (Johns et al., 2004).

John Cromby and I have argued that, rather than seeing paranoia as a kind of belief, it makes sense to view it as a kind of story that is embodied within us as a result of our life experiences (Cromby & Harper, 2009). It may help someone to make sense of a confusing world – where they feel influenced by forces beyond their immediate perceptions – to connect apparently unconnected happenings. It may be that, in its focus on whether supposedly delusional beliefs are *literally* true, reductionist psychiatry has missed the more important issue that many such beliefs may be *metaphorically* true, reflecting the influence on the person's life of a range of stressful experiences, including those resulting from social inequalities.[1]

So far, in this chapter, I have argued that the assumptive framework underpinning the psychiatric notion of paranoia presupposes: a naive realist model of the world; that paranoid beliefs are inherently pathological and abnormal; and that they are meaningless. But who is given the power to make these judgments and what is the basis for the legitimacy of their claims?

Who gets to decide what is 'normal'?

Of course, one of the key assumptions made when we say someone has a delusion is that this is a statement of *fact* rather than *opinion*. In his seminal social-constructionist analysis of delusions over 20 years ago, Heise (1988) argued that in the diagnostic interview one person's version of reality (the mental health professional's) is seen as more true than the other person's version of reality (the service user's) as the professional is granted, by virtue of their social position, the power to define reality. Eugenie Georgaca has investigated this empirically, using discourse analysis to examine interviews conducted with psychiatric service users considered delusional (2000, 2004). She argues that, contrary to received opinion, service users are able to provide evidence for their beliefs and to engage in discussion with others about them. The problem which arose is that, what some of her interviewees saw as persuasive evidence was not persuasive to her. Moreover, she noted that many of their claims were epistemologically ambiguous in that they would be hard to verify empirically and they were certainly impossible to test within the context of an interview (as occurs in most psychiatric diagnostic interviews). She argued that judging another's beliefs to be delusional was an interactional accomplishment, one in which the hearer of the belief (and their assumptions about the world) was important but ignored within the psychiatric literature.

The psychiatrist Suman Fernando has made a similar point:

> [I]n the process of making a diagnosis, judgments are hypothesized as symptoms and illnesses – as 'things' that exist in some way

separately from the people who make the judgments and from the people ('patients') who are said to 'have' them.

(Fernando, 1997: 16)

In other words, when we say that someone 'has a deluded belief', what we are *really* saying is 'that idea is implausible to me', 'I don't understand that idea' or even 'that idea is dangerous'. The process by which we come to these judgments occurs between people in conversation and it is likely to be influenced by all of the things that make us different from each other. There is one area of belief which throws this assumption into particular relief.

In a sense, when mental health professionals make judgments about whether beliefs are normal, they are making proxy judgments on behalf of all of us. But what is the standard against which they are judging beliefs? If this standard remains implicit, and if mental health professionals are actually significantly different from the general population, then this causes further problems for diagnosis. In fact, this is the case with religious belief where a number of surveys suggest that it is mental health professionals who are the 'abnormal' ones, statistically speaking. For example, Smiley (2001) asked British clinical psychologists about their religious belief and found that, whereas 61 per cent of psychologists reported having no religious belief, or were agnostic or atheistic, only 28 per cent of the population as a whole did.

Implications: Changing assumptions and changing society

We have seen how the 'assumptive framework' constructing paranoia influences both how it is experienced and how it is diagnosed by professionals. Here, I outline some implications of this analysis for practice, research and policy.

Practice

Therapists need to acknowledge that judgments about beliefs are social and cultural and so it may be more helpful to focus on the 'fit' between a person's beliefs and the lives they wish to lead rather than on the veracity of the belief. There could be a focus on the content and context of the belief, particularly its historical and biographical context, given that many of these beliefs appear to occur in late adolescence and/or following experiences of victimization. Therapeutic factors in alternative groups seem to involve helping the person to develop an explanation for their experiences which: makes sense to them; does not unduly distress them; puts them in contact with a community which shares those meanings since social isolation is generally anti-therapeutic; where there are often rituals, practices and other regular activities which ground the person in this community; and which allows them to lead the lives they wish to (Romme & Escher, 2000).

The development of paranoia support groups can help to combat the isolation that can be a consequence of some frightening beliefs and is an example of how people with distressing beliefs can help each other to cope (Bullimore, 2010; James, 2003; Knight, 2009). For those not able or willing to meet with others, the Internet can be a useful resource though this can become unhelpful if it begins to dominate the person's life.

Community psychology is another useful approach. May (2007) has discussed the development of community-based approaches for people having experiences others consider psychotic. Sue Holland's (1991) White City project developed a model of social action psychotherapy. She focused on women on a West London estate, offering a staged approach beginning with a number of sessions of individual therapy, leading into group work and then into collective social action. Of course, therapeutic work can only go so far and there is a need to influence researchers and policymakers too.

Research

An obstacle to research progress is the psychiatric diagnostic enterprise itself. I would argue that, certainly in the area of psychosis, diagnostic categories are actively unhelpful in that their use requires us to make many *a priori* assumptions about the nature of the phenomena they purportedly categorize. As Rogers and Pilgrim (2003) note, researchers attempting to trace the relationship between social disadvantage and mental health are often forced to use such categories as epidemiological data are structured by them. Fortunately, the availability of dimensional experience or symptom-based measures like the PDI provide an alternative.

We need, instead, to return to a focus on experience. What is it like to feel paranoid? Here qualitative research can be helpful in capturing the nuances of subjective experience. In particular it can be helpful to investigate experience outside of the clinic and to explore trust, mistrust and suspicion in a range of contexts, including the everyday (King et al., 2008; Willig, 1997). In trying to understand experience we need to use language but this, too, contains many presuppositions.

Indeed, Wallcraft and Michaelson (2001) have argued for the development of a 'survivor discourse' in order to reclaim the language used to describe their experience back from professionals. We need to rethink the language we use to describe paranoia and similar experiences. But what alternatives to the terms 'paranoia' or 'delusion' are there? The move from 'auditory hallucination' to 'voice hearing' in the 1990s was useful because it was behaviourally descriptive, carried little conceptual baggage and was open to different interpretations. The term 'paranoia' is challenged by some because it is thought to imply that such beliefs are inherently pathological – but this need not be the case and some survivors use it to describe their experiences since it is widely understood. There is much less agreement about the term 'delusion' or even about the term 'belief'. However, there is no obvious replacement. I do not think the term 'unusual belief' is necessarily better than delusion – unusual to who? Other alternatives abound (e.g. 'unshared beliefs', 'having an alternative sense of reality', 'heightened sensitivity to others' or Tamasin Knight's 'beliefs that might not be easily confirmable', see Hornstein, 2009b: 136).

Whatever words we use to describe paranoia, I would argue that we need to move research away from its focus on truth as a key factor given that it is rarely the key issue. David Heise made a similar point over 20 years ago when he argued that the 'factuality of belief' be discarded as a diagnostic criterion and the 'focus on sociality sharpened' (Heise, 1988: 270). If researchers were less enchanted by whether beliefs were true it might be easier to focus on the 'fit' between a person's beliefs and the life they wish to lead. What influences are there on that 'fit'? How do some people manage to live lives as 'mystics', 'eccentrics' or even 'extremists' (the subject of investigations by Peters, 2001; Weeks & James, 1997; and Ronson, 2001 respectively) rather than as psychiatric patients? If we begin to see 'delusions' as positions that people take up and/or are positioned in, what alternative modes of understanding might this open up in discourse? Fruitful avenues appear to be narrative (de Rivera & Sarbin, 1998) and dialogical models (Hallam & O'Connor, 2002). Indeed, how is it that some belief claims seem more plausible than others, or to some people than others?

Policy

[t]he more equitable the distribution of wealth in a country, the more trusting its people will be.
(Uslaner, 2002: 230 cited in Freeman & Freeman, 2008)

When mental health practitioners seek to influence policymakers there is a danger that they suggest solutions at the level of the individual – usually some form of medication or psychotherapy. Apart from being self-serving, this approach is too costly to be available for all those who might 'need' it and, moreover, it is ameliorative, rather than preventative. On the rare occasions that mental health services are involved in preventative efforts, the concern is often to target intervention on 'high risk groups'. However, Huppert suggests that this may be shortsighted as 'the majority who develop disorder come not from the high-risk group, but from the general population, simply because the members of the general population are so numerous' (Huppert, 2009: 109). Instead, Huppert makes a case for focusing interventions at the population level since 'a small shift in the population mean is associated with a substantial reduction in the prevalence of disorder' (Huppert, 2009: 109–10).

When we look at paranoia at the population level, it is hard to say whether we are 'more' paranoid than we were in the past (Freeman & Freeman, 2008) but, surveys show that levels of trust between people in Britain have been decreasing over the last 50 years. Moreover, neighbourhoods reporting low levels of overt mutual trust are the most disadvantaged and where there is most social disorder like crime, vandalism and so on (Ross, Mirowsky & Pribesh, 2001). What is interesting is that, at the population level, levels of trust appear to be correlated not with overall levels of income, but with the difference between the poorest and the richest in society – in other words, they are related to levels of income inequality. In The Spirit Level, Richard Wilkinson and Kate Pickett present persuasive evidence of this. In general, those countries with the lowest levels of income inequality (e.g. Sweden, Norway, Denmark and Finland) are also those countries reporting the highest levels of trust. Wilkinson and Pickett (2009) show that a similar pattern is also seen in the USA between States, which vary in terms of income inequality. Moreover, it appears that as inequality increases, trust decreases. Addressing such inequality requires action beyond the clinic.

When we use the notion of paranoia to diagnose others we may obscure the real causes of their distress, locating it instead in faulty brain mechanisms, rather than out there in a frequently hostile world. Likewise, when we experience paranoia we have the sense that we are the ones who know what is really going on in the world but paranoid ideas may simply mystify the causes of the real inequalities and victimizations we have experienced, transforming them into a dramatic personalized narrative (Harper, 2008). Perhaps we can 'decode' the

that do not (Rose, 1996a). In an entirely unremarkable example of this penchant for historicist fallacy, Magnavita's *Handbook of Personality Disorders* suggests that

> [p]ersonality and its disordered or dysfunctional states have been of interest to humankind since the early stages of civilization probably coinciding with the birth of consciousness.
>
> (2003: 3)

Although it is almost impossible, today, to conceive of a human being without the concept of personality, its development is a fairly recent one, stemming from the late nineteenth century (Healy, 2002). The notion of character had been in use for very much longer than that, but held different meanings from the modern meaning of 'personality' within psychology, defined by *Chambers Dictionary* (2003: 1122) as:

> [t]he integrated organization of all the psychological, intellectual, emotional, and physical characteristics of an individual, especially as they are presented to other people (psychol); the sum of such characteristics which make a person attractive socially.

Competing discourses in the late nineteenth century shared an essentialist conception of interior conditions: the 'soul' representing pure essence, formed an imaginary composite of the human interior; while the 'will' was associated with mind and reason, and was seen as amenable to being worked on, improved or controlled. Character began being used as a means of conceptualizing a link between interior and exterior (Rimke & Hunt, 2002). Corrupt souls were increasingly viewed as suffering from moral pathology or deficiency, which was understood as a form of disease. The medical profession therefore assumed the role of governing vices, which were seen to be growing alongside industrialization (Scull, 1979). Contrasting schools of thought accounted for so-called moral deficiencies: moral environmentalism's causal account cited impaired religious faith as well as a diminished capacity for self restraint; social environmentalism on the other hand cited adverse social conditions including low wages as causal factors. Within the former, excess was the key to morality. Hence, activating self-control was seen as key in the management of problem individuals who appeared to have no defect of reasoning. Krafft-Ebbing (1905) noted that moral insanity could be recognized by impulsive characteristics and certain social groups were represented as suffering from a regression in human evolution, such as paupers, criminals and the insane. Maudsley (1884) equated the terms antisocial and immoral, thus expanding the logic so that whole classes and races could be thought of as subject to degenerate tendencies rather than just individuals.

The medicalization of personality

What Magnavita describes as the birth of consciousness might be better described as the birth of academic psychology. The term personality was first used in a medical context in France in the latter part of the nineteenth century in relation to what is now referred to as Dissociative Identity Disorder (formerly known as Multiple Personality Disorder). Azam's (1876) paper *La dédoublement de la personnalité* described a patient who had two apparently separate states of consciousness that appeared to be unaware of the other. Following this, hypnotism began to be used as a treatment for patients diagnosed with hysteria. Bourru and Burot published *Variations de la personnalité* in 1888, describing a patient suffering from hysteria whom they had been treating with hypnotism when he began presenting with multiple separate states of consciousness, each aware of different portions of his life (Hacking, 1995).

Janet (1907) claimed that it was this work that prompted the establishment of the Department de Psychologie expérimentale et comparée at the Collège de France in 1888. Ribot was the first to occupy the chair of this department. His work *Les Maladies de la Personnalité* (1885) heralded the notion that personality represented an embodied entity that was prone to disease. Janet pioneered a treatment that involved working on memories to treat hysteria, which he saw as being caused by trauma, using hypnotic suggestion to convince his patients that their trauma had never taken place. Freud was also initially a proponent of hypnosis. Freud's psychoanalytic method was also initially predicated on a model of trauma-related aetiology, arguing that the cause of neurosis lay in sexual trauma. Freud abandoned the theory in 1897, replacing it with the idea that the management of constitutionally derived libidinous energy gave rise to human phantasies, which shaped a person's development. This forged a realm where the psychic could be thought of as distinct from moral functioning: the person was driven by hidden motives and memories, creating behaviours that lay outside of conscious control.

By the early twentieth century psychiatry had laid claim to the notion of personality in a form recognizable today. Kraepelin included the term personality as a psychiatric category in his textbook *Clinical Psychiatry*

(1904). The chapter titled 'Morbid Personalities' included the following description:

> We evidently have to deal with an instability of the will existing from childhood, and resulting in the want of all perseverance and all resistance to temptation. It seems as if those motives which arise from moral feeling had not developed in the patient ... [he] recalls his adventures with a certain degree of satisfaction ... the morbid want of self-control, which has made it impossible for him to win a place in life corresponding to the talents he possesses, is ... an evidence of degeneration ... We have before us a born swindler, who, in spite of many talents, is entirely destitute of the essential requisites for work – perseverance and a sense of duty ... Yet the physician cannot escape from the conviction that the patient has a congenital incapacity for a regular course of life, stronger than all education, experience and self control ... Our patient's grave heredity at one suggests the suspicion that this is a case of morbid personality.
>
> (Kraepelin, 1904: 281–2)

In later editions Kraepelin variegated the construct, suggesting six types: excitable; unstable; eccentric; liar; swindler and quarrelsome. In the early twentieth century statistical concepts also began to be used to individualize problem individuals who, despite the introduction of universal schooling, appeared unable to learn. Galton's concept of the normal distribution facilitated the development of intelligence tests by promoting the assumption that all qualities in the population vary according to a regular pattern, the characteristics of which can be established by cumulative acts of comparison in conjunction with the average figure for the population (Rose, 1990).

Schneider (1923) used these concepts to conceive of abnormal personality as that which deviated from the average. He advised against using nineteenth-century descriptions like moral insanity because of their 'social rather than clinical ring' (1958: 126). Instead he used the term 'psychopathy' to denote: 'abnormal personalities who either suffer personally because of their abnormality or make a community suffer because of it' (1958: 3). He categorized ten variants of the 'Psychopathic Personality': the hyperthymic; depressive; insecure; fanatic; attention seeking; labile; explosive; affectionless; weak willed and asthenic.

The consolidation of psychiatric expertise in matters of character was much advanced by the activities of psychiatry during World

War II. Psychiatry assumed an administrative role in the US military during the war; discharging soldiers who were deemed unfit to serve. The US War Department codified psychiatric disorders into a manual – *Technical Bulletin, Medical 203* – in 1943, to standardize and legitimize this role. A committee chaired by Brigadier General William C. Menninger authored the manual, which introduced the concept of 'Character Disorder' into an official nomenclature for the first time. Under the heading *Character and Behavior Disorders* the manual distinguished between: *Pathological personality types* – described as maladjusted individuals 'evidenced in lifelong behaviour patterns', who 'represent borderline adjustment states' between psychosis and neurosis; and *Immaturity reactions* – 'physically adult individuals, who are unable to maintain their emotional equilibrium and independence under minor or major stress, because of deficiencies in emotional development'

Much of the Technical Bulletin was taken directly from *Psychodynamics of Abnormal Behaviour* (1940) coauthored by Menninger's brother Karl and J. F. Brown, psychoanalysts at an inpatient hospital in Kansas – The Menninger Clinic. The 'Character Disorders' chapter introduces what it describes as the 'least developed' psychoanalytic field, opening with the following passage:

> In the category of character disorder we include a great many individuals whom the layman would consider simply queer or mean or unhappy or vicious or wicked. We include other individuals who seem superficially to be quite well adjusted but in whom on closer observation we find some disbalance or lack of proper integration between the various constituent parts of the self. Until recently such individuals were looked on as problems for the clergyman if their character defect was relatively mild or for the police court and the penologist if their character defect was severe. The normal individual is one in whom there is a proper balance between the forces of ego, superego and id and in whom the ego has a proper relationship to outside physical and social reality. Recently it has been shown that disbalance in these functions, which is not marked or severe enough to create actual psychosis, psychoneurosis, or perversion, creates character disorders or character neurosis.
>
> (Brown & Menninger, 1940: 384)

Bleuler and Brill's (1924) work was cited, which asserted that psychopaths suffer from the same anomalies as the insane but to a lesser degree and it was from this that the character disorder categories: paranoid, schizoid and cycloid were taken. Character disorders related to perversion, alcohol addiction and criminality were also listed as well as two categories taken from Reich's (1928) work: the compulsive and the hysterical.

Reich introduced to psychoanalysis the idea that character represents a stable organization of the libidinal economy of the person that is more or less rigid and is subject to the pressures of the drives and to social constraints as well as to the defences that they give rise to: 'character is in the first place a mechanism of narcissistic protection' (Reich, 1928: 158). He brought together various 'character traits' under the name 'character armor', which corresponded to the mechanisms used by the person to deal with the repressed material. Reich described specific forms of character disorder: the hysterical character, who was dominated by ostentation and sexual mobility; the compulsive character, marked by rigidity, retention and obsession for order; the phallic-narcissistic character, structured so as to resist passive-homosexual impulses; and the masochistic character, characterized by guilt and the desire for punishment (de Mijolla, 2005).

The army's diagnostic manual served an important 'medico-legal' purpose, in that it was used to determine whether problem individuals should be given an honourable discharge (the insane), dishonourable discharge (pathological personality types), or reassignment to a different battalion (immaturity reactions). The advantages of the dishonourable discharge system were that it allowed military commanders to exclude personnel thought to be bad for the morale of the group where it was felt that reassignment would not act as a sufficient solution, it discouraged unwanted behaviours and it relieved the army of responsibility for paying a pension to unsuitable recruits.

Following the war Menninger was appointed as head of the American Psychiatric Association (APA). He established The Menninger School of Psychiatry in 1946, which quickly became the country's largest training centre. This coincided with a hugely increased demand for psychiatrists to treat veterans returning from the war. *Time* magazine featured Menninger on its cover in 1948, celebrating him as 'Psychiatry's U.S. sales manager'. By 1948 three quarters of committee posts in the APA were held by analysts (Healy, 2002). The APA appointed a Committee on Nomenclature and Statistics, headed by Menninger, to develop a nosology that would standardize the diverse range of documents in use in the US at that time, leading to the publication of the first DSM. Much of the manual's chapter on character disorders is taken directly from Technical Manual, Bulletin 203. Both chapters begin with exactly the same paragraph:

> These disorders are characterized by developmental defects or pathological trends in the personality structure, with minimal subjective anxiety, and little or no sense of distress. In most instances, the disorder is manifested by a lifelong pattern of action or behavior ('acting out'), rather than by mental or emotional symptoms.
>
> (APA, 1952: 34)

Expedient constructions of the US War Department and essentialist psychoanalysts thus became permanent pathologies available for categorizing the population at large with the publication of the DSM. Having directed a new focus towards the personality of soldiers, the notion that a person could be alienated from their true self, or alternatively, maladjusted to society, emerged. Therapy was conceptualized as the solution to these problems leading to a profound shift in how people understood themselves (Healy, 2002).

After the war the concept of personality was also central to psychology's development as a scientific discipline. Eysenck combined large-scale factor analytic studies of personality with small-scale experimental studies of aspects of character and conduct – such as level of aspiration or sense of humour – to refine this factorization (Rose, 1990). In this way he grouped acts into habitual responses, which were in turn grouped into traits, and it was these that were claimed to form the general factors of personality. Eysenck claimed that personality determined the specific type of behaviour disorder observed, as well as predicting which factors would precipitate future problems.

The development of tests such as the Minnesota Multiphasic Personality Inventory (MMPI) after World War II have popularized the modern notion of personality as a structured whole. By 1960 the MMPI was the most widely used personality test in the world. Originally designed for use in a small hospital for mental patients in Minnesota, and employing a statistical techniques based upon the responses of a total of 724 white and mainly rural Protestant research subjects, Paul (2004) describes how the test was designed: the majority true or false answers given by the 'normal' subjects became the 'normal' answer, while the answer given by the majority of patients with a diagnosis of depression, hysteria or schizophrenia became the depressive answer and so on.

However, in the years following the test's initial publication problems emerged: rather than obtaining a single spike on a particular scale and thus eliciting a specific diagnosis, respondents often showed elevations on several of the scales. The test began to be conceived of as giving a complex profile or syndrome rather than a simple category or diagnosis. The original names of the scales were abandoned and replaced with numbers, allowing a test taker to be referred to by the sequence of numbers denoting elevated scales. The scales were taken to represent characteristics of a person, so for example somebody with elevations on what were the depression and hysteria scales was likely to be 'moody, insecure, and dependent, with a sensitivity to criticism and a tendency to play the martyr'. The Minnesota Normals formed psychology's major criterion for normality for the next 50 years.

In 1977 Millon developed an 'objective psychodynamic instrument' (Millon, 2004: 575), the Millon Clinical Multiaxial Inventory (MCMI), in order to identify and quantify the personality disorder constructs that had appeared in his 1969 book *Modern Psychopathology*. This constructed personality disorder on the basis of biosocial learning and evolutionary theories working on the premise that 'personality maladaptions ... represent partial expressions of evolutionary functions that have gone awry' (Millon, 2004: 535). At the same Millon was appointed to the Advisory Committee on Personality Disorders working on redefining the categories of the DSM. He recommended the use of a similar multiaxial system to that employed in his test, to separate off the personality disorders from the other mental disorders. Spitzer, who led the task force to transform the DSM in the late 1970s, had originally trained as a Reichian psychoanalyst (Lane, 2007). While his team expunged the psychoanalytic theoretical orientation of earlier editions of the DSM, replacing it with behaviourally based diagnostic criteria, he retained the Reichian psychoanalytic notion of Character Disorders, now rebranded as Personality Disorders.

Most of the personality disorder diagnoses in DSM 3 remained the same as those listed in DSM 1 and 2. Borderline Personality Disorder (BPD) was the most important of the new diagnoses; a study by Perry and Klerman (1978) found 104 different criteria identified in different texts for borderline disorder, with only one agreed on by all of the authors reviewed: that the patient's behaviour during interview appeared adaptive and appropriate (Wirth-Cauchon, 2001). Despite the heterogeneity of these criteria the DSM committee was successful in constructing a hegemonic meaning with clearly defined borders; controversy was smoothed over with a standardized definition. The Advisory Committee used Gunderson's description of borderline personality, which he primarily diagnosed in hospitalized women and which identified borderline personality as a manifestation of severe pathology (Kernber, in Cauwels, 1992). Millon formulated the borderline personality as 'a disintegrated mix of Histrionic, Dependent and Passive–aggressive personalities, in which the individual's personal cohesion and interpersonal competence were insidiously deteriorated' (Millon 1983: 812).

Hysteria, which had been the third most popular diagnosis in 1975, was an obscurity by the mid 1980s (Blashfield & McElroy, 1987). BPD was, instead, the most commonly diagnosed of the personality disorders by 1984 (Gunderson & Zanarini, 1987). The prevalence of BPD is now estimated to be ten per cent in outpatient mental health settings, 15–20 per cent in inpatient settings and 30–60 per cent among patients with a diagnosis of personality disorder (Skodol et al., 2002).

More recent developments

The essential ambiguity of the personality disorder construct has been put to use in policing deviance under a new guise in the last decade. The UK government created the term Dangerous and Severe Personality Disorder (DSPD) in 2001, which created a new class of individual defined – in law – by three criteria: that they must have an identifiable severe personality disorder; pose a high risk of causing serious harm to others; and for these two factors to be causally linked (Seddon, 2008). Such an individual is to be understood within the discourse of risk which 'dissolves the notion of a subject or a concrete individual, and put[s] in its place a combinatory of factors, the factors of risk' (Castel, 1991: 281). This strategy does not rely on concepts such as responsibility and guilt in punishing offenders; it involves the regulation of groups within the normal (non-offender) population as 'part of a strategy of managing danger' (Feeley & Simon, 1992: 173). The assessment of risk with the use of standardized tools is central to this venture, creating a numericized quantum of risk and constituting a relationship between a network of expert assessments to form the patient's dossier (Rose, 1996b). The preventive, potentially indefinite, incarceration of unpleasant, but only *potentially* dangerous, characters who have not necessarily been charged with – let alone been convicted of – any offence has thus, by the application of a veil of psy 'science', been legitimated in the name of public safety. The seriousness of this demands a more detailed analysis of the cloudy conceptual status of the concept.

Conceptual issues in the 'diagnosis' of BPD

The central ambiguity inherent in the personality disorder construct seems to hinge on volition. Is a person choosing to act the way that they do, or does their behaviour result from some deficit or illness or other process that is beyond their control? With its close conceptual relationship to notions of intentionality, or *mens rea*, this is, self-evidently, a moral – not a medical – question. It is the answer to this question that warrants, or not, the ascription of blame and culpability for conduct. That is, the issue of volition is crucial to the legal consequences of the diagnosis: people with a personality disorder are fully responsible for themselves and often held to be *more* culpable for their actions than people without the diagnosis:

> Personality disorder is unlikely to impair cognition and volition substantially, and therefore people with personality disorders rarely are considered nonculpable for their acts … If the personality disorder is not severe enough to be a mitigating factor in forensic decision making it may be considered, somewhat ironically, an aggravating factor, something that can be used to argue for harsher punishment or imposition of long term social controls.
>
> (Livesley, 2001: 556)

Volition has been central to the construct since its nineteenth-century ancestors, moral insanity and moral defectiveness. Will, mind and reason were causally linked in nineteenth century discourses on moral pathology, which stressed the need for such people to be worked on, improved or controlled. Diagnosis within this model was explicitly based upon moral judgement. The *explicit* moral judgement was removed by twentieth century 'medical' developments in the construct, but its conceptual bedfellow, volition, was left behind together with the implicit moral condemnation essential to the very idea of flawed character from which it evolved.

Schnieder replaced the moral aspect of the construct with the concept of a normal/abnormal continuum in the 1920s. This consolidated the shift of conceptual moorings from a social to a clinical domain, medicalizing the construct within a statistical and normalizing discourse. This purportedly transformed the diagnostic judgement from a moral one, concerning right and wrong, to a medical one, concerning what is normal or abnormal. Implicitly, however, the position of the diagnosed person remained largely unchanged, as volition was retained as conceptually central to Schnieder's system.

Reich's work on character analysis in the late 1920s, which produced the templates for many of our modern personality disorder categories, was based on a radically different stance towards the issue of volition. In Reich's theory, character neurosis represented a stable pathological organization of libidinal energy that was more or less rigid. This was a thoroughgoing medical discourse: 'the usual treatment of such individuals through punishment and threat avails very little because these ... characters are actually sick' (Brown & Menninger, 1940: 392), and took an antithetical position on volition from the normalizing discourse promoted by Schnieder. Since the person's character is derived from their unconscious conflicts, and since those conflicts are theorized as occurring prior to the Oedipal phase of development, personality pathology is constructed as *essentially* unresponsive to traditional psychoanalytic approaches (Basch, 1981). Conceptually, here the person's control is severely diminished, since the person's actions issue from the very deepest part of their unconscious, formed in the earliest phase of psychic development. It is from here that the PD construct acquired its essentialist nature; the problem is now stable, rigid and life long, as well as being beyond the person's conscious control.

The amalgamation of the competing psychiatric conceptions concerning volition, or will, and the essentialist psychoanalytic discourse that produced *Technical Bulletin Medical 203*, and subsequently the DSM, thus blends fundamentally incommensurable positions on the issue of volition. This conceptual double bind remains unresolved today. Although the moral dimension of the concept has, notionally, been removed, the retention of volition means that the act of moral judgement has been repressed rather than expunged. This is evidenced by patients' experiences: people with a personality disorder diagnosis have been described as 'difficult to tolerate let alone treat' (Reiser & Levenson, 1984: 1528). Yet the essentialism inherent in the construct makes it very difficult, conceptually, for a person to change: their problems are pervasive, enduring and inflexible.

A further rarefaction of this essentialism took place with DSM 3, which theorized personality disorders as representing the enduring context within which more transient elements of disorder unfold. Axis-I disorders are constructed as illnesses (transient and treatable), personality disorders are constructed as the context in which these illnesses manifest, characterized as being both enduring and prosaic. This paves the way for the person 'with personality disorder' to be conceptualized as *being the disease* rather than *having a disease*. Thus the UK Home

Affairs Select Committee recently described personality disorder as: 'essentially a developmental disorder, it is the person and it is not, so to speak, treatable in the same way as an illness' (2000: 176).

Clinically this led to a dead end. People with a personality disorder diagnosis had a developmental disorder, rather than an illness, and could not therefore be treated, leaving personality disorder primarily as a diagnosis used to exclude people from services. In the past few years this has begun to change. Some of this change seems to have come about as a consequence of clinical developments and successes, with dialectical behaviour therapy and mentalization based treatments both publishing results of good clinical outcomes with patients diagnosed with borderline personality disorder, for example. However, some of the shift has been politically driven, with the changes to the definition of 'mental disorder' and the removal of the treatability test from the *Mental Health Act* (2008) and government's drive – through NIMHE guidance and additional funding – to provide treatments for people given this diagnosis. Although this has cleared the way for more people with a personality disorder diagnosis to receive treatment, conceptually it leaves them in the same conceptual cul-de-sac with respect to understanding their situation and experiences.

A way out of the conceptual cul-de-sac? – shame

There are a number of reasons why shame seems to be the (unspoken, and largely untheorized) conceptual underbelly of the PD construct. The notion of volition logically demands that a person experiences and expresses guilt for their actions and, subsequently, changes their behaviour. After the 'normalization' of the PD diagnosis, guilt could no longer be explicitly discussed, since what is ostensibly at stake is not right or wrong but normality and abnormality. However, since the notion of volition is retained, the expectation of guilt also remains tethered to the construct. When PD took on its essentialist framework the now unspeakable expectation of guilt was transformed into shame. Shame differs from guilt in that it is linked with the violation of ideals rather than specific prohibitions, and it affects the whole self rather than a specific part of the self (Teroni & Deonna, 2008).

A relationship between shame and personality disorder diagnoses has been discussed in the literature; Crowe (2004), for example, has suggested that the way of being-in-the world that is called BPD might be better understood as a chronic shame response. In reviewing the literature she draws attention to the large body of research that has identified the impact of childhood abuse in relation to this diagnosis, as well as studies that have identified a connection between a history of abuse and overwhelming shame responses (Andrews & Hunter 1997; Grilo et al., 1999). She suggests that

> it may be that those individuals who experience the features of BPD may be experiencing an overwhelming shame response linked to an impairment in the development of those interpersonal skills necessary to integrate the shame affect into their self-image. These skills normally develop at a preverbal stage of development which therefore situates the shame response as a corporeal response.
>
> (Crowe, 2004: 330–1)

It seems plausible that some people who are diagnosed as having a personality disorder have suffered abuse during their early development, and that associated shame may be productive of what are seen as their adult 'symptoms'. However, the diagnosis of personality disorder seems to be a source of shame in itself. Teroni and Deonna (2008) suggest that while guilt is usually oriented towards others (one feels guilty towards another for having done something to them), shame is a social emotion that is usually oriented towards the self. Leeming and Boyle (2004) similarly see shame as a social phenomenon: an emotion that results from social interaction (Kemper, 1987). The personality disorder construct provides a professionally sanctioned meaning making system that shapes social interactions between doctors and patients. It provides social norms that shape individuals' emotional responses to different situations through the use of a shamed identity role. Shame, although experienced on an emotional level, may be seen the product of a socially sanctioned mechanism for positioning people who behave in certain ways as shameful, rather than as a dispositional attribute that exists outside of the person's ongoing relationships within which they are embedded (Gergen & Gergen, 1988).

Although personality structure is often employed to explain apparent differences in individual susceptibility to shame, it is culture that seems to determine the criteria against which to judge failure (Lewis, 1993). The homosexual, labelled as a pathological personality type, and given a dishonourable discharge during World War II, may have found it understandably difficult to resist attributing failure to their whole self. Once positioned in a shamed identity, shame may affect people in markedly different ways. Gilbert and McGuire (1998) note that angry and assertive behaviours may function to avoid a submissive or shamed identity. Morrison (1989) has written about shame in relation to narcissism, suggesting that defences against shame may manifest in clinical contexts such as rage, envy or contempt, which function to obscure the underlying emotion. Seu (1998) argues that self-blame and isolation, the very things that characterize shame, are accentuated by constructing relational phenomena as individual problems, as happens with the use of constructs such as PD. Understanding oneself as shameful implies that responsibility is ascribed to one's own flawed nature, or at least that a person will refrain from resisting this (Leeming & Boyle, 2004).

Shamed roles may have an important social and cultural function, that of policing and upholding a particular moral code. The 'passive–aggressive' soldier of World War II, who shows hostility and disrespect, can be described as displaying one of the 'Immaturity Reactions' and is, thus, positioned as shameful in order to protect the army's moral code (Hodge, 1955: 87) thereby maintaining authority through the mechanism of shame. Similarly the invocation of a shamed role for 'difficult to treat' patients may function to protect certain truths or professional statuses: Reich's undoubted lack of success with 'PD' cases led him to develop the conception of 'character armor' and 'character neurosis' (de Mijolla, 2005) and this claim, that personality disorders or extreme personality traits are responsible for interfering with treatment outcome in psychotherapy, pharmacotherapy, or even electroconvulsive therapy of Axis-I syndromes (Cloninger & Svrakic, 2008), functions to protect those therapies from being seen as failed treatments. Rather, placing the patient into a shamed role, ascribing a flawed nature to them, locates responsibility within the individual and deflects attention from theoretical and therapeutic inadequacy.[1]

The future of the construct?

Confucius is said to have said: when we see men of contrary character, we should turn inwards and examine ourselves. It seems important for the psy professions to reexamine both its concepts of, and it 'treatments' for personality disorder.

The shift to a dimensional concept of personality disorder is looking likely to be the next development in the genealogy of the construct. This is intended to provide a solution to the empirical problems that the construct suffers from. A dimensional approach would replace the categorical system of the DSM that assumes that a disorder is present if sufficient diagnostic criteria are met. This would remove the problem of adequately (and reliably) demarcating the boundaries of the individual diagnoses, replacing categories with a version of the Schneiderian system, which would assume that personality disorder is an extreme position on a dimension of normal personality (Millon, 1981). A dimensional approach, then, shifts from *diagnostic categories* to an *analysis of dysfunction* based on multifactorial models of normal personality. This would make personality disorder or extreme personality variation a much more complex, scientific-seeming construct and the issue of reliability would be transformed into a technical one with a complex statistical solution.

This shift would reposition the domain of personality disorder away from psychiatry, which has long eschewed it anyway, and towards clinical psychology, by foregrounding clinical psychology's tools for measuring personality. However, the central assumption that further understanding 'normal' personality would elucidate dysfunctional personality is entirely at odds with historical precedent. According to Rose:

> Our vocabularies and techniques of the person, by and large, have not emerged in a field of reflection on the normal individual, the normal character, the normal personality, the normal intelligence, but rather, the very notion of normality has emerged out of a concern with types of conduct, thought, expression deemed troublesome or dangerous.
>
> (Rose, 1996a: 26)

As we have seen, the newly minted DSPD diagnosis employs a dimensional approach to administer the most extreme end of personality variation; DPSD is defined by a combination of factors of risk and dissolves the notion of a concrete individual (Seddon, 2008). Risk is the defining feature of the diagnosis. A conceptual shift to a dimensional approach for the (non dangerous and severe) personality disorders would shift the whole construct to a risk discourse.

It was Bleuler's concept of a dimensional model for 'types' of insanity that gave rise to many of the personality disorder constructs in the first place. As time has gone by, these 'disorders', initially representing a lesser degree of pathology, have become severe and enduring phenomena. Millon's concept of personality as being the contextual dimension of the Axis-I disorders was, we are lead to believe, conceived with the best of humanist intentions: not wanting anybody to suffer in silence from an unacknowledged psychiatric problem. The effect though has been to vastly increase the number of people whose behaviour has been pathologized. A further dimensionalization and rarefaction of the notion of PD would open a space where a person could be judged to be 'vulnerable' to PD, part way towards an extreme personality variation, risking pathologizing behaviour and experiences that lie outside of what would inevitably be a more narrowly defined range of 'normal' behaviour.

The personality disorder construct has already been said to obscure the potential aetiological factors of psychological distress (Shaw & Proctor, 2005). A conceptual shift to extreme personality variation would do nothing to remedy this obfuscation. It would do nothing to facilitate a better understanding of the very high correlation between childhood sexual abuse and diagnosis with BPD in adulthood (Castillo, 2000). Indeed, Johnstone (2000; this volume) suggests that the 'symptoms' which are used to define 'conditions' such as BPD might be better understood as adaptive reactions to relational traumas that occurred in childhood; 'symptoms' may be more meaningfully understood when viewed as complex attempts to maintain personal survival and integrity when faced with past and current trauma.

A dimensional reconceptualization of PD maintains the focus on the individual and intrapsychic and is devoid of historical, social or contextual dimensions. This decontextualization locates dysfunction firmly within the individual and 'responsibility' with the reified disorder: the person is distressed and difficult because they have BPD, rather than viewing their conduct and experience as resulting from abuse and oppression, thus obstructing an exploration and understanding of aetiology (Linnet, 2004; Shaw & Proctor, 2005). This protects and reinforces the status quo while further invalidating the experiences of survivors of abuse and, hence, renders potential voices of discontent impotent (Ussher, 1991). This decontextualized approach also obscures the effects of inequality on mental health. The World Health Organization notes that socially inequitable distribution of resources has been found to causally affect mental health. Friedli suggests that

> both health-damaging behaviours and violence, for example, may be survival strategies in the face of multiple problems, anger and despair related to occupational insecurity, poverty, debt, poor housing, exclusion and other indicators of low status'. The report suggests that a focus on social justice is currently particularly important following an overemphasis on individual pathology.
>
> (Friedli, 2009: iii)

Adopting a dimensional approach will do nothing to support a focus on social justice or an understanding of the aetiology of distress. The extreme personality variation concept would continue to position people given this diagnosis in a shamed identity as the construct continues to rest on the dual – and incompatible – notions of a flawed identity and of personal responsibility.

Personality disorder and the wider culture

The personality disorder construct is explicitly based on a value judgement: it is 'behaviour that deviates markedly from the expectations of the individual's culture' (APA, 2000). What is meant by the 'expectations of the individual's culture' is left to the discretion of the diagnostician. Central to current cultural expectations are the prescriptions of the neoliberal economic and social order that has risen to ascendance throughout the world, with particular virulence in the US and the UK since around 1980, coinciding with an exponential rise of research and clinical interest in the personality disorder construct. During that time psychiatry had become a highly regarded profession, largely as a result of the success of the highly individualistic chemical imbalance theory of psychiatric disorders, which situates aetiology in neurotransmitter abnormalities. This model of psychiatry has 'helped to create the social and cultural milieu favoured by neoliberal policies' (Moncrieff, 2008b: 235) and those polices have fostered the hegemony of both biologically oriented psychiatry and psychotherapeutic approaches which prescribe talking cures as the interactional equivalent of medication.

The notion of individual responsibility is central to our culture. If you are one of society's losers, if you are struggling – that is your problem. And of course, the other side of the neoliberal economic and social order has been increased inequality and labour insecurity, coupled with raised expectations fostered by the conspicuous consumption of celebrity culture. It has been neoliberalism's losers for whom discontent has been medicalized. Limited, culturally available alternative ways to make sense of distress and difficulties has minimized resistance to biologically oriented psychiatry (see Coulter & Rapley; Smail, this volume). But the patients who do not 'get better' when given pharmacotherapy are problematic. A solution has been the development of a second class of patients, patients who are constructed not as having a *neurochemical* imbalance but a *personality* imbalance. Moncrieff (2008a) suggests that the chemical imbalance model requires people to locate the source of their troubles in themselves rather than in their environment, leading people to seek medical rather than political solutions. The difficulty posed by the second class of patient is that they do not initially locate the source of their troubles in themselves.

As such, people 'with' PD are notorious for failing to seek medical solutions (Livesley, 2001). In order to be persuaded to locate the source of their troubles within themselves, and to seek medical solutions to them, these patients have to be shamed into so doing: they need to be persuaded that their problems result from their flawed nature, that they have failed to meet the expectations of their culture, that their failure is attributable to their whole self, and that this is their fault. This, then, is the self-appointed project that psy has undertaken and, as evidenced by recent legislative change in the UK, continues successfully to pursue.

If, as Rose (1996) argues, our definition of what is normal emerges from our theories of those that we find troublesome and dangerous, it is essential to neoliberal culture's expectations of individual responsibility to keep notions of trouble, danger and disorder centrally bound up with the concept of dysfunctional *persons* rather than dysfunctional (social) *systems*. Indeed, in furthering this project, Livesley et al. (1994: 12) suggest that the proposed reformulation of personality disorder under a dimensional approach should define normal personality as 'the individual's striving to attain long-term strategic goals'.

Such a redefinition of the 'normal' would ascribe disorder to those who are unequal to the task, who give up on the struggle, or for whatever reason fail to attain (socially sanctioned) 'long-term strategic goals': a growing number of people living in appalling social conditions in an increasingly unequal world.[2] In this formulation, then, responsibility for their condition lies with them, the individuals, not with the sociocultural system. Those with little power are accountable for their 'disorder' while it's very existence as *explanadum* allows those with power to act with impunity. Mental health professionals should consider carefully whether their constructs benefit those that they claim to serve.

7

Medicalizing Masculinity

Sami Timimi

The rate of diagnosis of childhood psychiatric disorders has undergone a steep rise in many Western countries. Among school-age children (particularly in primary schools) there is a strong gender bias, with boys about three times more likely to be diagnosed with a psychiatric disorder than girls, and even more likely to receive drug treatment for this. Furthermore, these diagnoses (such as Attention Deficit Hyperactivity Disorder, Autistic Spectrum Disorder, and Conduct Disorder) do not concern themselves with boys' emotional lives, but instead focus on their perceived unruly and nonconformist behaviour. Mainstream child-psychiatric theory and practice appears to offer little explanation for, or discussion of, this gender split: instead these diagnoses have become reified. They are widely viewed as being caused by a biological dysfunction, with treatment being dominated by the use of psychopharmaceuticals. In this chapter I introduce key debates about what is happening to the space of 'boyhood' in modern Western culture (by referring to the nonpsychiatric literature), and follow this with a look at the evidence base that supports (or rather doesn't) the use of medication for 'treating' these boy problems.

Constructing masculinity

We live in an era of modernist Western culture, where discourse about children can be characterized by polarized anxieties about the risks they face and the risks they pose (Timimi, 2005; Miller, 2008). These anxieties have a strong gender bias, with girls being viewed as 'at risk' and boys as posing risk (through unruly, violent and impulsive behaviours). This moral panic about boys has attracted much debate in the media and among academics, with three models of the changes facing boys, and how we respond to these, emerging.

The first model, often referred to as the 'Boys will be Boys' perspective, starts from the assumption that boys and girls are biologically different. In this view boys are 'programmed' (for example via the effects of testosterone on the developing brain) to excel at visuospatial tasks but not at verbal–emotive skills. Furthermore, boys, as evolutionary 'hunters', are more easily distractible (scanning the environment), impulsive risk takers, and more active and aggressive. As our societies have changed, these 'natural' states have become pathologized and viewed as threatening. In addition, instead of having role models to help boys channel these traits in healthy directions, the increase in fatherless homes and a feminized education system that is more geared to the learning style of girls, means these tendencies are all too often acted out in destructive ways (see e.g. Gurian, 1999, 2001; Sommers, 2000).

The second model is known as the 'Boy Code' model. This model emphasizes the dominant cultural beliefs about what it means to be a 'man' and how this effects growing boys' socialization. Dominant cultural beliefs in the West require men to be encouraged to show stoicism, physical strength and aggression, and bravado; while discouraging overt displays of affection and/or distress. With such a 'code', boys learn that they should not appear sad or afraid, but instead should be able to 'tough it out'. Similarly any display of warmth, tenderness, and empathy should be suppressed (at least publicly), leading to feelings of shame surrounding boys' emotional life and with anger as the only emotion which is allowed in 'public'. As boys grow up, this code leads them to suppress their emotional life (with all the attendant consequences for their emotional well-being) until eventually they become 'disconnected' from this inner experience. Boys' emotional life then stays buried deep behind superficial social masks, apart from occasional (and sometimes extreme) eruptions in the only acceptable emotion – anger – often accompanied by violence and cruelty (see e.g., Kindlon & Thompson, 2000; Pollack, 1998).

The third model posits a more complex interaction between culturally constructed models of masculinity. In this 'Multiple Masculinities' model, it is argued that an increasing number of culturally constructed models of 'what it means to be a man' are available, however, they are always relative to the dominant model. The dominant model (i.e. the hegemonic model of masculinity) remains that which I have outlined above (revolving around bodily abilities, non-display of emotions, control, aggression etc.). This is the model associated with the 'patriarchal dividend', that is associated with men being in a more powerful and influential position than women. Having other available models causes great anxiety, as a defined role or 'way of being' becomes diffuse and ambiguous, as well as threatening men's position of privilege. Thus, while men may depart from this hegemonic masculinity and take up other identities (from 'bookish' to 'geek' to 'gay'), such a contravention carries risks. Boys who stray from the hegemonic model frequently become targets for bullying, teasing and exclusion by their male peers (see e.g. Connel, 2000, 2002; Kimmel, 2004).

Engaging with these perspectives would seem to provide a rich contextual backdrop through which we may find new ways of understanding the very recent phenomena of a rapid rise, mainly North American, North European and Australasian countries, in rates of diagnosis of boys with psychiatric disorders, particularly Attention Deficit Hyperactivity Disorder (ADHD) (active, impulsive, inattentive, risk taking boys with anger problems) and Autistic Spectrum Disorders (ASD) (shy, isolated boys who don't express their emotions – apart from anger). Sadly, instead of taking such analysis seriously and incorporating ideas from such perspectives into clinical practice, the discourse in child psychiatry over the last couple of decades has ignored these perspectives and instead focused on a biodeterministic view, seeing diagnoses such as ADHD and ASD as belonging, pretty much completely, to the realm of brain-based dysfunction. This neurocentric model has not only discouraged a more context-dependent view of children, but in addition has allowed for the mental-health professions to act as if the share price of the pharmaceutical industry was more important than the well-being of children under their care.

Child psychiatry and drug 'treatments' for boys

There is a long history in psychiatry of exorbitant claims being made for a variety of practices from insulin comas to radical brain surgery such as lobotomy. Each new 'advance' brought enthusiastic claims of 'miracle' cures, which, over time, when subjected to rigorous objective research, were shown not to be as effective as first claimed with risks having been unduly minimized. In recent decades, waves of optimism about 'curing' and 'treating' mental illness through modern psychopharmacology has popularized the use of psycho-pharmaceuticals changing the prescribing habits of doctors and the health seeking behaviour of patients. Sadly, closer scrutiny of the scientific evidence reveals that the new age of the mass use of psycho-pharmaceuticals is more the result of good marketing than of good science, through a confluence in the interests of neoliberal politics, the profit motive of pharmaceutical companies, and 'guild' interests of psychiatrists (Moncrieff, 2008b). Closer scrutiny of the science shows that, as in previous eras, physical treatments for psychiatric disorders and claims for the curative properties of psycho-pharmaceuticals have been exaggerated and their dangers minimized (Whitaker, 2002; Moncrieff, 2008b).

The treatment of children with psychiatric drugs is even more con-tentious than that of adults as many of the drugs now being used on children are meant for, and have only been researched in, adults. In a context in which no objective tests exist to verify the 'diseases' being diagnosed, pharmaceutical companies realize that a bigger market for their product can be created by 'disease promotion'. Here the task of the pharmaceutical company becomes that of convincing the medical profession and the public that young people's emotional and behav-ioural problems are the result of underdiagnosed and undertreated 'brain' disorders, which of course sets the context for their products to be marketed as 'treatments' for these alleged physical disorders. They do this by a variety of methods including sponsoring or producing material for doctors' waiting rooms that alert the medical and lay community to the existence of these conditions, producing 'educational' material for parents and teachers, and funding parent support/campaigning groups (Moynihan, Heath & Henry, 2002).

One favoured means of promoting new illnesses is for pharmaceuti-cal companies to invest in consumer support groups. For example, the US-based National Alliance for the Mentally Ill received over US $11 million from 18 pharmaceutical companies between 1996 and mid-1999 (Medawar & Hardon, 2004). It is cost-effective for pharmaceutical companies to invest in such groups without any direct promotion of their product, as support groups can increase the number of patients who present to doctors with ready-made diagnoses. This also allows them to present what they are doing as a 'service'. However, the prob-lem is not just that of the profit motive of pharmaceutical companies, as it is a problem of professional identity, which makes child psychiatry vulnerable to manipulation, and which must also be owned by the profession. Child psychiatry should sit at the confluence of many dif-ferent systems of knowledge: medical, psychological, social, paediatric, anthropological, cultural and so on. The move towards favouring bio-logical models and physical treatments has been attractive to sections of the profession that wish to carve out a clearer territory that bolsters a more 'doctor-like' image of what they do, rather than the more diffuse, hard to define role a more complex approach that spans several disciplinary territories provides.

The above dynamics (pharmaceutical company marketing and profiteering combined with some child psychiatrists' willing collusion with this) has subsequently distorted the evidence and ultimately practice for all psycho-pharmaceuticals currently used with children. For the purposes of this chapter, however, I will highlight the evidence base supporting (or not) psychiatric drug treatment for the two disorders that have become the most commonly diagnosed (mainly in the English speaking countries) child psychiatric disorders – ADHD (Attention Deficit Hyperactivity Disorder) and ASD (Autistic Spectrum Disorders). In both cases the diagnosis and prescriptions are given primarily to boys and pharmaceutical treatments are aimed at modifying the child's unruly and nonconformist behaviour. I start with the example of the most widely used psycho-pharmaceutical in children.

Stimulants for ADHD

In November 2004, an article, containing several interviews, was published which highlighted the fact that questions about the scientific credibility of psychiatric drug research of stimulants were widespread (Hearn, 2004). Gene Haislip, the now retired director of the US Drug Enforcement Agency (DEA), set production quotas for controlled substances such as the federally restricted stimulant Methylphenidate. During that time, he fought hard to raise public awareness about the drug's high rate of nonprescription use/misuse and about its long-term health impact on young patients. He notes:

> When I was at the DEA, we created awareness about this issue. But the bottom line is we didn't succeed in changing the situation because this – prescribing methylphenidate, for example – is spiraling ... A few individuals in government expressing concern can't equal the marketing power of large companies.
>
> (quoted in Hearn, 2004)

Haislip suspects that the marketing tactics of big pharmaceutical companies supported by a small group of prolific researchers in ADHD, whose work is funded by corporate producers of ADHD drugs, fuelled the spiralling use of stimulants. He is also concerned about links between some of the ADHD patient advocacy groups and the pharmaceutical companies that produce stimulants.

William Pelham, a prominent ADHD researcher and former member of the scientific advisory board for McNeil Pharmaceuticals, was also interviewed for the article (Hearn, 2004). Between 1997 and 1999, he was paid by McNeil to conduct one of three studies used to get US Food and Drug Administration (FDA) approval for a long-acting slow-release version of methylphenidate. But Pelham says the studies were flawed and claims made on the basis of their data that stimulants cause low rates of side effects, including appetite, sleep and growth problems, are misleading because the studies started with children who had already been taking the drug and who had experienced no significant side effects – children who exhibited side effects were not included in the study to begin with.

In the world of ADHD advocacy, Children and Adults with Attention Deficit hyperactivity Disorder (ChADD), a large US-based parent-support group, engages in lobbying and claims to provide science-based, evidence-based information about ADHD to parents and the public. Pharmaceutical companies donated to ChADD nearly $700,000 in the fiscal year 2002–3 (Hearn, 2004). Pelham, listed by ChADD as a member of its professional advisory board, came face to face with what he says are the group's glaring conflicts of interest. In 2002, after he received the ChADD Hall of Fame Award, he was subsequently interviewed for 'Attention!' the organization's magazine. In the interview, Pelham said, among other things, that stimulant drugs have serious limitations. Eight months later, 'Attention!' published Pelham's interview but with a large part cut out, particularly his comments about the limitations of the stimulants.

In a world run by those with the power to buy media attention, it is not uncommon for single studies to become the basis on which practice develops. One such study was the Multimodal Treatment Study of ADHD (MTA), a large multicentre trial in the USA testing the efficacy of the stimulant methylphenidate (MTA Cooperative Group, 1999). This publication led to widespread publicity claiming that the results show that we should be treating children who have ADHD with stimulant medication as the first line and possibly only treatment. In the years since the publication and popularization of this study there has been a sharp rise in the rates of stimulant prescription in all over North America, Northern Europe, Australasia and beyond (Timimi & Leo, 2009). In the UK this had resulted in a prescription rate for stimulants of over 550,000 per annum by 2006 (Department of Health, 2007) a staggering rise of over 7000 per cent in a decade.

The MTA study (MTA Cooperative Group, 1999) compared four groups of children who were given medication only; intensive behavioural therapy only; combined behavioural therapy and medication; and standard community care. The study lasted 14 months and concluded that the medication-only and combined behavioural therapy and medication groups had the best outcome, with the 'combined' group having only a marginally better outcome than the medication-only group. A closer look inevitably brings up important questions of methodology and the hidden question of conflict of interest as many of the researchers were found to have extensive links with the pharmaceutical industry (Boyle & Jadad, 1999; Breggin, 2000). Methodologically this was not a placebo-controlled double-blind clinical trial, and the parents and teachers who participated were exposed to pro-drug literature at the start of the study, thus potentially putting them in a mindset of positive expectation for change in the children receiving medication. There are also many question marks with regard to the selection and recruiting process, the behavioural interventions used, the placebo effect of the active medication arm continuing until the end of the 14 months but the behaviour therapy component finishing many months prior to 14 months, the lack of attention to the number of children experiencing side effects, and the dismissal of some reported side effects as probably being due to non-medication factors (Breggin, 2000). In addition, two-thirds of the community-care group were also receiving stimulant medication during the study, yet the community-care group was the poorest outcome category (Timimi, 2005).

The three-year outcome for the MTA study was finally published in 2007 (Jensen et al., 2007) – eight years after the results of the study at 14 months were published. All the advantages with regard to symptoms of ADHD for the medication-only and 'combined' groups had been lost, whereas the improvements in the behavioural-therapy-only group had remained stable. At the end of the original 14-month study, participants had been free to pursue whatever treatment they wanted. Some children had started taking medication and others on medication had stopped. The therapy-only group remained the group with the lowest use of medication. When the researchers analyzed outcomes for those who had used medication in the previous year they found that they had a worse outcome than those who had not. Furthermore, those who had taken medication continuously had higher rates of delinquency at three years, and were significantly shorter (by an average of over 4 cm) and lighter (by an average of over 3 kg) than those who had not taken medication. The likelihood of ending up being prescribed medication was not related to initial severity of symptoms. The three-year outcome data, therefore shows that the study that is repeatedly quoted as providing the scientific basis for prescribing stimulants to children (MTA Cooperative Group, 1999), actually demonstrates that there is little advantage (compared to behaviour therapy) associated with its use, but considerable risks. According to Pelham, who is on the steering committee for the MTA studies,

> [n]o drug company in its literature mentions the fact that 40 years of research says there is no long-term benefit of medications [for ADHD]. That is something parents need to know.
>
> (Pelham, quoted in Hearn, 2004)

The children in the MTA study have been followed up for eight years. Although details for these outcomes have not been published, it seems that outcomes for the 'medication management' group continued to deteriorate. Reporting on a recent conference presentation by James Swanson (another member of the steering committee for the MTA studies), Mytas (2009) notes that Swanson reports that

> [t]he medication management group functioned better at 14–24 months, but was associated with worse functioning and greater need of additional school services at 36, 48, 72, and 96 months.
>
> (Mytas, 2009: 23)

Thus we come full circle. The study that was most widely quoted as the study that 'proved' that ADHD should be treated with medication as a first line treatment has found that such a treatment (when compared to nonmedication based first line treatments) is associated with the worst outcomes and the greatest need of extra school support. This adds to the accumulating evidence on stimulants for ADHD, which, despite being the most researched drug treatment for a child psychiatric disorder, has failed to find long-term benefits accruing from their use. Systematic reviews of ADHD medication treatment (Jadad et al., 1999; Klassen et al., 1999; Schachter et al., 2001; McDonagh & Peterson, 2005; King et al., 2006) have noted the inadequate reporting of study methodology, possible publication bias, limited reliability of results, inadequate data regarding adverse events, and the lack of Randomized Control Trial evidence of any long term benefit from taking stimulants. In the face of such findings it is impossible to continue to claim that using stimulants for treatment of ADHD is evidence-based with the benefits outweighing the risks. Unfortunately practice is already so strongly established in some countries that reversing this trend is proving very difficult to achieve. Hopefully, preventing the uptake of such nonevidence based approaches will be easier to achieve in parts of the world where such practice has yet to take root, although the might of the drug companies still means this is an uphill battle.

The above example shows the extent to which the so-called scientific literature on the use of psycho-pharmaceuticals for childhood behavioural and emotional problems has demonstrated that it is unreliable and compromised – in particular by conflict of interest issues. Psychiatry appears to be the top 'offender' among medical specialities with regards use of, and sponsorship from, drug companies. Perhaps this is not surprising given the enormous potential markets that can be (and have been) developed if psychiatry is successful in medicalizing peoples' emotional responses and behaviour, in a field so reliant on subjective interpretations of normalcy and deviance. Child psychiatry seems particularly vulnerable (Timimi, 2008), with, most recently, an influential group of child psychiatrists at Harvard, extensively involved in research promoting the use of psycho-pharmaceuticals (particularly for ADHD and paediatric bipolar disorder), found to have received millions of dollars of income from pharmaceutical companies most of which they had not disclosed (Harris & Carey 2008). These types of problems have resulted in a growing distrust of the claims made for the use of psycho-pharmaceuticals with children, not only in the general public, but also within the medical profession more generally. For example, an editorial in 2008 in one of the world's oldest and most respected medical journals concluded:

> We know little about the long-term effects of psychiatric drugs in children. Side-effects of anti psychotics include shaking, damaged bones, reduced fertility, obesity, and increased risk of heart attack, diabetes, and stroke. Stimulants can damage the heart and stunt growth. Antidepressants can increase the risk of suicide in children. Do these drugs work? Evidence is often scant – and, where it exists, is largely discouraging ... Many patients have argued for years that psychiatric drugs are often more harmful, and less effective, than doctors believe. Increasingly, these patients are seen to be right. If psychiatry is to retain its claim to rationality, it must allow patients, including children, to be heard, and not merely drugged.
>
> (Editorial, *The Lancet*, 2008: 1194)

Anti-psychotics for autism

As far back as 1973, Ornitz commented that

> [A]lmost every conceivable psychotropic medication has been used with autistic children. The classes of medication have included sedatives, anti-histamines, stimulants, major and minor tranquilizers, anti-depressants, psycho-mimetics and anti-Parkinsonism drugs ... As with psychotherapy, behaviour modification, special modification and speech therapy, no single medication or class of modification has made an autistic child any less autistic. Nor has any medication or class of medication proven successful in removing any particular symptom of the autistic syndrome.
>
> (Ornitz, 1973: 40)

These decades' old observations are as true today as they were then, despite his comments referring to a much narrower group of children, as this was prior to the broader concept of 'Autistic Spectrum Disorder' (ASD) taking root. However, this is not the impression you get if you observe current practice in child and adolescent psychiatry. A good example of this comes from an editorial entitled 'Antipsychotic drugs in children with autism' that appeared in 2007 in the highly influential *British Medical Journal*. Use of antipsychotics, particularly risperidone, for 'treating' children with autism who have concurrent behavioural problems has become popular in recent years and well before any evidence for the safety and efficacy of such practice was available. Studies in this area appear to have the purpose of trying to justify an already established practice.

In this article, 'opinion leaders' Susan Morgan and Eric Taylor (2007) take an apparently moderate stance suggesting that antipsychotic drugs should not be used indiscriminately in children with autism but reserved for those with more 'serious' behaviour problems. This apparent moderate position is still worrying however, as it effectively sanctions the use of antipsychotics for 'aggressive' behaviours in those diagnosed with autism, without presenting sufficient evidence that such practice is either safe or effective, yet the article is written in a style that suggests the recommendations are both evidence based and cautious. They state that 'we consider off label use [of anti-psychotics] is justified when other approaches fail or are unfeasible' (Morgan & Taylor, 2007: 1069). This effectively leaves the door open for the continued increase in the use of (off-label) antipsychotics as the reading doctor is left to wonder what other approaches to use and for how long before deciding they have failed (an important point, particularly bearing in mind what Ornitz, above, had to say about the lack of efficacy for any treatment in autism). Furthermore, unfeasibility of other approaches is near universal as the increasing popularity of the diagnosis of autism, together with this diagnosis becoming more often than not the responsibility of busy community paediatricians, means 'other approaches' are thin on the ground. They further recommend that 'diagnosis should distinguish between aggression and other seriously challenging behaviours (which may justify an antipsychotic agent) and lesser levels of irritability (which may not)' (Morgan & Taylor, 2007: 1069). However, they don't explain how a clinician is supposed to differentiate between what one should consider 'seriously' challenging behaviour and 'irritability'. Not only is the conceptual basis of the article shaky, but the evidence presented also does not clearly support their recommendations.

In support of their recommendation to use antipsychotics for challenging behaviour they refer to two studies only (McCracken et al., 2002; Shea et al., 2004). A critical review of these two studies reveals anything but encouraging news for this practice. Firstly, both studies were of only eight weeks in duration, far from the many years that drugs' prescribed to pacify behaviour are usually used for. Secondly, one of the studies (McCracken et al., 2002) reviewed their subjects at six months and found a familiar pattern seen with drug treatment for behavioural problems – that of diminishing returns, with less than half of the group that had received risperidone (the antipsychotic) now rated as 'improved' (interestingly they do not provide the data for how the placebo group were doing after six months: see also Double, this volume). Thirdly, a decrease in challenging behaviour in those receiving an antipsychotic at a sufficient dose is really a foregone conclusion, after all, antipsychotics are not classified as 'major tranquilizers' for nothing. Whether this is viewed as a therapeutic effect or side effect depends on your perspective. Reflecting this fact, both studies rated high levels of somnolence (sleepiness or drowsiness), for example, Shea et al. (2004) recorded a 72 per cent rate of somnolence in the group receiving risperidone, leading to the rather peculiar scenario where arguably the same pharmacological effect is simultaneously rated as therapeutic (decrease in aggressive behaviours) and an adverse effect (somnolence) – after all you can't get up to much mischief if you're drowsy.

What is most worrying, however, is that the editorial pays little attention to minimizing of the serious adverse effects of the antipsychotics, which were prevalent in both studies. To give just one example, both studies found the group receiving risperidone put on more weight than the group with the placebo; in McCracken et al. (2002) this was an average of 2.7 kg in the drug-treated group compared with 0.8 kg in the group taking placebo, and in the Shea et al. (2004) study drug-treated children gained an average of 2.7 kg compared with 1.0 kg in the placebo group. Remember this was after only 8 weeks of 'treatment'. Thus these children were being put at a greatly increased risk of serious illnesses such as cardiovascular disease and diabetes.

As noted by Morgan and Taylor, Janssen-Cilag withdrew their application for risperidone to be licensed in the UK for use in behavioural problems associated with autism. However, the editorial recommends the continued off-label use of antipsychotics to control the behaviour of children with autism. As influential clinicians and researchers writing in an influential journal, their position encourages the use of powerful, risky medicines, with unproven long-term efficacy, for a group of citizens (children) who have never really had a say in what is being imposed upon them and with scant evidence to back up the validity or utility of such practice, but sufficient evidence to demonstrate that such practice exposes children to significant risks.

Conclusion

There has been a rapid increase in diagnosis of psychiatric disorders in children and adolescents in most Western societies, particularly for behavioural problems and, among these, particularly for boys. Childhood problems are increasingly medicalized resulting in an apparent 'epidemic' of several psychiatric disorders in children in the West and a rapid rise in the prescription of psychotropics to the young. I have summarized the problematic nature (in terms of lack of evidence for a biological substrate, high comorbidity, lack of cross-cultural validity, boundary issues, marginalization of certain types of evidence, and lack of evidence for effectiveness of medications used) of current popular child psychiatric diagnoses elsewhere (Timimi, 2002, 2004, 2005, 2007, 2008; Timimi & Maitra, 2006; Timimi & Leo, 2009). In this chapter I have first contextualized this issue by referring to the nonpsychiatric literature on the perceived crisis with boys in the West and then I have concentrated on the way evidence (or rather lack of it) for the safety and efficacy of using psychotropics for children diagnosed with quintessentially 'boy' disorders, has been distorted to increase the potential market and bolster a more 'doctor-like' image for child psychiatrists.

The increasing popularity of diagnoses like ADHD and ASD, owes more to social, political and economic processes than to scientific breakthroughs (see also Rapley & McHoul, 2004). The popularity of these diagnoses can act as a barometer for cultural attitudes toward boys and how to deal with them. Those countries with high rates of diagnosis and high rates of medication use for essentially social control purposes demonstrate their lack of tolerance or wish to understand and engage in the emotional lives of boys. In that way they replicate the dominant cultural discourses rather than challenge them. In doing this they contribute to the processes leading to the 'boy crisis', rather than help ameliorate them and improve the emotional well-being of boys and men in our culture.

8

Can Traumatic Events Traumatize People? Trauma, Madness and 'Psychosis'

Lucy Johnstone

Over a decade ago I wrote a critical review of the literature about family influences on 'schizophrenia' under the title *'Do Families Cause "Schizophrenia"? Revisiting a Taboo Subject'* (Johnstone, 1999). The controversy has recently resurfaced in a slightly different form, in relation to the debate about the role of trauma and abuse in the development of 'psychosis'.

To make my own position clear, I welcome this research and admire the rigour and determination with which John Read, a leading figure in the debate, and others are pursuing this controversial agenda. At the same time, I believe there are possible pitfalls in some of their arguments that could result, yet again, in the neutralizing and defusing of the situation in which 'the entire construct of schizophrenia receives arguably its largest challenge since its inception' (Read, 1997: 4).

A summary of recent findings

John Read is a New Zealand-based psychologist who has, singly and alongside others, published a series of papers on the relationship between trauma and 'psychosis' (Read, 1997; Read et al., 2003; Read & Haslam, 2004; Read et al., 2005; Morrison et al., 2005; Kilcommons & Morrison, 2005; Read, Rudegeair & Farrelly, 2006; Larkin & Morrison, 2006; Moskowitz et al., 2008).

Trauma, in this body of work, refers mainly but not exclusively to events in childhood, and includes physical and sexual abuse and general neglect; and 'psychosis' includes 'schizophrenia' and 'bipolar disorder' as well as specific 'symptoms' such as delusions and hallucinations. The themes have been taken up by a number of other researchers (see Larkin & Morrison, 2006 for an overview).

The findings of this body of work can be summarized as follows:

- There is a general relationship between child abuse and adult pathology of all types, but this has typically been ignored or downplayed in relation to 'psychosis'.
- Childhood abuse and neglect is at least as strongly linked to 'psychosis' as to other psychiatric conditions, and the link appears to be a causal one.
- There is some evidence linking particular kinds of abuse experience with particular 'symptoms' (for example, childhood sexual abuse seems to be a stronger causal factor than childhood physical abuse for auditory hallucinations).
- The content of 'delusions' is often closely related to actual experiences of childhood abuse.
- Cognitive theories suggest that unintegrated memories of abuse may lead to cognitive misattributions (for example, about where voices come from). 'Delusions' may be a defence against overwhelming feeling.
- We need a 'traumagenic neurodevelopmental' model which incorporates recent evidence that adverse early events confer biologically based sensitivity to stress.
- 'Psychotic' clients should be offered the same range of psychological therapies as any other clients with a history of abuse.

The researchers also acknowledge various caveats:

- The relationship between trauma and 'psychosis' is complex.
- Trauma is not relevant in all cases of 'psychosis'.
- Other factors also contribute to the development of 'psychosis'.
- Self-reports of abuse may be unreliable.
- Little is known about the mechanisms by which trauma results in 'psychosis'.
- It is important to distinguish between correlation and causation, although evidence of a dose-dependent relationship between severity, number, and number of types of abuse and the probability of breakdown, suggests the latter. In fact, the severest abuse raises the risk of psychosis by up to 48 times.

(Janssen et al., 2004)

Despite these reservations, two papers and an editorial in *Acta Psychiatrica Scandinavica* were summarized in rather sensationalist terms in the *Guardian* daily newspaper by psychologist and author Oliver James (2005):

> The psychiatric establishment is about to experience an earthquake that will shake its intellectual foundations ... Physical or sexual abuse has been shown to be a major, if not the major, cause of [schizophrenia] ... Read's earthquake may trigger a landslide.

So why is the issue so controversial? The answer to this is fairly obvious. The abuse debate is a rerun of a dialectic that dates back to the origins of psychiatry: is madness a meaningful and understandable response to life circumstances? Or is it simply the manifestation of a biologically based illness, with life events operating, at most, as 'triggers' of a meaningless disease process? Much of the debate has centred around the status of 'schizophrenia' – in Szasz's words 'the sacred symbol of psychiatry' (Szasz, 1976) and in Boyle's words 'the prototypical psychiatric disease' (Boyle, 2002a). What is at stake, however, is not just the status of 'schizophrenia-as-a-disease', but rather the whole set of biomedical assumptions on which psychiatry is based, and the vested interests therein (from politicians and drug companies downwards).

What makes this recent manifestation of the debate even more contentious, if possible, is the explicit link to another equally explosive issue – the widespread occurrence of child abuse. This, like the alternative understanding of madness, is something that we seem to have to rediscover at regular intervals: As Calder (2005: 122) notes: 'child abuse has always been known about and talked about [but] the willingness amongst public and professionals to do something about it has waxed and waned through the years'. In her classic book *Trauma and Recovery*, Judith Herman reminds us that 'the knowledge of horrible events periodically intrudes into public awareness but is rarely retained for long. Denial, repression and dissociation operate on a social as well as an individual level' (Herman, 1992: 4).

So, neither of these issues is at all new – in fact the link between sexual abuse and madness was made by both Freud and Jung. Nor, from a clinician's perspective, is it very surprising to be told that many of our 'psychotic' clients have a history of abuse. The new aspects are the attempts to link particular 'symptoms' with particular types of abuse experience and the availability of technology to detect the effects of trauma on the developing brain.

What are the likely responses?

In the light of the above, Read was absolutely right to 'anticipate a degree of outrage, from biological psychiatrists and people acting as spokespersons for relatives' groups' (Read, 2002: np). As an example, a spokesperson from the mainstream UK mental health charity *Rethink* commented: '[T]he mental health field has been here before. The antipsychiatry movement of RD Laing rejected the concept of schizophrenia as an illness and set out to blame the parents ... [Let's not] resurrect a sterile 40-year-old debate' (Pinfold, 2005: 17). There have also been some slightly more sophisticated, but equally misguided, responses.

Response number one

This response seeks to integrate the findings outlined above within an existing 'vulnerability–stress' model, which privileges the 'biological' and by so doing reduces other factors ('stresses') to the lesser status of 'triggers' of the underlying 'illness', thus divesting them of their personal meaning and preserving biomedical assumptions relatively intact. This is a familiar manoeuvre within the family management literature (which holds, in brief, that family dynamics are not significant in themselves, but are merely non-specific precipitants of the disease process, via levels of Expressed Emotion; Johnstone, 1993). Boyle (2002b) summarizes the situation thus:

> The vulnerability-stress hypothesis ... has proved to be an extraordinarily useful and effective mechanism for managing the potential threat to biological models ... Its usefulness lies in its seeming reasonableness (who could deny that biological and psychological and social factors interact?) and its inclusiveness (it encompasses both the biological and the social – surely better than focusing on only one?) ... while at the same time it firmly maintains the primacy of biology ... by making it look as if the 'stress' of the model consists of ordinary stresses which most of us would cope with, but which overwhelm only 'vulnerable' people. We are thus excused from examining too closely either the events themselves or their meaning to the 'vulnerable' person.

Read (2005: 597) is fully aware of this danger suggesting that, despite the superficial promise of a synthesis of models, it is rather 'a colonisation of the psychological and social by the biological'. Examples of this predictable manoeuvre are not hard to find, for example:

> The research must not be interpreted as evidence of a cause of psychosis ... It may indicate that those who are genetically predisposed

to schizophrenia ... may be more likely to go on to develop the disorder at a later stage compared to those who have no abuse history.

(SANE, 2002)

Not many people would want to go as far as Palmer (1994, in Read, 1997) and suggest that you can be genetically predisposed to being abused. However, even the weaker version of the vulnerability–stress model carries the blaming and insulting, implication that service users' experiences of abuse are not enough in themselves to justify their distress; in other words, that if they had not been in some sense biologically defective, they would have coped. This might well be experienced as insulting and blaming by survivors of abuse.

As an alternative, Read calls for a genuinely integrated bio-psychosocial model which includes recent evidence about the effects of trauma on the developing brain, but which does not make unwarranted biological assumptions, or prioritize biological factors over psychosocial ones (Read, Rudegeair & Farrelly, 2006.) This version of a mixed model would lead to mainly psychosocial interventions (more use of psychotherapy and less of neuroleptics) and would neither justify, nor rely upon, the medical model of distress.

Response number two

This response preserves the concept of 'schizophrenia' and its associated biomedical assumptions by re-diagnosing those who turn out to have a history of trauma, and thus separating them off from those who 'really' have the biologically based illness. There are historical precedents for this in the emergence of the diagnosis of 'shellshock' during World War I; the very obvious role of extreme stressors in soldiers who broke down at the front made it implausible to diagnose a mass outbreak of 'schizophrenia'. A similar situation arose after the Vietnam War, resulting in the new diagnosis of PTSD (Van Putten & Emery, in Read et al., 2005).

Typical examples of this response are:

There may be at least two pathways to positive symptoms of schizophrenia. One may be primarily endogenously driven ... The other may be primarily driven by childhood psychosocial trauma.

(Ross et al., 1994)

There appears to be some consensus in the literature that there may be two different aetiological pathways to psychosis ... The first is ... primarily endogenous, driven by biological factors ... whereas the second is largely trauma–induced.

(Kilcommons & Morrison 2005)

A similar argument is put forward for the existence of a subsection within the 'schizophrenia' spectrum, which should be called 'traumatic psychosis' (Callcott & Turkington 2006). Such tactics may account for the massive rise in cases of 'Borderline Personality Disorder' in people who would surely have attracted the diagnosis of 'schizophrenia' a decade ago – and often did.

The reasoning here seems to be thus: 'it can't be a proper case of schizophrenia because they had good reason to break down'. This, of course, begs the question of whether *all* cases of 'schizophrenia' occur for 'good reasons', even if these are not immediately obvious to professionals. It is also a form of circular logic: 'why is this called PTSD/BPD/traumatic psychosis and not schizophrenia?' 'Because there is a history of trauma'. 'How do you know there aren't equally good reasons for breakdown in schizophrenia as well?' 'Because otherwise we would have called it PTSD/BPD/traumatic psychosis'.

Once again, Read (1997: 4) is well aware of this manoeuvre:

In practical terms, a change of diagnosis, once abuse is identified, from schizophrenia to one that identifies the role of trauma, such as PTSD, may have significant advantages for the individual. It may increase the chances of psychotherapy being offered to address the effects of the abuse ... There is, nevertheless, what might best be described as a backwards circular logic at work here that both negates the possibility of considering whether abuse may be causally related to psychosis and protects the biomedical assumptions about the causes of schizophrenia from critical analysis based on the relevant data.

So much for the responses. However there are, in my view, some aspects of Read's own, and others' research into the area, which could help to undermine its radical implications just as effectively.

Problematic aspects of Read's and others' work – the concept of 'psychosis'

There are potential problems with the uncritical use of the word 'psychosis' in this research, as in titles of books and papers such as *Trauma and Psychosis* (Larkin & Morrison, 2006); *How Does Trauma*

Lead to Psychosis? (Read et al., 2005); *Relationships between Trauma and Psychosis* (Kilcommons & Morrison 2005); and many other examples.

The term 'psychosis' has recently emerged as an alternative to the decreasingly credible concept of 'schizophrenia'. As one sign of this, perhaps, the UK branch of the *International Society for the Psychological Treatments of Schizophrenia and other Psychoses* voted this year to remove the word 'schizophrenia' from their title. 'Psychosis' can be seen as a more user-friendly and less stigmatizing diagnosis. However, a moment's thought shows that it is equally, if not more, problematic in terms of reliability, validity and so on, while its woolliness serves to disguise and defuse fundamental critiques about the nature, purpose and consequences of psychiatric diagnosis. Mary Boyle, in an analysis of the recent literature on psychosis, puts it well:

> The shift to 'psychosis' appears to involve fundamental conceptual change, particularly through the application of 'normal' psychological theory ... and through a (limited) focus on the content as well as the form of 'delusions' and hallucinations. But there is also much evidence of 'psychosis' being used in ways which may perpetuate the problems of the concept of schizophrenia, including the continued use of a discourse of deficit and chronicity ... privileging biological over psychological and social theories.
>
> (Boyle, 2006: 2)

In other words, the term is used in different ways by different authors, with, in some cases, a welcome emphasis on 'meanings' rather than just 'symptoms'. However, reifying the concept of 'psychosis' as something separate from, and additional to, the reaction to a traumatic event, sets the scene for the reintroduction of the vulnerability–stress model with all the problems I have already identified. Thus Mueser et al. (2002: 127–8) suggest that 'our model is an adaptation and extension of the stress-vulnerability model developed for schizophrenia ... Psychobiological vulnerability ... can be increased by stress'.

The argument then runs that there is a 'psychosis' of some kind, over and above the natural reaction to a trauma, a disease process 'triggered' and made worse by the trauma. This bizarre logic may be more apparent if we draw an analogy with another common trauma, bereavement. Contrast the following two causal explanations:

§1.   She was badly abused – and we now think that is what led to her psychosis and in fact made it worse.

§2. Her husband died – and we now think that is what led to her grief, and in fact made it worse.

It would be even odder, to pursue the analogy, to argue that some people are biologically vulnerable to, are genetically predisposed to develop grief, and to attempt to find its 'real', biological cause, the death of a partner being merely the 'trigger'.

This logic also leads to confusion about whether a person's reactions are the 'symptoms' of a 'disorder', and therefore in need of 'treatment', or normal and rational responses and beliefs which are an inevitable part of coming to terms with a very painful experience. Compare the following:

§1. Negative beliefs about self, world and others (such as 'I am vulnerable' and 'Other people are not to be trusted') have been shown to be associated with the development of psychotic experiences.
                                                    (Morrison et al., 2005)

§2. Negative beliefs about self, world and others (such as 'I am lonely'and 'My husband is never coming back') have been shown to be associated with the development of grief.

We might note in passing that Morrison's apparent assumption is that people *are* trustworthy and individuals are *not* vulnerable, which shows a remarkable degree of optimism in the face of the evidence of widespread abuse that his paper has just summarized. Maybe the task of the therapist is not to try and change these 'dysfunctional beliefs', but to help abused clients come to terms with the truth that is expressed in them – even if it is not the whole truth?

This type of logical mistake has been characterized as a 'category error' (Ryle, 1948). Ryle illustrates the error by describing visitors looking around Oxford University – the colleges, the libraries, the lecture halls – and then asking 'But where is the university?' The main point of Read's research is that there is growing evidence that the experiences that service users report (unusual beliefs, distressing voices etc.) are, in many cases, a reaction to the abuses they have been subjected to. There is the abuse, and there are the responses to the abuse. There is – like 'the university' – nothing else, no *additional* 'psychosis' that needs explaining.

Category errors abound in psychiatry; indeed, the DSM is composed almost entirely of them. This faulty thinking inevitably leads to excruciatingly complicated questions about the possible relationships between 'psychosis' and other reifications such as dissociative disorder, PTSD, SMI ('severe mental illness') and so on. An example of the resulting intellectual contortions that these reifications engender is provided by Mueser et al. (2002: 128 ff.)

> In our model ... we hypothesize that PTSD is a comorbid disorder which mediates the relationships between trauma, increased symptom severity, and higher use of acute care services in persons with a SMI ... We hypothesize that PTSD can both directly and indirectly increase symptom severity, risk of relapse, and use of acute care services in patients with a SMI. PTSD symptoms can directly affect SMI through the avoidance of trauma-related stimuli, distress related to reexperiencing the trauma, and overarousal. Common correlates of PTSD can also indirectly influence SMI ... and so on for another 10 pages.

This could be rendered more simply as follows: 'People are often very badly affected by abuse.' Then we could get on with working out how best to help them, instead of being distracted by the theoretical equivalent of a wild goose chase.

Problematic aspects of Read's and others' work – the concept of 'trauma'

There are also potential problems with the indiscriminate use of the term 'trauma' to summarize the huge range of painful and damaging experiences that can be inflicted on children and adults. While the word does at least put psychosocial causal factors on the map, at the same time it shifts the focus away from wider issues such as poverty, classism and racism, all of which have been linked to 'psychosis' as well. It also fails to account for 'the importance of more mundane but also very damaging experience ... complex and long term interpersonal and relational patterns ... such as serious communication problems and enmeshment in families' (Boyle, 2006: 6). These, of course, were precisely the kinds of family environments described so controversially by Laing, Bateson and others.

The word 'trauma' also takes the focus off the abusers and places it onto their victims. Of course, it is vitally important to find ways of helping the latter – but there seems to be a surprising lack of social or professional curiosity about the vast numbers of perpetrators who are helping to fill our psychiatric hospitals. This is in marked contrast to high levels of concern about action to address causal factors in other medical 'epidemics' (e.g. obesity, heart and other smoking-related diseases; diabetes).

Finally, "trauma", as a neat summary word 'can also sanitize people's experiences because it needn't involve spelling out the troubling and sometimes shocking experiences people have actually had' (Boyle, 2006: 7). What all this amounts to is 'a striking reluctance to keep people's life experiences at the forefront of our theories' (Boyle, 2006: 10). The passionate desire to reintroduce these painful realities to our consciousness is what is most admirable and most needed about Read's work. Here, for example, is one instance described by Read et al. (2003: 12) of how the content of someone's 'delusions' related to their actual experiences:

> Another's chart read 'Sexual abuse: Abused from an early age ... Raped several times by strangers and violent partners'. This person believes they are 'Being tortured by people getting into body, for example the Devil and the Beast ... At one stage had bleeding secondary to inserting a bathroom hose into self, stating wanting to wash self as people are trying to put aliens into my body'.

This kind of 'delusional belief' can be seen as an example of the tell/don't tell dynamic described by Herman (1992: 4): 'People who have survived atrocities often tell their stories in a highly emotional, contradictory, and fragmented manner which undermines their credibility and thereby serves the twin imperatives of truth telling and secrecy'. As she also notes, 'Witnesses as well as victims are subject to the dialectic of trauma. It is difficult for an observer to remain clear-headed and calm, to see more than a few fragments of the picture at one time, to retain all the pieces, and to fit them together. It is even more difficult to find a language that conveys fully and persuasively what one has seen'. With this in mind, it is vitally important to be aware of the conceptual traps that would allow such disturbing knowledge to be concealed and lost, yet again, behind a mountain of individualizing and pathologizing psychiatric theories. Hence the importance of being clear about the most helpful questions to ask from this point onwards.

Helpful and unhelpful questions

I suggest that unhelpful questions are ones that are based on category errors, such as: *Can trauma cause psychosis?* Since a trauma is usually defined as an event that 'involves direct threat of death, severe bodily harm, or psychological injury which the person ... finds intensely distressing or fearful' (Mueser et al., 2002: 124), traumas are, by definition, 'traumatic'. This means that the question, without the category error, actually translates as: *Can traumatic events traumatize people?*

The key issue here, then, is whether (much of) 'psychosis' is actually better understood as a reaction to trauma and abuse. Better questions, therefore, would be: What are the ways in which people (can) react to trauma? Do these (routinely) include some of the experiences we refer to as 'hallucinations' and 'delusions'?

Helpful questions will be about trauma and abuse, in the widest sense, as well as other types of damaging experience, and about specific experiences such as hallucinations, not about 'psychosis'. Other examples might be:

- What factors influence whether people develop one form of distress rather than another?
- How do people experience and understand their distress, and what helps them to cope with it?
- How does all this relate to the structure and functioning of the developing brain?
- Should psychiatric services be based on a trauma model, not a biomedical model?

Some services have already answered the last question in the affirmative. In the USA it is much more widely acknowledged that 'trauma survivors are the majority of clients in human service systems', leading to the establishment of 'trauma-informed services' in which 'service delivery is influenced by an understanding of the impact of interpersonal violence and victimization on an individual's life and development' (Elliott et al., 2005: 3).

A further consequence of moving away from individualizing assumptions about 'psychosis' being caused by some combination of dysfunctional thoughts and genetic vulnerability, rather than by trauma itself, is that we will be forced, as a society, to take some action about the epidemic of child abuse in our midst. It will not be easy to acknowledge this epidemic of abuse in our midst. In Read and Haslam's (2004: p. 133) words: 'bad things happen and can drive you crazy'. I would put it even more strongly: people do terrible things to each other, and this can drive you crazy. The consequences of accepting this are profound, both for psychiatry and for society as a whole.

9
Children Who Witness Violence at Home

Arlene Vetere

> Interpersonal violence, especially violence experienced
> by children, is the largest single preventable cause of
> mental illness. What cigarette smoking is to the rest
> of medicine, early childhood violence is to psychiatry.
>
> (Sharfstein, 2006: 3)

The effects of witnessing violence in their own homes are well documented to have adverse effects on the psychological development of many children (Vetere & Cooper, 2005). Moffitt and Caspi (1998) estimated that over 2/3 of assaults in the family home are actually witnessed by children, and the risk of direct harm to children is estimated to be four–nine times higher than if they live in homes where violence does not occur. It can be argued from therapeutic experience that children always know, even though they might not know the details. In our experience of working systemically in our domestic-violence project, it is often the children who call for help during an attack, and who take on responsibility for family safety, beyond their years and their maturity. Such children can often develop social, moral and interpersonal competence in this context, alongside other potentially deleterious emotional effects, such as the risk of traumatic responses.

And this will be the point of this chapter – to explore how trauma responses in children may not be recognized by family members, education and mental health professionals, either because they are masked, hidden, or not easily understood. And there lies the rub, as these trauma responses may then be misinterpreted, and this could lead to children and their families not receiving trauma services but, rather, being diagnosed with some variety of 'childhood mental disorder'. One of the well-understood impacts of living with chronic fear and the threat of violence and actual violence is that traumatized parents may not be able to listen to their children, who may be trying to speak of their emotional state. This is not because they may not *want* to listen, but that it is very hard to hear children's accounts of trauma, both because it can retrigger a parent's trauma, and because, in order to fully empathize with the child's experience, the parent needs to enter it at some level, and most of us find that hard. Similarly, we could argue that we all carry a wish for denial – a tendency to minimize the effects of aggression and violence born of a wish that such things could not happen in children's lives. So this chapter is written in the spirit of a wish to illuminate the intergenerational effects of fear, sadness, shame and worry in our lives, and a parallel wish to celebrate the spirit of resilience, adaptation and coping that we see in so many of the children and families with whom we work.

Trauma is here defined as an exceptional experience of powerful and dangerous stimuli that overwhelm the child's capacity to regulate their emotions. Children show the same signs of distress when they are witnesses to violence as when they are assaulted themselves (van der Kolk, 2005). In addition, the frequency and intensity of physical conflict between the parents is linked to worse behavioural outcomes for children. It was this consistent research finding that influenced the UK government in 2005 to change existing child-protection legislation, to include child witnesses to domestic violence as a child-protection issue.

What are children learning when they live in households where fear is a daily experience?

Trauma theory, attachment theory, social-learning theory and systemic theories can all contribute to our understanding of the short term and longer term effects of living with domestic violence on children's development. For us it is an ethical issue of accountability in our practice that we do not rely on one explanatory model for how violence in intimate relationships develops, happens and continues over time and across generations. Browne and Herbert (1997) use a social learning framework to summarize what children are learning when they are exposed to physical and emotional violence in their households. It may teach them aggressive styles of conduct in relation to interpersonal influence and control; it can both reduce restraint and increase arousal to aggressive situations, making it harder to learn self-control and to self-soothe; it can desensitize children to violence so that they come to see it as normal or trivial; and it potentially distorts their views about conflict resolution in intimate relationships with family and friends. Repeated exposure to others' aggression and violent behaviour can reinforce expectancies about how others will behave, and form the basis on which children learn to make predictions about how relationships 'work'. Children who develop tendencies to behave in the above ways often come to others' attention because their behaviour is seen as worrying, or as a nuisance as it involves the infringement of others' rights. These behaviours are sometimes clustered as 'externalising' behaviours and seen as a problem of the child. This can lead to diagnosis from mental health professionals and to individualized therapeutic responses, which risk missing the context of fear that may be at the heart of the problem. Unless child-mental-health practitioners ask children what is happening at home, and in their communities, in detail and with gentle persistence, a child's behaviour patterns could be misdiagnosed and the child's safety might not be at the forefront of the work. Clearly there are ethical, moral and theoretical issues here for training, supervision and practice, but we still find that domestic violence awareness and practice remains patchy in the UK.

Attachment theory suggests that most children learn to understand, name and regulate their affect in the social and developmental context of the family. Constant exposure to fear and intimidation interferes with the child's capacity to learn to calm themselves and to self-soothe. If the adults looking after the child are frightened and/or frightening the child cannot predict consistent caretaking, and it is likely that secure attachment is compromised (Crittenden, 2006). This poses a developmental dilemma for children. It can lead to confusion, hyper vigilant behaviour, and poor emotion regulation with no clear behaviour strategy for responding to stress. In more extreme circumstances, trauma theory suggests that children develop coping strategies of splitting, denial and dissociation, that can persist into adulthood and make the development of satisfying intimacy in adult relationships harder to achieve, unless exposed to corrective life experiences and relationships along the way (van der Kolk, 2005). Some children may seek an illusion of safety by identifying with the aggressor and seeing aggressive behaviour as a way of feeling powerful in the face of unpredictable and inconsistent and/or frightening forms of care giving (Balbernie, 2001). Balbernie also suggests that children learn to mentally 'dodge', as a way of avoiding having to think about what is happening – to avoid contemplating that the person whom they love or is looking after them, means them harm. It is not difficult to see how this pattern of responding overlaps with diagnostic categories of behaviour, such as ADD, or ADHD.

Chronic and repeated fearful experiences, with little opportunity for seeking comfort and reassurance, may make it hard for a child to learn to trust, and they may internalize models of relationships that leave them vulnerable: vulnerable to feeling themselves unworthy and undeserving of others' attention and care, and that others are unresponsive, inaccessible and not interested in caring for them. For some children, this can lead to risky and sexually promiscuous behaviour as they seek warmth and affection from anyone who might be perceived to give it. Similarly, we have talked to men who watched their fathers beat their mothers, and then promise themselves they would never do that when they grew up, only to break their promise to themselves by beating their own wives. Problems with affect regulation can continue into adulthood. Attachment fears and jealousy, and the tendency to feel shame and perceive humiliation from a partners' behaviour, whether intended or not, with such sensitivity perhaps deriving from their own fathers' attempts to shame and humiliate them as children, can contribute to overwhelming emotional experiences in adult intimate relationships, often expressed as explosive rage, and thus masking fear, loneliness and sadness. Such experiences, repeated over time, continue an intergenerational legacy of the effects of witnessing early childhood violence, and reinforce men's sense of unworthiness and powerlessness, making it more likely they will respond with aggression the next time when aroused and emotionally overwhelmed, in fear of rejection, shame and abandonment.

The effects on children of exposure to violence

The emotional and social effects on children of direct and indirect exposure to family violence are mediated by a number of interacting factors. The effects are never straightforward, and thus every child and their family needs to be understood and helped in their own right. However, it is helpful to be mindful of those factors that can influence the effects on children, as they may be amenable to intervention. The main point here is that families need to be offered help and support as much as the children do.

The characteristics of the violence need to be taken into account, such as the severity, the duration and the frequency of attacks. Clearly, the more severe the attack and the greater the fear and feelings of helplessness, the more the child will suffer. These effects can be moderated by the child's ability to be proactive and get help for the victim of violence. Similarly, if the children themselves do not have a significant emotional connection to the attacker, for example, a transient boyfriend of their mother, the emotional trauma might not be as overwhelming as if this was their father who was violent, a person to whom they have an emotional connection and with whom they might wish to identify. It is in these more extreme cases that some children cope by creating an illusion of safety and control through identifying with the aggressor.

The age and developmental phase of the child is significant in relation to how the child understands the violence, takes a moral position, and the extent to which they can access psychological and social resources to help them cope, for example, by having friends in whom they can confide or being involved in safety planning with family and professionals. Proximity to the violence is important in whether the child tries to intervene on behalf of the victim, or watches helplessly during an attack. The response to violence exposure by extended family, school and neighbours, can influence how children fare, for example in terms of the support offered, the concern for safety, and in not colluding with secrecy. If significant people in the child's social support network hold the perpetrator responsible for their behaviour, there is clarity for the child in support of their own moral development.

Descriptions of children in our work

When working on behalf of children and their families, either in our therapeutic practice or in writing reports for court, it is helpful to include descriptions of the following factors and influences when children witness interpersonal violence. We need to draw out how the abuse of power and constant use of intimidation and humiliation in the home affects children's sense of themselves, as agents, as loveable people, and so on; and similarly how their trust has been betrayed in a context where adults have not taken responsibility for safety. In all of this, children have no choice or chance to consent. It takes time for children to learn to make social comparisons and some developmental contexts preclude possibilities for reflexive contemplation. In more extreme circumstances, where the adult means the child harm, it is developmentally difficult for children to reflect on the fact that people they turn to for support and protection want to hurt them (Fonagy & Target, 1995). Children might cope by developing major distraction behaviours, such that they never sit still long enough to contemplate this terrible fact. This in turn can affect educational engagement and the capacity to stay focused and on task. We need to help other professionals understand the wide range of violent, intimidatory and bullying activities involved in abuse, and the chronic, continuous and likely intergenerational patterning of violent behaviour. It is important that we illuminate the child's perception of threat, either spoken or unspoken, and their ways and means of coping. Finally we need to pay attention to the development of resilience, and the ideas and beliefs that children hold about safety and protection.

We need to ask what helps children develop a sense of entitlement to their own safety and a commitment to the safety of others. If they are regularly pushed and shoved about, how do they develop a sense of entitlement to personal space? Under what circumstances can a child's empathic capacity be supported and developed? How has fear been created in the household and what has been the power of secrets in the child's life? If the child was involved in the adult's abusive behaviours, how did that occur? I worked with a family where the older boys were encouraged to laugh at their mother and to kick her when she cried during an assault by her male partner. This left them guilty, confused and very afraid. In another example, I worked with a man who beat his wife, and who beat her harder when she cried during his attack. He could not understand why he beat her and why he beat her harder when she cried. We learned that as a boy he hid behind the settee and watched helplessly while his father, whom he loved, tortured his mother, whom he also loved. His own wife's tears during his assaults triggered trauma memories that overwhelmed him, and it seemed he beat her harder in an attempt to shut her up.

How can we help?

In our work as practitioners, trainers and supervisors we need to prioritize safety at all times, both seeking signs for safety in family living, and in creating safe spaces for people to talk, think and reflect, before inviting them to take emotional risks (Vetere & Cooper, 2005). We draw on the community-based work of Osofsky (1999) in this regard. We can support family-friendly practice that knows how to talk to young children and their parents/carers, and that supports traumatized parents in listening to their children. The first task is to help the child feel safe and to understand their worries for their family members' safety. Such anxiety might be expressed indirectly or be masked. Helping re-establish routines as part of the safety work enables children to settle. We need to work to support and strengthen relationships by, for example, providing post-adoption consultation to new adoptive parents who care for a traumatized child. When carers better understand the impact of trauma on a child's attachment strategies, and ways of coping, they are themselves better able to avoid unhelpful conflictual interaction with the child and coercive battles for control. If the child's strategies were developed in order to defend themselves and survive, it is unrealistic to expect children to accept the love of alternative carers, such as foster carers, without the passage of time in which they can learn to feel safe with the help of reassurance, empathy, acceptance and predictable responding. When foster carers can recognize when to help the child soothe and calm and contribute to a low stress environment by not taking the child's responses so personally, as a rejection of their care, for example, traumatized children are helped to accept new rules for relating and to adapt their internal working models of relationships.

Our contribution to raising awareness of the effects of domestic violence on children in schools, communities and within professional networks should not be underestimated. Children benefit from reassurance and encouragement, and knowing that they are safe and do not have to worry about the safety of family members. In trauma work, the opportunity to explore, express and process their feelings and experiences is crucial. Some young people value meeting other children in similar circumstances and in realizing they are not the only ones (van der Kolk, 2005; Osofsky, 1999). Children need opportunities to disclose their experiences of abuse to someone they know and trust, and similarly children need help to talk with their non-violent parent about what has happened. These are sensitive and necessary tasks in the resolution of trauma experiences, that help children and their families settle down again. The capacity for empathic responding is developed when we support family members in being able to listen to each other, in spite of their own distress – the ability to really listen, when you too are upset demands attunement, the capacity to suppress your own needs temporarily, and the recognition that the other is similar to you. In our therapeutic work with children and families we seek signs of resilience and we look for positive role models in people's past and present lives – people who have shown kindness and taken an interest, can be a source of encouragement, hope and inspiration. In this regard our work challenges unhelpful gender stereotyping, such as machismo values, and challenges the idea that violence is trivial, normal or to be tolerated. Such work demands that the practitioner take up a clear moral position in relation to violent behaviour among intimates, and is prepared to acknowledge their own moral dilemmas around the acceptability of violent behaviour in a multilayered social context where we are all subject to the same social discourses. Children and their families may need help in dealing with behaviour problems and help to catch up and perhaps reintegrate with school. Contact with the perpetrator of violence may be possible, if the children want this, but with safety in mind at all times, as women and children are more at risk at times of separation and divorce, and with custody disputes. In my experience it is not uncommon for some children in the family to want contact, and some not. This has ramifications for sibling relationships and relationships with the non-violent parent, as complex loyalties intersect with needs for affection and gender identification.

How can we help small children?

Osofsky proposes the following advice for carers of small children. Children need reassurance that they will be protected and kept safe. Listening to children's worries and giving simple answers to their questions is necessary, and this in turn helps children to play and talk about their feelings. Play is a very useful context to help children name and identify their feelings. Follow the child's lead as best you can, so if the child wants to be picked up, do so. Try to maintain the child's usual routines with eating, sleeping, play time, and so on, and as best as possible try to be flexible in how the child's needs can be accommodated. If the child responds to trauma with 'clingy' behaviour, be patient, as it will take the child a while to learn they can trust that their new context is safe.

How can we help school aged children?

Osofsky offers the following advice for carers of school-aged children, six–11 years. Similarly be patient, and give additional attention as needed. As best you can, clarify any distortions and misconceptions the child may have. Give straightforward and realistic answers to their questions. Offer support and reassurance around post-trauma symptoms they may be experiencing, help them maintain their routines, and set gentle and firm limits for acting-out behaviour. All of this occurs within a context of age appropriate activities and non-demanding tasks at home.

How can we help young people?

Osofsky suggests that carers of adolescents should, again, give factual answers to questions. Encourage discussion of events or trauma experiences with peers and adults, and help link behaviours to feelings.

Involve the adolescent in safety planning, and encourage involvement in community activities. Set clear limits and address any reckless or aggressive behaviour. As above, all of this occurs within a context of resumed community activities, physical activities and school events.

How can we help families?

Family members may need help to resume and maintain their normal routines, and to develop a sense of self-efficacy. Help them appraise their safety in their environment, their economic concerns, issues of relocation, and address their losses. Support their faith and spirituality, and help them best use available community supports. Family members may need more traditional mental health supports and specific help with their trauma responses and aids to recovery. Signpost interventions to help with longer term problems with mental health, behaviour, school attendance, and overall adjustment.

Involvement in safety planning

Teachers and other community workers may find themselves in a position to develop a personal safety plan with a child, when that child is still living with risk and uncertainty in their family households. When developing a safety plan, adapt it to the age and understanding of the child, and consider the following: identifying a safe place to go if there is further violence; identifying a person they can go to if necessary; making sure the child knows how to contact the emergency services; and making sure the child knows it is neither safe, nor their responsibility, to intervene to try to protect their mothers or other family members during an assault (Hester et al., 2000).

In assessing the child's safety, some of the following questions may be helpful:

- How often do violent incidents occur?
- What was the most recent incidence of violence/abuse? What are the details of this incident?
- Were any weapons used or threatened to be used? Have any weapons been used to harm or to threaten, in the past?
- Was their mother/other family member locked in a room or prevented from leaving the house? Has this happened before?
- Was there any substance misuse involved?
- Have the police ever come to the house? What happened?

- What does the child do when there is violence? Does the child try to intervene? What happens?
- Where were the child's siblings during the violence? (Hester et al., 2000).

Similarly, in circumstances where you might suspect a child is living in a household where violence takes place, but you cannot be certain, Hester et al. (2000) suggest some of the following questions:

- What happens when your mother/father (stepmother/stepfather) disagree?
- What does your mother/father do when she/he gets angry?
- Did you ever see or hear your father hurting your mother? What did you do?
- Did you ever see or hear your mother hurting your father? What did you do?
- Who do you talk to about things that make you unhappy?
- What kinds of things make you scared or angry?
- Do you worry about your mother and father?

An example of hidden trauma

We use the following example to illustrate how trauma effects can remain hidden if professional staff does not ask about a child's experience of witnessing violence, such that the child's behaviour can be misattributed to other causes. We were asked by the family court to assess whether it was safe for two girls (aged 11 and 13 years) to have contact with their father, following his release from prison for attempting to kill their mother during a sexual attack. The father, Mr Blue (a pseudonym) had applied to the court for permission to meet with his daughters on a regular basis and, as they had initially refused to see him, we were asked to do a safety assessment for the court. In addition, we were asked to assess the mother's competence in caring for the two girls, as Social Services had concerns about the quality of her care.

In conducting the assessment, we met the father on his own, the mother on her own, the two girls alone and together, and the mother with the two daughters. When talking to the father about safety, we asked him about repeated violence, the contexts of previous violence, boundaries around anger management, his capacity for empathy, and capacity to reflect on experience. In addition, we looked for evidence of the ability to work cooperatively with professionals, to see professionals as potentially helpful, to take responsibility for behaviour that harmed others by acknowledging there is a problem and by recognizing that harmful behaviour has deleterious consequences in relationships. In talking with Mr Blue, he maintained that he was not responsible for the attack on his wife, blamed his wife for provoking the attack and stated that her description of the attack was exaggerated. He maintained that serving his prison sentence exonerated him from any moral responsibility for the attack and its effects. Mr Blue did not accept any responsibility for the consequences of his behaviour for the well-being of his daughters, nor for the impact on his relationship with either of them. He claimed not to understand why his daughters did not want to see him.

The two girls, Anna and Maria, were living with their mother. We met them for an introduction first with their mother, then separately and then together. The girls had been in the house during the attack and overheard it. The younger girl, Anna, had gone into her older sister's bedroom at the start of the attack. We were surprised to discover that no one had asked the girls about what they might have overheard, and what effect it had on them. Similarly, when their father was released from prison, no one had informed the family, and the first they knew of his release was when Anna saw him seated in his car, parked at the end of the road, as she came out of school. It was at this time, that Anna began to exhibit 'bizarre' behaviour, according to social services, that was blamed on the mother's poor care, such as tying rope around her bedroom window to seal it. In addition, someone had been stealing from the mother's purse, and cutting up the mother's clothing. Everyone assumed Anna had done this. Anna also made accusations of harsh and bizarre punishments against school staff, her mother, and her mother's best friend, such as being kicked by school staff and put in a cupboard, and being tied to a tree in her front garden by her mother. The accusations could not be substantiated, but social services were sufficiently concerned that they placed Anna into foster care for three months, with six different families, finally returning her to her mother's care as it was obvious she would not settle into foster care.

In talking to Anna, she spoke of her fears that her father would repeat the attack. She told us of her strange sensations in her stomach, and she told us of hearing a gruff voice, telling her to cut up the clothing. When we asked, we found that Anna had witnessed much physical violence from her father to her mother over the past few years, had been exposed to sexual material in bondage magazines left in the bathroom by her father, and had witnessed sexual advances from her father to her mother. Maria had similarly been exposed to these experiences, but one crucial difference for the two girls was that during the attack, when Anna went into Maria's room for shelter and comfort, she had wanted to rescue their mother. Maria had held her and put her hand over Anna's mouth to stop her from crying out. Maria admitted to us that she was the one who had been stealing from her mother's purse.

Mrs Blue told us she had been physically and sexually assaulted by her husband over the years, that no one had asked her about this as a possibility, neither about the effects on her of the recent attack, nor how this impacted on her authority as a mother. We asked Mrs Blue about potential trauma effects and found that she suffered from sleeping difficulties and nightmares, anxiety attacks, and low mood. Mrs Blue talked about how she struggled to look after her two girls in this context, without help, understanding or support.

The two girls were adamant with us they did not wish to see their father now, or in the future. They maintained this position in conversation with other professionals. We recommended that it was not safe to start contact now, because of the wishes of the two girls, and because Mr Blue would not take responsibility for the effects of his behaviour on his two girls and on his relationship with them. Had he been able to take some responsibility, we could perhaps have helped him, as a father, to think about how he could begin to heal his relationship with his daughters in such a way that it might pave the way for contact in the future. Mr Blue refused any offer of help.

We recommended that the mother and her two daughters be referred to a child and family psychology service, so they could be helped individually and as a family. We recommended trauma therapy for all of them, and support for Mrs Blue in redeveloping her sense of confidence and competence as a mother.

When we contacted the family six months later, as part of a follow up assessment, they were making progress in talking to each other more openly about their hopes and fears, and working in cooperation with child and family services. The psychologists had been able to improve relationships with social services and the family, and had recommended a change of social worker.

Conclusion

As practitioners, when we meet children and families and conduct (psychological) assessments, we need to pay attention to the broader familial and social context, and to consider whether interpersonal violence in the home might be the cause of psychological distress and difficulties. Thus a picture of unexplained somatic 'symptoms', a sudden lack of interest in activities, and/or a high activity level (constantly moving about and being highly distractible), emotional numbing and a lack of ability to self-soothe, repetitive play that appears to re-enact trauma themes, and post-traumatic problems, such as difficulty in sleeping, nightmares, behaviour changes and the development of new fears that are developmentally unexpected, might indicate that the child lives with fear, and with parents/carers who are afraid and/or frightening. Recognizing these 'problems' for what they are – entirely sensible and understandable responses to terror – and not 'symptoms' of 'mental disorder' is crucial: assisting children to survive and resolve the developmental dilemmas inherent in living with fear is of the greatest concern as the manner of its resolution may well dictate the child's well-being, and that of future generations.

10
Discourses of Acceptance and Resistance: Speaking Out about Psychiatry

Ewen Speed

This chapter considers the different ways that are available to people to talk about mental health, mental illness and psychiatry in general. This may seem like a strange point of departure, and it certainly begs the question – 'but surely people are able to talk about these issues in whichever way they choose'? I would argue that this is not the case. It is more accurate to say that a range of possible discourses exist that enable people to construct and imbue meaning into talk about mental health, mental illness, psychiatry or anything else for that matter. For example, phrases such as 'nutter', 'schizo', or 'psycho' draw from negative, stigma laden discourses of mental health, whereas 'service user' or 'consumer' are attempts to move towards more neutral characterizations of people who are using mental health services.

These different ways of talking can be regarded as indicative of wider social and political struggles in regard to the positioning of people with psychiatric diagnoses, and mental health itself, within Western countries. Some of these linguistic systems of classification can be seen to work in tandem with medical discourses. The starkest example of this would be the classification of 'patient'. The ways of talking and sense making that this patient type offers to people are passive and work to endorse the medical model, whereby biological aetiology is privileged over any social or environmental aetiology. In this context, the patient can be regarded as drawing from discourses of acceptance, in that it does not offer the 'patient' a chance to resist or problematize the medical interpretation of their distress. Counter to this would be the 'survivor' type, which is explicitly political, can draw heavily on the disability rights movement, and actively resists and rejects the medicalization and psychiatrization of emotional distress. I shall talk more about these specific examples later in the chapter.

A third type (and there are many others which I don't consider here) or position from which it is possible to talk about psychiatry is that of the healthcare consumer. The healthcare consumer is a relatively recent addition to the discursive canon (Speed, 2007) but it is one that dominates, particularly in a health policy context. We can see consumerism and consumption across a range of healthcare policies and practices, the most visible being the so-called choice agenda that has proliferated in the UK NHS (Forster & Gabe, 2008). Here I explore some of the implications and contradictions of invoking patient, consumer and survivor discourses in talking about psychiatry.

A word on discourse

This chapter takes a broadly Foucauldian approach to conceptions of discourse (Howarth, 2000). The approach I adopt means that the analytical focus is on talk and text as a system of representation. What people say, or how things are written in policy documents, can be regarded as systems of representation that reflect wider systems of meaning within society. For the analyst, the interest lies not in *what* somebody said, but in *how* they said it. Furthermore, interest lies in how, what they said might be understood – in terms of wider issues they may be representing (intentionally and unintentionally) in their talk. Howarth (2000) describes how discourse analysts are 'concerned with how, under what conditions and for what reasons, discourses are constructed, contested and change' (131). So the change from the 'mental patient', to the 'health service user', to the 'consumer', can be read as examples of how discourses are constructed, contested and change. This chapter explores some of these processes and the implications for the person with the psychiatric diagnosis.

Additionally, these types, for example patient and survivor, can be usefully characterized as 'subject positions' (Foucault, 1982; Hall, 1997; Howarth, 2000). This concept describes the 'author function', whereby emphasis is placed on the 'discursive conditions that make knowledge possible' (Howarth, 2000: 80). Under this conception of subject positions, individual actors are regarded as 'little more than ways of speaking within a particular discourse' (Howarth, 2000: 80). In this regard, the psychiatric patient becomes a subject position: the patient position becomes a way of speaking within a psychiatric discourse. This patient–subject position can be defined by how it differs from the survivor subject position or consumer subject position (these are all different ways of speaking, within a psychiatric discourse). The discourse analyst is not primarily interested in the individual person who may say they are 'psychotic'. The discourse analyst is much more interested in the possibilities opened up (and shut down) for this person by talking about themselves in this way. For example, to describe oneself as 'psychotic' is different (and offers different possibilities) to describing oneself as a 'voice hearer'. The argument here is that 'it is discourse, not the subjects who speak it, which produces knowledge' (Hall, 1997: 55). What this means is that it is the discourses of and around mental health that set the conditions of possibility for talking about mental health. It is not the person who uses the discourse, but it is rather the discourses that are available to be used that set the parameters of talk about psychiatry. So the medical discourse versus the legal discourse versus the empowerment discourse all construct or present different subject positions from which it is possible to speak about self and others. To quote from Hall (1997: 131) again: 'subjects may produce particular texts, but they are operating within the limits of the *episteme*, the *discursive formation*, the *regime of truth*, of a particular period and culture'. Thus discourses of power and knowledge are intrinsically bound up with what comes to be the *episteme*, the *discursive formation*, the *regime of truth*. The dominance of the discipline of biomedicine is indicative of the power that this particular epistemological position has in current healthcare settings.

The implications of this dominance are wide ranging. If the service user draws from a medical discourse to explain their situation (invoking a chemical imbalance in the brain, for example, as the reason they have auditory hallucinations) then it becomes very difficult for that same person to blame, for example, poverty or abuse they experienced as a child. These explanations draw from different subject positions (one which favours nature over another which favours nurture) that advance different discursive formations or regimes of truth for understanding mental illness or social inequality. One invokes science while the other points to social and environmental factors.[1] An important point here is that subjects do not choose which discourse to use based on a thorough appraisal of all possible discourses (through a rational choice process identifying which discourse gives them maximum benefit). The discourses it is possible to use are delimited by social and political processes and forces (such that a reductionist medical explanation is the current hegemonic discourse for understanding mental illness). I expand on the implications of this perspective in the following section.

Patient/consumer/survivor

The medical 'patient' enjoyed a prolonged period as the dominant subject position with regard to medicine. The patient, after the rise of the clinical gaze (Foucault, 1973), came to be seen as a repository of pathology (Armstrong, 1983). The rise of medicine and the development of pathology (whereby corpses were dissected and physical abnormalities located within the physical body) meant that the body came to be regarded as the site and locus of health (both good and bad). Illness, with the rise of the anatomical atlas, came to be associated not with the environment that the person might live in, but rather came to be seen as a property of their individual body. Once illness is located within the individual body, that body is furthermore required to be passive, such that medicine can act upon it, to correct the abnormality. In order to explore these issues I want to present a number of excerpts from interviews with mental health service users in the Republic of Ireland that demonstrate the different subject positions. To be clear, I am stating that there is a patient subject position in regard to psychiatry and that this subject position is characterized by an acceptance of biomedical reductionism.

The patient discourse

Excerpt 1: Example of patient discourse

Harry: which I found out later the psychoanalysts thought that paranoia was a symptom of hatred for others.

Int: mhhm.

Harry: whereas the psychoanalysts think that paranoia not psychoanalysts … but the psychiatrists think that it's because of a chemical imbalance.

Int: mhhm and what would you make of the chemical imbalance argument.

Harry: I definitely agree with it I agree with the chemical imbalance imbalance very much you know.

Within this extract, Harry deploys the subject position of the patient ('I agree with the chemical imbalance'). Harry talks about psychoanalysis and psychiatry and compares their different assessment of his symptoms. One reading available to the analyst is that the psychoanalytic perspective (as it is represented) involves Harry taking on some of the responsibility for the diagnosis, he, himself, is recruited into the paranoia, such that it is characterized by something he does (*he* hates other people, he is subsumed into the explanatory model). Conversely, the psychiatric perspective does not involve him in the explanation, the cause (again, as it is represented) is purely and simply attributable to his biology being out of balance, therefore he cannot be held to account for his situation, it is beyond his control and therefore it is not his responsibility. It thus becomes the responsibility of psychiatric science (probably through medication) to correct the imbalance.

By implication, through accepting the biological model, it becomes difficult (though not impossible) for Harry to invoke other causative agents in his sense of the situation. The subject position of patient obviates Harry from voicing any disquiet he may have about, for example, side effects from his medication. If he wants to absolve himself of responsibility, he needs to accept a baseline medical aetiology, which prioritizes the medical over the environmental, and is characterized by a passive patient subject position.

I will not immediately turn to the consumer discourse. It is the most complex of the three and as such, it makes more sense to consider the survivor discourse first. The survivor discourse can be regarded as antithetical to the patient discourse. I would characterize the survivor discourse (in the UK at least) as a development of the antipsychiatry movement (as championed by Laing and Cooper). In a discursive context, it can be considered a reaction against the passivity of the patient, characterized by way of an active engagement with the politics of madness (see Crossley, 1999). Whereas the patient subject position may be characterized by the patient being the repository of pathology, the survivor subject position is a repository of resistance. Where the patient may be subjugated before – and by – medicine, the survivor actively resists any medical categorization. Excerpt 2 offers an example of this.

The survivor discourse

Excerpt 2: Example of survivor discourse

> *Int*: ehhm so how do you who would you see yourself in relation to psychiatry now then

> *John*: well for a start, for a start I no longer class myself as Schizophrenic ... I class myself just as John Knox ... I just classify myself as myself again ... ehh diagnosis means nothing I don't even really I I don't actually believe that it exists I don't even actually believe there's any scientific proof to ... to back up a diagnosis of

schizophrenia it's a process of the medical model ... and the medical model is a reductionist model so therefore ehh its its ehh I suppose its an easy way of them tagging a label into somebody.

Within John's talk there are a number of instances, a number of ways of talking, where he openly and actively resists a medical categorization of his situation. He describes how he resists classifying himself through a medical lens. He describes how he sees himself as someone outside of and away from medicine and medical understandings or discourses. He sets out an alternate subject position to that of the patient, one which offers him different ways of talking and thinking about emotional distress, mental health, psychiatry, science or medicine. He problematizes the scientific basis of psychiatry, arguing it signifies a process of the medical model (that it is constructed) rather than signifying an underlying scientific principle. He goes on to reduce this further, stating it is nothing more than a labelling process. This for John might be regarded as the key point, this to him is the primary function of 'scientific' psychiatry.

This labelling critique implicitly draws upon the work of people like Szasz (1961) and Scheff (1984), suggesting that it is nothing more than a process for dealing with social deviance. This is the key point. The 'survivor' subject position, as set out here, locates emotional distress and the ways in which it is dealt with, in a *social* context, *not a medical* context. By invoking the social in the subject position, it becomes possible to counter (or resist) the totalizing hegemonic force of the biomedical model. If the medical 'causes' are problematized, it becomes necessary to look around for other ways of making sense of the situation. John asserts that a diagnosis of schizophrenia is a label, deployed as a means of dealing with those who deviate from social norms.

This brings us to consideration of the consumer. As I already mentioned, the consumer subject position is the most complicated of the three outlined in this chapter. The patient and the survivor can almost be used to define each other. The consumer subject position offers a different approach to the others. It is perhaps most easily demonstrated through reference to an excerpt.

The consumer discourse

Excerpt 3: Example of consumer discourse

Int: I mean well what's your attitude to medication then if I mean you've kind of medicated yourself it would seem right the way through all of this ehhm would you still see medication as something that was necessary

Ian: well you have to understand me what I'm saying is that's all we have ... in the society we are living in

Int: but for you yourself ehhm if you had the choice between taking medication and not taking medication what would your choice be

Ian: but we don't have the choice because there's nothing else there at at the moment if you know what I mean

This example demonstrates an uncomfortable tension between the patient and survivor poles. The consumer position is neither accepting nor resistive. It accepts the medical frame while almost simultaneously rejecting it. The subject position is one that is neither passive nor active but one that vacillates between these positions. It is a discomfiting position. Ian talks about a lack of choice, but this assertion of a lack of choice is incongruent with his choice to self-medicate which preceded the talk presented here. It is indicative of a position that accepts the medical model as the best system of making sense of his situation, but is also rejected by him because of the passive patient role it requires. He is not prepared to act as the passive supplicant, but rather seeks to adopt and adapt the patient position into one that affords him, or appears to afford him, a higher degree of control.

I have written about these positions previously (see Speed, 2002, 2006, 2007). The different positions (patient, consumer and survivor) can be characterized in relation to how they typify issues of emotional distress.

Subject position exemplars

Patient: 'I am a schizophrenic'

Consumer: 'I am a person with schizophrenia'

Survivor: 'I am a person who hears voices'

Taking these in turn, it is apparent that the patient position has no room for anything other than diagnosis. It is the diagnosis that solely defines the person, such that any sense of subjectivity is subsumed under the diagnosis. The survivor offers a place for subjectivity, as well as a rejection of medical understanding, such that the medical frame can be resisted. The consumer sits somewhere in the middle, still drawing from a medical frame, but it is a position which attempts to impute some subjective positioning into the agent, such that they are not defined solely through the diagnosis.

These subject positions do not just relate to the ways they are utilized by Ian, Harry and John: they are ways of speaking within discourses of psychiatry. I want to explore these positions in terms of the bigger social projects that they might be aligned with in terms of their discursive genealogy. I have already indicated the medical genealogy of the patient, and the anti-psychiatry genealogy of the survivor. Without the 'patient' we would not have medicine. The survivor position is part of the antipsychiatry social project. What social project(s) can the consumer be aligned to? It is in addressing this question that the remainder of this chapter will be concerned.

The genealogy of the consumer

As a point of departure for this exploration, I want to assert that the consumer subject position can be partly read as the historical outcome of the incongruence between the patient and survivor positions. Chronologically, the consumer discourse follows the development of the survivor discourse, but discursively, the picture is different. The consumer represents the midpoint between the other two, in what is a contested field of identity politics (see Barnes, Mercer and Shakespeare, 2000, for a discussion of identity politics in relation to issues of disability).

It is within this identity politics field that it becomes possible to delineate the social project that the consumer is aligned with (or perhaps more accurately, the social project that the consumer has come to be aligned with, see Mold, 2010). In order to do this, it is necessary to locate identity politics within a wider social context, and this context is best typified as civil society.

Civil society as a social project

Powell (2007) outlines the ways in which civil society has been utilized in contemporary political contexts. It is in many ways a contested terrain, desired by the left and the right, and this means discourses abound in trying to label and define it. Generically, Wedel (1995) states that civil society can be seen to exist when individuals are free to form organizations that function independently and can mediate between citizens and the state. Characterizing these at a broad general level, non-governmental organizations (NGO's) such as the Hearing Voices Network, MIND or Rethink would be good examples of civil society organizations within a mental health context. Broadly defined, civil society can be characterized as those voluntary civic and social organizations that exist outside of market and statutory considerations. Civil society organizations are neither statutory bodies nor are they market-based. Having said that, the boundary between civil society organizations and the state is becoming harder to delineate as more and more voluntary organizations move into tendering for, and providing, statutory services.

Kaldor (2003) in addressing these changing relations identifies five different versions of civil society. These are as follows:

  i. societas civilis
 ii. bürgerliche gesellschaft
iii. activist
 iv. neoliberal
  v. postmodern

Kaldor characterizes *societas civilis* as a version of civil society based on the rule of law and civility. *Bürgerliche gesellschaft* encompasses all organized life between the state and the family. A conception of an *activist* civil society is described through reference to the activities of social movement organizations (SMOs) and civic activists (e.g. the 'disability' movement, or organizations such as the 'hearing voices network'). Social Movement Organizations as discussed in this chapter correspond to the definition offered by Tilly (2004). Social movements in this context can be defined as a series of contentious performances, displays and campaigns by which ordinary people make collective claims on others. Social movements are a major vehicle for ordinary people's participation in public politics. They represent concerted action for political change outside of the realm of formal representational politics (Tilly, 2004:3). Kaldor aligns a *neoliberal* conception of civil society with third sector organizations and charities. The last, *postmodern*, Kaldor associates with nationalist and fundamentalist movements. In terms of the current chapter, the two most pertinent types of civil society are the activist and neoliberal types.

Taking Kaldor's (2003) characterizations as a framework, the survivor subject position sits most comfortably within the activist conception. The survivor is openly political and is concerned with effecting change in the ways services are set up and provided (and indeed with changing the very ontological and epistemological foundations of psychiatric practice). The survivor position can be characterized by close association with social-movement organizations and civic activists, which often have political agendas.

The consumer subject position sits most comfortably within the neoliberal formation of civil society. Within the activist framework, the boundaries between the state, the market and the activist are stark. This distinction becomes much more blurred in the context of the healthcare consumer. That is to say the healthcare consumer marks a fundamental reconceptualization of the relationship between the state and service users.

Consumers, markets and the state

Just as the patient is a constitutive component of the medical project, I argue here that the consumer is a constitutive component of the neoliberal project of healthcare reform. Newman and Clarke (2009) assert that the 'neo-liberal project' has all-too-readily been accepted by critics and supporters as just that, a unique and distinct project. This uncritical acceptance does much to essentialize a programme of neoliberal reform, affording it more power and kudos than it might command were these assumptions interrogated. For example, Klein (2001) demonstrates very clearly how the neoliberal reforms of the Thatcher government in the late 1980's and early 1990's actually required an increased level of state involvement to guarantee the 'success' of the reform programme. This increase in the role of the state would appear anathema to the neoliberal doctrine of marketization necessarily leading to reduced levels of state intervention. As such it is a crude and useful demonstration of this problem of uncritical acceptance in regard to neoliberalism. I accept and agree with Newman and Clarke in this regard, but I still find it difficult to reject the purchase that discourses of neoliberalism have in terms of making sense of processes of change and reform within public service provision within the last 20 years. The rhetoric of neoliberalism as a means of implementing economic processes of exchange, founded on a sovereign, choosing consumer persists and is an incredibly useful mode of explanation. I am not interested (in the current context) in pursuing the veracity or accuracy of neoliberalism as a category of reform (see Harvey, 2005). I am interested here in the ways in which rhetoric or neoliberal talk of healthcare reform opens up or creates opportunities for new subject positions available to providers, the state and the service users.

Without the neoliberal healthcare consumer we would not have had the 'choice agenda' in the UK NHS, nor would we have had the 'Next Stages Review', 'World Class Commissioning' or any of the other recent policy initiatives in UK healthcare. Without the neoliberal healthcare consumer the reform of public services, and healthcare in particular, would have taken a different course. The neoliberal consumer makes it possible to invoke responsibility in any talk of rights (contrast this with the activist model, where responsibility is more readily ascribed to the state: the position being that it is the state's responsibility to ensure that people's rights are legally protected). The discourse of the neoliberal consumer pushes responsibility, or responsibilization, onto the individual consumer. It is an atomizing and individualizing process, which functions to make health status something for which individual consumers are expected to take responsibility. Health becomes a commodity determined by lifestyle choices (how much we smoke, drink, eat or exercise), rather than anything more enduring or extra-individual, such as an issue of social equity and social justice.

The healthcare consumer also makes it possible to employ, and adapt, market mechanisms to engender competition between healthcare purchasers and providers. It is in this context that I argue the real utility of the consumer becomes most apparent. The insertion of a consumer role, into what was previously a two-way relation between the state (as purchaser) and medical practitioners (as provider), is intended to tip the scales in the favour of the state. In this context, the role of the consumer (with a heightened sense of entitlement compared to the patient) can be seen as a command and control mechanism deployed by government to hammer professional providers (for more on this process see Speed, 2010). By invoking the consumer, the healthcare exchange becomes contractual. The market needs to provide or qualify the goods that are available for the consumer to 'choose' from.

It is in this context that we see the proffering of various choices in healthcare: choose and book, choice of provider, choice of time, choice of procedure, are all offered, but they are all tightly delimited and tied back to stipulated sets of tariffs. The healthcare consumer, in this context, is used by the state to exercise a command function over health professionals. This process is intended, I argue, to enable a tighter control on expenditure by these professionals. It should be noted that the responsibility/rights/entitlements of the consumers do not feature centrally within these policy considerations. All markets need consumers but the market, in this instance, is not primarily about meeting consumer needs, it is more concerned with meeting the state's needs in limiting healthcare expenditure.

It is not my intention, however, to imply all consumers are 'dupes'. I want to argue that while a lot of bottom-up activists have used, and indeed continue to use, the consumer frame and discourse to effect real social change, the key beneficiaries have been, and indeed continue to be, the state, on two counts. Firstly, the consumer frame invokes biology rather than social or environmental factors as the main causes of ill health, allowing for the persistence of deprivation and social inequality. If poor quality housing is held up to be cause of poor mental health, then the housing situation needs to be addressed. If the person who lives in the poor quality house is regarded as having a chemical imbalance in their brain, then it is the imbalance that needs to be tackled, not their living conditions. This is an ultimately cheaper solution to the problem. Secondly, by raising the sense of entitlement among these consumers, by emphasizing their consumer rights, it becomes possible to undermine the autonomy of professionals by instituting national guidelines 'intended' to provide a higher standard of care for consumers.

Consumerism, rather than resisting the clinical gaze, is a subject position that works *with* medicine. There is much less potential within the consumer position for resistance. In the context of the state, consumerism arises from the programmes of neoliberal health and welfare reform, through the first Griffiths report in 1983, the *Working for Patients* inspired reforms of 1989 onwards (DoH, 1989), the new Labour programmes in 1997 and 2002 and so forth. These reforms are marked by attempts to systematically retrench the state provision of statutory healthcare. In effect the state reduces the amount of state supported direct involvement in healthcare provision (through provision of free-at-the-point-of-delivery health services). Instead, this free-at-the-point-of-delivery service is offered by a growing band of providers, many of them non-statutory, who compete against each other for healthcare tenders.

This is in effect a quasi-privatization of healthcare provision. To admit to such a programme would be political suicide, as such, these reforms need to be presented in such a way as to accentuate the positive. Hence the role of the healthcare consumer, whereby the choices available are presented as increased, not decreased, by these reforms. The rhetoric is one where competition can only be seen to impact positively upon the provision of services. Responsibility for what services are available is laid at the feet of the market, rather than the state. The myth that the market will provide is bolstered, while the policy makers argue their concern is with making sure the consumers get the best deal possible.

In this respect there is a troubling contradiction. In this model, policy makers' claims of consumer centredness are intrinsically tied into processes of reduced service provision (on the part of the state provider). A brief note of clarification is required here. Provision works in this example at different levels. There is the micro-level conception of provision, whereby it is the local healthcare community that provides health services to a local purchaser. This is not the level I am interested in at this point. I am interested more in the macro level, in the idea of the state as provider, where the state is regarded as the political distributor of resources to cover the costs of free-at-the-point-of-delivery healthcare. The state provider utilizes programmes of increased consumer choice as a means of limiting what services are available. For example, increased choice can be negative because it often means fewer services are offered, but that they are offered by more providers (in effect, a confounding or paradoxical increase in choice opportunities).

In this context, increased choice can be seen as negative, not positive. A decrease in available services has to be regarded as a negative for the consumer. As consumers, we might have more choice of whom we can go to for care, but less choice of the types of care we can receive. We can buy more orange juice in more retail outlets but we have less choice in terms of the types of juice (organic, smooth, not from concentrate etc.) we might be able to buy.

To bring the discussion back to the civil society context, these processes also mark an expansion of regulatory governance frameworks into more and more areas of civil society. The rise of consumerism and choice means that the state is now looking for alternative providers of statutory services. As soon as the voluntary organizations or the NGOs decide to tender for these services, then they must become accountable to means and processes of regulation. I am not arguing here that this should not be the case. All organizations that offer services for vulnerable children and adults alike must be subject to regulation. My concern is that this process marks the steady creep of the state into areas of civil society where previously it could not go. By extension this process marks a fundamental realignment of the boundaries between civil society and the state. Couple this to the consumer rhetoric and market logics that underpin these programmes of reform and they can also be read as marking a fundamental realignment of the boundaries between markets, the state and civil society. These reforms can be read as processes that are fundamentally reconfiguring civil society. They may mark a very real shrinkage in the opportunities available to activists to resist hegemonic discourses of medicine.

These regulatory and expansionist processes most readily align themselves with Kaldor's (2003) conception of a neoliberal civil society. Within this model, charities, voluntary organizations, and NGO's come to be identified not as civil society organizations, but as third sector organizations. In this context, 'third sector organisation' has to be read as an apolitical alternative to more 'activist framed' civil society descriptions, such as social movement organization, which has a much more political frame of reference (and is aligned with Kaldor's (2003) *activist* model). Again, I offer a word of qualification. It is not my intention to criticize third sector organizations. I am exploring the possibilities that these different ways of talking about civil society have for the constituent actors.

The third sector as a neoliberal social project

This chapter was originally drafted before the UK coalition government took office in May 2010. It draws on source material from the Cabinet Office website which has since been archived by the new government. However, it is not anticipated that the change in government will lead result in too much of a change in the increased regulation of civil society or third sector organizations. Indeed the Conservative party is defined by a historical preference for voluntary organizations to fulfil more of a role in the provision of help and support, so there is no need to think that this process will be reversed under a new government, indeed it may increase. However, at the current time of writing it is not possible to explore this in any detail, simply because there has not been sufficient activity in this sector by the coalition government. To return to the historical source material, in setting out the role of the Office of the Third Sector, the Labour administration Cabinet Office (CO) stated in February 2010:

We deliver on our aims by:

- Driving cross-government action to improve partnership working and ensuring better terms of engagement between government and the third sector.
- Investment in programmes to support the sector's development and promotion.
- Ensuring a good policy and regulatory environment for the sector.

- Developing a strong evidence base and analysis to better inform the work of the Government and third sector.
  http://webarchive.nationalarchives.gov.uk/+/http://www.cabinetoffice.
  gov.uk/third_sector/about_us.aspx (Accessed May 2010).

The emphasis in this Cabinet Office text is on principles of mutualism and partnership working. However, this emphasis is problematic. It cannot be an equal partnership, as there are clear and distinct power differentials between the voluntary organizations and the state. Take the state requirement for regulation as part of the statutory service arrangement; this marks a clear distinction between provider and client. The lesser partner is beholden to the stronger partner. This corresponds with Kaldor's (2003) neoliberal typification of civil society. If the government is the dominant partner, and if this realignment marks an encroachment of regulatory processes into what was the civil sphere, then these changes function to limit the capacity for civil society organizations to resist these regulatory processes. An emphasis on partnership, and adapting civil society organizations to become statutory provider organizations undoes much of the radical potential of civil society groups.

Under Kaldor's (2003) and Wedel's (1995) definitions there is the clear need for a degree of autonomy or independence between the state and the voluntary sector. The example I pursue here illustrates a clear case of policy being designed around regulation and partnership (with unequal partners). It is difficult to find the gap between what civil society organizations might offer and what the government might offer. It is in this context that these changes are best regarded as examples of the neoliberal conception of civil society. They have to be read, in this context, as attempts to extend the arm of government into previously inaccessible areas of civil society. The dominant mode of organization in the government sector is a market competition model, as such, the rise of the need for strong regulation of non-statutory providers (offering previously denied statutory provision) must be read as marking an expansion of the principles of neoliberalism into the third sector (nee civil society). The introduction of the capability to provide statutory services is inherently bound to the processes aimed at promoting competition (choice) between providers, such that the local purchasers can secure the best price. The inclusion of civil society organizations in this context is simply an opportunity to introduce more providers in order to increase competition.

As an example of this process, I want to compare the statement, as taken from the Cabinet Office archive, with material taken from the website of the Hearing Voices Network (HVN), which I would characterize within the current context as an activist social movement organization. In a excerpt taken from their website, they set out their aims and objectives. These are as follows:

- To raise awareness of voice hearing, visions, tactile sensations and other sensory experiences
- To give men, women and children who have these experiences an opportunity to talk freely about this together
- To support anyone with these experiences seeking to understand, learn and grow from them in their own way

We try to achieve our aims through these objectives:

- Promoting, developing and supporting self-help groups
- Organizing and delivering training sessions for health workers and the general public

http://www.hearing-voices.org/ (accessed May 2010).

Compare and contrast the capacity for social action across the two contexts (the Cabinet Office versus the Hearing Voices Network). The HVN website demonstrates actions intended to reconfigure medical aetiology, offering an alternative framework within which to understand it. There are implicit efforts to ignore the stigmatizing effects of these issues (mention is made of ability to talk freely). There is also a stated desire to engage in processes of education for service providers and the wider general public (which can be read as evidence of a civil society project aimed at promoting a degree of social change).

Conclusions

In much the same way that patient, consumer and survivor offer different subject positions from which people can talk about how they experience their mental illness, mental health or emotional distress, so too, these typifications of neoliberal third sector versus an activist civil society represent different contexts in which it is possible to talk about the activities of these different groups. The neoliberal third sector model involves a degree of partnership working between voluntary organizations, and statutory services providers. It offers an opportunity for service user organizations to become centrally involved in the provision of 'mainstream' services, but at what cost? The rise of regulatory frameworks brings into question the role that voluntary sector organizations ought to pursue within contemporary society. This neoliberal model represents (at best) a choice of working within the confines of what already exists, accepting it and working to change/adapt it from within.

The second, activist model evokes a much more resistive frame of action, and offers a range of possibilities to the activists. The key difference is the way in which this different (perhaps less compromised) model conceives of, or offers a different conception of civil society. Within this less compromised model, the capacity for resistance, to both professional norms and to regulatory, governmental norms remains more intact. There is still a clear distinction between state, the market, and the voluntary sector.

In terms of the current health and social care landscape, there is clearly a need for both of these typifications, as they clearly perform different functions. The key issues to consider, and this brings me back to my opening title about voices of acceptance and voices of resistance, is the capacity that each of these typifications have for resistance, and what they might offer the service user in terms of their deployment.

Acceptance and resistance

Resistance can take many forms, from coordinated and collective political engagement with government through to self-management of prescribed medication (to name but two). Just as the patient might be best characterized as an essential constitutive component of the medical project, then the consumer might be best characterized as an essential and constitutive component of the neoliberal project of health reform. The survivor might be best characterized as a precondition of a more activist-oriented civil society project. In this sense, the consumer can be seen to work with rather than against the medical model. This means it has less capacity than the survivor model to resist the medicalization of emotional distress. In turn it has less capacity for resistance in terms of the stigmatizing processes of psychiatric labelling (Speed, 2002). If the service user wants to actively resist the psychiatrization of their experiences, then they need to be fully aware of the implications and limitations of drawing on different ways (different subject positions) of talking about mental health, mental illness or emotional distress. The use of terms such as emotional distress, voice hearer and suchlike mark explicit attempts to resist medical dominance and the psychiatrization of experience. The argument presented here calls for very careful thought to be given to the use of the term consumer.

Whatever positives this label carries with it for service users, and the service user movement, it also carries a lot of negatives. My analysis has highlighted how the consumer subject position is part of a range of social projects, with wide ranging implications for how we think about the role of professions, the state and service provision within contemporary Western society. Many of these processes do not locate the service user at the centre and may be more limiting in terms of the potential they offer to service users wishing to effect a degree of political change. Indeed many of these consumerist contexts may be regarded as creating conditions that are detrimental to the service user.

11
The Personal *is* The Political

Jacqui Dillon

The recognition that the personal cannot, ever, be other than politically developed from the women's liberation movement of the 1960s (Hanish, 1970). It was an acknowledgment that the experiences, feelings and possibilities of our personal lives are not just a private matter of personal preferences and choices but are limited, moulded, defined and delimited by the broader political and social context. They feel personal, and their details are personal, but their broad texture and character, and especially the limits within which these evolve, are largely systemic. This concept is very relevant to contemporary mental health but, before looking at the political, I need to start with the personal. I would like to go back, right to the very beginning.

The personal

I grew up in Hackney in East London. Aged 5, I was already hearing voices. My early years were filled with terrifying and disturbing experiences that literally shattered me into pieces. My family was involved with a group of organized paedophiles, who abused children and took part in extreme sadomasochistic practices. The consequence of such extreme and sustained abuse is devastating. Its effects are all-consuming, encompassing every aspect of experience. To be betrayed and exploited by those who are meant to protect you leaves a profound sense of terror, isolation and shame.

I inhabited a dual world. In one, I was a normal schoolgirl with normal parents, a gifted child who went to school, won writing and drawing competitions, played with her friends, and liked wearing clips and ribbons in her hair. In the other world, I was a dirty little bitch, evil and unlovable, treated with cruelty and contempt by anyone who could get their hands on her. Everything I got I deserved. I was repeatedly threatened that if I ever told anyone about what was happening I would be put into prison because I had done terrible things, or everyone would think I was mad and they would lock me in an asylum forever and throw away the key; no one would ever believe me. Or my abusers would find me, they would always find me, they would hunt me down and they would kill me, my children, anyone or anything that I ever loved. However much I yearned for it, I had no place of safety, no saviour to rescue me, so I did what many children have to do. I survived the best way I could.

Survival techniques

The survival strategies that I unconsciously developed as a child created an illusion of control, an illusion that I had some agency over what happened to me. Despite my abject helplessness, I utilized all the resources available to me at the time – my mind, my body, my spirit – and I fought for my life.

Mind

I have heard voices for as long as I can remember: voices in my head that talked to me, talked about me to each other, who comforted me, protected me and made me feel less alone. One of my early voices and one that has been there for me throughout my whole life is that of 'the great mother'. She is a very powerful maternal figure, who is beautiful and kind, a beneficent figure who has always been there comforting and soothing me. She has been central in enabling me to survive with my humanity intact and she has also enabled me to be a loving and compassionate mother to my own daughters.

Body

My body became the locus of my horror and my need; I began self-harming at an early age. Cutting myself, banging my head against the wall and tearing at myself were ways I discovered of safely releasing my anguish. I drew no attention to myself. I hurt no one else. No one could touch me. My relationship with food became a mysterious journey of adventure in which I discovered many special powers. By controlling what I ate, overeating, forcing myself to vomit and starving myself I was the creator of many marvellous tricks, sleights of hand that made me feel more in control in a world that was filled with terrible, inescapable, arbitrary cruelty. For once, I had control of my body. I could do what I liked to it. I was mistress of my own universe.

Spirit

My creativity extended beyond my body into the world. I loved writing stories and poems, drawing and painting, reading as many books as I could get my little hands on. Books allowed me access to other worlds, worlds where there were endless possibilities. In my imagination the characters and stories in books captivated and entranced me, became meaningful to me to the extent that I internalized them so that I felt less alone and the world still held some magic and wonder. My sense of justice burnt inside of me the whole time. I knew that what my abusers were doing to me was wrong. I began to dream of a world where one day I would be safe and free and loved.

The abuse ended when I was 15 but its consequences lived on inside me for many years. Despite this, I managed to develop a successful career in the media. I was still hearing voices and self-harming throughout this time but I hid it well. I was adept at inhabiting different worlds and used to keeping secrets locked inside me. My abusers' threats echoed in my mind long after the worst had already happened, reminding me of what they would do if I ever spoke about what had happened, so I remained silent.

Breaking the silence

The birth of my first daughter, when I was 25, freed me to break the silence. My daughter was planned and much longed-for and the day of her birth is one of the happiest in my life. But it unlocked terrifying secrets from the past. My voices multiplied and intensified, saying things that disturbed and frightened me. I began seeing horrifying images of abuse, torture and death. I could feel it in my body. Marks and bruises appeared on my skin like stigmata. My self-harming spiralled out of control and I became convinced that someone would try and hurt my daughter and me. I became intensely paranoid; terrified to leave the house in case someone tried to abduct us and kill us.

I felt like I was going mad. Again I inhabited a dual world. I was a devoted mother, with a close and intimate bond with my baby, breast-feeding her on demand, yet I feared contaminating her with all of the poison that swirled around inside of me. I started to feel as if there was no escape from the horrors of the past. I began to think that the only way out was to end my life. In desperation, I called my GP who urgently referred me to a psychiatrist. I was admitted to the local psychiatric hospital that afternoon. It felt like the end of the world.

Psychiatry

Despite the threats that my abusers had made, I did start to try and talk about what they had done to me. I was desperate to get home to my little girl and I knew that what had happened to me as a child was the cause of my distress. The first psychiatrist I tried to tell assessed me on admission. We sat in a small consultation room which had two chairs, a table and a filing cabinet. I began to try and talk about what had happened to me as a child. I was shaking at the time and after a few sentences the psychiatrist stopped me and said: 'Jacqui, we have had other people in here reporting similar kinds of incidents but when we have invited their families in, and we all sit and talk about it together, they begin to see that this is a part of their illness. These things didn't really happen – this is part of your illness.' I remember looking at him in astonishment. I had a surge of adrenalin and the image of lifting up the filing cabinet behind him and dropping it squarely on his head filled my mind. Fortunately I didn't do that, as I would probably still be in a secure unit now. Instead I told him that I didn't feel well. I left the room, walked down the corridor to the bathroom, locked myself in the toilet and banged my head against the wall.

I knew then that I had to get out, so I did what a lot of people do to get out of psychiatric hospitals. I lied. I started to say that I was feeling much better, the rest had helped and that I was ready to go home. And because I was a good actress, and because I was articulate and because I was white, they let me go.

The clear message I received from the mental health system was that I was ill. *Everything* that I said and did was caused by my illness. The abuse never happened – even thinking it did was part of my illness. If the abuse did happen (one psychiatrist did believe me) then, in his words, 'Pandora's box should never have been opened'. Because I was ill I needed to take medication. The fact that I didn't want to take medication was because I was ill. If I wanted to get better, I must accept my diagnosis and take medication and then they would give me benefits and a bus pass. I wouldn't ever recover. I would always have this illness. I wouldn't be able to work. I didn't know what was best for me. I lacked insight. As mental health professionals, they all knew what was best for me, because they were the experts.

As far as I am concerned, I am not sick. What my abusers did to me was sick. I have had a perfectly natural, human response to devastating experiences. Living with the knowledge of what was done to me, and the way in which psychiatry has added insult to injury by blaming me, is enough to drive anyone mad. My first psychiatric admission in 1993 was my last. I knew then, and I still know now, that to be in such a desperate state in such an unsafe environment was potentially lethal. Ironically, the place that was meant to provide sanctuary for me became the place that nearly drove me over the edge.

Finding a new way to make sense of the personal

I was very fortunate to have other people in my life who didn't deny what had happened to me. They believed that some adults do terrible things to children. They believed that I was more than the bad things that had happened to me. They were willing to listen to me, and my voices, and to support me in making sense of what my voices were trying to communicate to me.

I worked closely with a counsellor and later with a therapist, who believed in me and had faith in my ability to recover. With their support and that of my partner and closest friends, I started on a long winding, road, back to myself. It has been an internal process of truth and reconciliation, of listening, bearing witness and of facing horrors.

A starting point was creating a new sense of myself, which honoured my resilience and capacity to heal. I wanted a way of understanding, which enabled me to listen to my voices safely and make sense of my experiences. I read a vast amount of material and became better informed of the many ways to understand human experience. I researched dissociation and began to appreciate the extent to which I had utilized this capacity in my own survival. I also read a lot of attachment theory. I began to comprehend the impact of my early experiences as well as understanding conceptually, what a 'good enough' parent was.

Discovering the work of Judith Lewis Herman (1992) in *Trauma and Recovery* had a profound effect on me. Suddenly, my own experiences were put into a wider context. I was not alone in feeling outraged by the damage done by society, in pathologizing survivors of abuse. The personal became political. I began envisaging a brighter future. I was a woman on a mission. One day, I would show them all.

Recovery

Herman describes the need to establish safety before the work of remembering and mourning the trauma can properly begin. This wasn't a linear or prescriptive process for me but something that emerged and unfolded organically and intuitively over time. Sometimes I felt as if I were walking on a tightrope, in the dark without a safety net but slowly, hesitantly, I began to trust the process and glimpsed something powerful in me that was guiding my healing. As I was determined never to return to the psychiatric system however desperate I felt, I had to actively work at keeping myself safe. I wrote a list of 20 things to do when desperate and kept it by my phone; I learned self-hypnotic techniques that helped me go to a safe, internal place (Dolan, 2000); I used mantras, grounding exercises, meditated, drew and painted images that haunted me. I did everything I could to get the trauma safely out of me and replenish myself with nourishing, restorative experiences.

Having the space and safety to find a language to describe what had happened, in the presence of an empathic witness, was essential. Through therapy I discovered that I wasn't alone in quite the same way that I had always been. I experienced the restorative power of truth telling – to tell and to be believed was an enormous relief, tremendously comforting and liberating. I wasn't crazy. My responses were normal in abnormal circumstances. Despite feeling a mess, I was ok. I made sense. I began to believe that recovery was possible. Others had recovered – if they could do it so could I. I began to ask for and accept support as an act of courage and commitment to life and the future rather than as a sign of weakness. All of this strengthened me sufficiently to begin to truly mourn for what I had lost as a result of abuse and deprivation. I never knew it was possible to cry so many tears. I am summarizing in a few lines a complex, arduous, life changing process that has taken me many years to accomplish, work that continues to this day.

From me to we

The most profound realization dawned gradually, becoming apparent incrementally over time. And then one day I suddenly knew what I had always known. My voices were more than just voices. They were different selves, with different names, ages, experiences, feelings, identities; dissociated selves that had became internal representations of my external world. There were many selves, children and teenagers, who held the memories of the trauma. There were also those who held the memories of the abuse from the perspective of perpetrators, selves created to handle the abuse. There were deniers and blamers, comforters & protectors, including the great mother. I discovered intellect guides, strategists, free from feeling which is always useful in a crisis. The spiritual ones, those with a connection to a higher power, to nature, a healing force, beauty and truth, the one who says – 'love is my religion'! Rather than trying to eradicate these different parts of me I tried to transform my relationship with them. Each was part of the whole of me. I learned that I needed to listen to them and understand them and the context in which they had emerged – and to greet them with compassion and understanding. I began to honour them as they had helped me to survive. We each worked towards supporting and understanding each other, which increased our sense of connectedness and wholeness. Over time, life has become a shared, mutual collaboration. Gradually I felt less ashamed about who I was and began to marvel at how creative I had been in surviving such monstrous abuse. I became excited by what my mind had managed to invent. At times it felt like I had created a work of art.

The survivor mission

Herman (1992: 197) says that 'helplessness and isolation are the core experiences of psychological trauma. Empowerment and reconnection are the core experiences of recovery'. For me, reconnection incorporated a number of different activities but the most significant has been what Herman calls finding a 'survivor mission' (1992: 207). I wanted to become part of a collective voice demanding change in a world that often made no sense to me, a corrupt and crazy world, which frequently exploits the vulnerable and protects the powerful. I saw that there are many complex forces at play and that the mental-health system is part of a larger system of denial operating within our society. With all that I knew I could not just stand by and let that happen. If I was to reconnect with the world then I would do what I could to make it a place I could actually inhabit: 'survivors also understand that those who forget the past are condemned to repeat it. It is for this reason that public truth telling is the common denominator of all social action' (Herman, 1992: 208).

The political

I first became involved with the Hearing Voices Network when I began working for a community mental health project in East London, my first paid job since having my first daughter. I was working with adults deemed to have serious and enduring mental health problems. Many of the people that I worked with had received a diagnosis of schizophrenia, many of them had spent years in and out of psychiatric hospitals and all of them were on large doses of neuroleptic medication. Despite their suffering and their plight these people were without pretentions, warm and real in a way that touched me deeply. I felt a real affinity with them. I saw how my life might have turned out very differently if I hadn't found alternative help for myself, if I hadn't had people in my life who had loved and believed in me. I believed in these people. I contacted the Hearing Voices Network after reading about their work and feeling excited and inspired by their revolutionary approach (e.g. Romme & Escher 1990) which – in stark contrast to traditional approaches – encouraged people to listen to their voices, make sense of their meaning and saw voice hearers, many who had been diagnosed with schizophrenia, as the experts in the experience. 'Mad' people as the experts? This was something I wanted to be a part of.

The Hearing Voices Network

The Hearing Voices Movement was founded more than 20 years ago, following the groundbreaking research of Professor Marius Romme and Dr Sandra Escher who advocated for a radical shift in the way we understand the phenomenon of hearing voices. Rather than taking the approach favored by biological psychiatry, which views voices as a product of brain and cognitive faults, their research has firmly established that voices make sense when looking at the traumatic circumstances in life that provoked them (e.g. Romme & Escher, 1989a, 1990, 1993, 2000). Romme & Escher's research shows that at least 77 per cent of people who hear voices have had some traumatic experience connected with hearing voices. Subsequent research confirms their findings and attests what many of us with first-hand experience of madness have always known – bad things that happen to you can drive you crazy (e.g. Read & Ross, 2003; Read et al., 2005; Read & Gumley, 2008; Johnstone, 2007; Hammersley et al., 2008; Moskowitz & Corstens, 2008).

Since its launch in 1988 the Hearing Voices Network (HVN) has become an influential grass-roots movement that openly critiques the traditional psychiatric relationship of dominant, expert clinician and passive, recipient patient. HVN is a network of people who hear voices, their friends and relatives, carers, support workers, psychologists, psychiatrists and others, who work together, to gain a better understanding of hearing voices, seeing visions, tactile sensations and other sensory experiences and we work to reduce ignorance and anxiety about these issues.

HVN creates safe spaces to share taboo experiences. People are free to share and explore their experiences in detail including the content of what their voices say, without the threat of censorship, loss of liberty or forced medication, a common feature of disclosure in traditional psychiatric settings. As a consequence, Hearing Voices Groups and the 'Hearing Voices Approach' have now become accepted within mainstream mental health services. A recent Healthcare Commission report, *The Pathway to Recovery: A review of NHS acute inpatient mental health services* (2008), commended mental health trusts which provided hearing voices groups as offering 'appropriate and safe interventions' in acute settings.

Living with Voices

Living with Voices is an anthology of 50 stories of voice hearers who have learned to live with their voices through accepting them. It has contributions from voice hearers from all over the world. Several key themes have emerged from the testimonies in the anthology that illustrate how it is possible to live a fulfilling life with the experience of hearing voices.

Living with Voices: Key themes

Voices are a survival strategy. They point at real life problems in the past and the present, they often use metaphorical language that can be translated into real life challenges, they are split off feelings – feelings that are unbearable, they are awful messages about terrifying past experiences. Voices are both an attack on identity and an attempt to protect or preserve identity.

All 50 contributors linked their voices with traumatic life experiences: descriptions of the causes of hearing voices as reported by contributors to were: sexual abuse, 18 (3 with physical abuse); emotional neglect, 11 (3 with sexual abuse); adolescent problems, 6; high stress, 4; being bullied, 2; physical abuse, 2; unclear, 7. Those people who are 'unclear' about what caused them to hear voices, whose experiences do not fit so neatly into a category of trauma, raise the importance of developing our understandings of the huge range of painful and damaging experiences that can be inflicted on children and adults (Johnstone, 2007).

By listening to people's stories and looking at the rapidly emerging evidence in the field, it is clear that the impact of trauma, particularly experiences like child sexual abuse, are frequently at the root cause of 'psychosis' (Janssen et al., 2003; Read & Ross, 2003; Read et al., 2005; Read & Hammersley, 2006; Whitfield et al., 2005; Johnstone, 2007; Hammersley et al., 2008). However, other more mundane and less obvious experiences can also be profoundly affecting like serious attachment difficulties, enmeshment in families, the consequence of intergenerational trauma, the long-term impact of racism and other social inequalities are all significant factors in the development of 'psychosis' (see Bebbington et al., 2004; Bijl et al., 1998; van Os, 2004; Bentall, 2006; Morgan et al., 2006; Campbell & Morrison, 2007). Crucially, voice hearers' experience suggests that *recovery is not about getting rid of voices* but about the person understanding their voices in relation to their life experiences and person changing their relationship with their voices so that the voices become harmless and/or helpful.

Furthermore, recovery is *only* possible outside of the traditional, biological model of psychiatry. To illustrate this I quote from one of the stories in the anthology – this is an extract from Audrey Reid:

> I was first admitted to hospital when I went to see my GP and told them to take me in. I believed that I had an implant in my head. I was having a lot of migraines so I had a lot of pain in my head and it felt like there was something just above my brow which was the root of the pain and I was dopey with the drugs so it made sense to me. I did feel very controlled and like a lot of people were out to get me. Doctors do have a lot of power over you especially if you feel like you are cracking up. Doctors can take all your power away. I had a real go at my GP saying, 'you are part of a conspiracy and take this fucking implant out of my head'. This was a sure way of ending up in hospital!
>
> I was back in after about 3 months. It all seemed so pointless. Nothing changed, nothing got better. It was just a place to go when things got out of control. The 2nd time I was admitted I was so angry. I went in voluntary because otherwise they would have sectioned me. Again I was feeing very angry and fearful, I had been sleeping with knives under the bed. They sent me on an anger management course which just made me fucking furious! Why wasn't I allowed to be angry?
>
> The drugs made me sleep so much and the small times when I was awake I was cracking up and it was a really despairing time. I was 26 years old and I was asking, 'what am I doing with my life?' Going

round in circles and not going anywhere. It was very frightening and I felt such hopelessness. No one in the psychiatric services gave me any hope, in fact, it was the opposite. In one week I had 2 appointments and on the Tuesday they told me that I had manic depression and on the Thursday they told me it was schizophrenia. What do you do with that? They are completely bizarre words that don't mean anything. I can't even spell schizophrenia so what are you supposed to do with these bizarre diagnoses?

Like every single person whose story appears in the anthology, Audrey's recovery began once she had escaped the psychiatric system and was free to start making sense of her own experiences of abuse, madness and survival in a way that made sense to her. She now lives a content and productive life – which includes living with the experience of hearing voices.

Like many of us, Audrey found the Hearing Voices Network after becoming seriously disillusioned with the approaches taken by traditional psychiatric services. Despite the fact that the current mental health system has appropriated the term 'recovery' if we compare the biomedical recovery model with approaches taken by HVN and others, it becomes apparent why real recovery is only possible outside of traditional psychiatry (see Blackman, 2007).

Recovery – The biomedical version

Crisis

Crises are understood as being caused by a biomedical abnormality. Biological and genetic theories abound and millions of pounds have been spent trying to determine the biogenetic causes of mental illness. Even if social factors are implicated in the person's distress, they are still seen as having a genetic predisposition to being vulnerable to stress. This is despite the fact that there is no proof of genetic determination in mental illness. As Bentall has said: 'it would seem that schizophrenia is an illness that consists of no particular symptoms, that has no particular outcome, and that responds to no particular treatment. No wonder research revealed that it has no particular cause' (Bentall, 1990).

Denial

Denial is a literal denial of the experience of hearing voices and what may have caused it in the first place. Patients are instructed to ignore their voices, to use distraction techniques and to act as if the voices are not there because they are not 'real' (see Leudar & Thomas, 2000). Mental health workers have traditionally been trained not to 'collude with' or 'encourage delusions' by allowing patients to talk about their voices or visions. Exploration of what may have triggered the voices originally, or of the actual content of the voices is strongly discouraged: their content is deemed meaningless. Many former patients have described to me their frustrated attempts to talk to nurses on acute psychiatric wards about voices tormenting them only to be met with the response, 'let's play Scrabble'! I have also heard numerous stories of people attempting to disclose histories of abuse which they linked to their own experiences of distress only to be told that it's 'all in the past' and they need to 'move on and start dealing with the fact that they have a serious mental illness'. Patients, particularly female survivors of childhood sexual abuse, who refuse to be silenced and persist in raising experiences of abuse, run the risk of being diagnosed with a 'personality disorder' (see Bourne, this volume). Despite the growing acknowledgement within society of the widespread abuse of children, I have seen a correlative increase in the number of women receiving a diagnosis of borderline personality disorder.

Denial is aided by the suppression of distressing emotions via the widespread use of neuroleptic medication. There have been many critics of the unethical relationship between psychiatry and the pharmaceutical industries who promote the idea that mental disorders are caused by 'chemical imbalances' (e.g. Breggin, 1991; Moncrieff et al., 2005; Moncrieff, 2006, 2007; Breggin & Cohen, 2007; Stastny & Lehmann, 2007). Some critical psychiatrists note that 'the ubiquity of the industry's message pushes psychiatry into a biological straitjacket' (see Moncrieff et al., 2005; Moncrieff, Hirsch & Healy, this volume). There is increasing awareness and growing concern about the damaging side effects of long term use of neuroleptic medication (Jacobs, 1995;Whitaker, 2004; Hall, 2007; Holmes et al., 2008).

What is less widely known among the general public is that for many years psychiatrists have accepted sponsorship and funding for research from pharmaceutical companies with only selective, favourable, results being published. Psychiatrists accept drug company hospitality and gifts, funding for ongoing study, travel to conferences, and so on, leading even a former president of the American Psychiatric Association to state that psychiatry's 'accept[ance of] kickbacks and bribes from pharmaceutical companies [is] leading to the over-use of medication and neglect of other approaches' (see Sharfstein, 2005).

Insight

Within the biomedical context, insight means that the person accepts that they are ill and that the cause of their distress is biomedical in origin. This most usually means that 'help' is in the form of reliance on, and compliance with, long-term use of psychotropic medications and other interventions that professionals deem to be useful for the person's rehabilitation including mandatory, ongoing psychiatric intervention. People will be encouraged to reduce their expectations for the future to take account of their illness. They may be 'too ill' to work or study again, 'too ill' to live in their own homes and may now require residential care, 'too ill' to look after their own children anymore, 'too ill' for therapy which will only make them relapse (see below).

Recovery

Recovery is – in the traditional approach – inextricably tied to the person's acceptance of their experiences as being biological in origin. Hope is proffered via the potency of medications, which are meant to alleviate 'symptoms' and the ability to recognize experiences as signs of a mental illness (see Blackman, 2007).

Relapse

Relapse frequently occurs, as the underlying issues that precipitated the initial crisis have not been addressed. As well as this, the person now has additional problems including hopelessness, loss, stigma, social exclusion and the toxic effects of medications and associated problems of lethargy, weight gain, sexual dysfunction and secondary health problems to content with. Many former patients have described to me the terrifying experience of forced hospitalization and sedation, which have further traumatized them and engendered profound feelings of shame, despair and alienation.

Cost

There is an enormous long-term cost to both society and to individuals within the current system, in which a biomedical model dominates. As a society, we are investing time and money in creating chronic, revolving-door patients through the self-prophesizing medical model, which sees people as helpless victims of a chronic illness. The long- term financial cost of repeat inpatient admissions, visits from assertive outreach and crisis resolution teams, a care coordinator, social worker, medication, healthcare for secondary problems caused by the long term use of neuroleptics, disability-living allowance, housing and council tax benefit and free bus passes cost billions of pounds annually. In 2007 mental healthcare in England cost £22.5 billion pounds with an additional £26.1 billion in lost earnings (see McCrone et al., 2008).

Of course the biggest cost is the appalling personal cost to individuals. People face a lifetime of chronic 'illness', passivity and dependency, condemned to lives dulled by drugs and blighted by stigma, and offered no opportunity to make sense of their experiences. As well as this, research has shown that long-term psychiatric patients are at greater risk of losing their lives to suicide, heart disease, respiratory disease, stroke, hypertension, diabetes, bowel cancer and breast cancer. People with serious mental health problems are not only more likely to contract such diseases but also more likely to get them at a younger age and die of them faster resulting in a life expectancy some ten years less than that of people without such difficulties (see Disability Rights Commission, 2006).

Recovery – the Hearing Voices Network's version

At the Hearing Voices Network we support individuals on a meaningful journey to understand, learn and grow from their experiences, in their own way. HVN creates sanctuary for people – safe spaces where there are real possibilities for healing and growth.

Crisis

Our starting point is that the crises that people experience are real, and that they are happening for reasons directly connected to the person's life and their experiences. We endeavour to support people to make sense of the real things in their lives that may have precipitated their crisis. We show a genuine interest in the range of peoples inner, subjective experiences. When people describe experiences that are deemed 'psychotic' we look for the meaning in their madness. Sometimes people are using metaphorical or symbolic language to convey their realities and sometimes they are talking literally about things that have happened to them. However crazy someone appears, we believe that what they are experiencing is a meaningful attempt to survive maddening experiences and makes sense in the context of their lives.

Acknowledgment

Contrary to traditional approaches, we see voice hearing as significant, decipherable and intimately entwined to a person's life story. Consequently, we encourage and support people to listen to their voices and acknowledge their reality in order to better understand their meaning. We acknowledge that people are having normal reactions to abnormal stress. Instead of asking people – what is wrong with you? We ask people – what has happened to you? On a daily basis we hear stories of abuse – physical, sexual and emotional abuse, the impact of neglect and poverty on people's lives, as well as the impact of racism, sexism and classism. We show respect for the reality of the trauma and suffering that people have experienced, and a keen awareness of how these may limit their expression of feelings, ability to think clearly and so on. A key part of our role is to magnify the voices of people who are not normally listened to, by emphasizing the belief that each person has a deep wisdom and expertise about ways of managing and dealing with problems. We show validation and support for people's resilience, creativity, stamina and emotional strengths, even when they themselves doubt these exist.

Insight

Acknowledgment enables people to develop true insight into their own distress and suffering which leads to an increasing sense of meaning and purpose in their lives. We are interested in people's subjective experiences – including their altered states of consciousness, unusual perceptions, ideas and ways of seeing and experiencing the world. When your own feelings, thoughts, bodily sensations and so on begin to make sense to you, insight is a natural consequence. When you understand your own 'symptoms' as meaningful and essential survival strategies, a more respectful and loving acceptance of yourself begins to emerge.

Recovery & growth

We recognize that recovery is an ongoing process with no fixed end point and that each person's recovery is unique as each and every one of us is unique. Crises may occur again because recovery is an evolving process, an expansive process not a reductive one which seeks to control and maintain people. We have faith in people's inherent right and capabilities to heal, to make mistakes, to learn and to grow. We know that there is much about human experience that we still do not understand and we remain humble and curious and open to new ways of seeing the world. We are not interested in complying with social control or in servicing normality. 'Instead of being a list of symptoms, with side effects on top, we are people who hear voices and see visions, have unusual thoughts, passionate feelings, intense experiences' (see Dillon & May, 2002). We celebrate our differences.

The personal is political

It is a scandal that in the twenty-first century, every week in the UK, intelligent people are expected to accept discredited diagnoses for fear of being labelled as 'lacking in insight' and having treatment forced on them. Every week thousands of people are coerced into taking medication that they don't want and which frequently does more harm than good. Every week, people are incarcerated against their will, sectioned under the mental health act, 'for their own good'. The Human Rights Act is exempt for those who are of 'unsound mind'. Fighting for the rights of people deemed mad, many who have already suffered more than enough, is the last great civil rights movement.

It is time for a paradigm shift in the way that we conceptualize and respond to experiences currently defined as mental illness. As Mary Boyle has said:

> The claim that there exists a biologically based diagnosable disorder called schizophrenia has been the focus of intense and persistent criticism and been shown to be scientifically bankrupt. But the label is also morally problematic. It is imposed on people in the absence of any evidence base and used without their informed consent (informed that is, of the controversies surrounding it). The label also appears to justify drugs as the major intervention as well as a vast and very unsuccessful research programmes searching for biological and genetic causes. But schizophrenia is much more than a label. Behind it lies the medical model – the claim that emotional distress and problem behaviour are pathological symptoms of illness or disorder rather than meaningful responses to serious problems and adversity in people's lives and relationships.

> (Boyle, nd)

The development of DSM 5 and ICD11, due for publication in 2011, provides an opportunity to develop more accurate, specific and acceptable terminology as part of broader efforts to reduce stigmatization and to address the real things in people's lives that make them 'psychotic'. The Campaign to Abolish the Schizophrenia Label (CASL), a broad alliance of psychiatric survivors, service user activists, academics and clinicians, is demanding the abolition of psychiatric diagnosis and a return to ordinary language which is meaningful, morally acceptable and firmly rooted in peoples lived experience (Bullimore et al., 2007). Rather than pathologizing individuals, we have a collective responsibility to people who have been maddened by their experiences to support them to get the help that they need, to make sense of their experiences and to heal their suffering. We must expose the truth and not allow further injustices to be perpetrated; otherwise today's child abuse victims become tomorrow's psychiatric patients. Individualizing and pathologizing people who display normal responses to trauma conveniently focuses the attention on the supposed deficits of victims but also colludes in protecting abusers from being held accountable for their crimes, from families being supported to heal their distress, from society dealing effectively with its ills. We have to take collective responsibility for the endemic trauma in our society – how widespread abuse is, how cruel human beings can be to each other, how insane the world really is. Otherwise we become bystanders – our silence gives consent. We become complicit, colluding in the further oppression of people who have already suffered enough meanwhile providing huge profits for pharmaceutical companies with their voracious appetite for the control of human experience.

Despite the horrendous abuse I experienced as a child and the pain it has caused my loved ones and me, I consider myself one of the lucky ones. I have a lot of love in my life. I have a voice. I have my freedom. In many ways, I am blessed. Although I live in a world that often makes no sense to me, I do what I can to make it a better place. I am proud to be a part of a collective voice demanding a paradigm shift in the way we understand madness and distress. Improving all of our personal experiences means that we must collectively address oppressive political structures. This for me is why the personal is political.

12

'I'm Just, You Know, Joe Bloggs': The Management of Parental Responsibility for First-episode Psychosis

Carlton Coulter and Mark Rapley

The moral and political landscape

Eekelaar uses the term 'moral duties' to refer to the responsibility that parents have to care for their children, and suggests that legislation in this area is usually considered to 'give force to a pre-existing moral obligation' (1993: 51). Over the last two decades a massive volume of legislation and policy has been introduced in the UK 'giving force' to these obligations and placing ever-greater emphasis on the responsibilities of parents for, and towards, their children. The *Children Act* (1989), *Child Support Act* (1991), *Family Law Act* (1996), and *Child Support, Pensions and Social Security Act* (2000) have provided a legislative framework under which parental responsibilities have been specifically identified and enshrined in law. At the same time, these parental responsibilities have been underpinned by the *Supporting Families* green paper (1998) and the aptly titled *Children's Rights and Parents' Responsibilities* white paper (1999) both of which set out the government's policy regarding parenthood.

In parallel with the above, legislation such as the *Crime and Disorder Act* (1998) and additional policy documents such as the *Respect and Responsibility – Taking a Stand Against Anti-Social Behaviours* white paper, and the *Every Child Matters* green paper (both 2003), have introduced the means by which parents can be held legally accountable for the conduct of their children. For example, parenting orders have been introduced as a vehicle by which the state can take action against parents for the antisocial behaviour of their children. Thus, parents of children whose conduct is deemed to be socially unacceptable may now find themselves in weekly counselling and guidance sessions. The justification for such measures was summarized by the former Home Secretary, David

Blunkett: 'parents are accountable for the actions of their children and set the standards they are to live by ... Where families and parents are failing to meet their responsibilities ... we will work with them until they do' (Home Office, 2003: 4).

Both the volume and content of such policy and legislation has led some commentators to conclude that what has taken place over the last 20 years in the UK is a significant transfer of responsibility for moral development from the state and church to parents (Such & Walker, 2005). Yet, through the creation of new powers to hold parents accountable, the state also stands ready to judge parental performance, and to pass sentence when bad parenting is held to be responsible for behaviour that is unacceptable to the rest of society. It is against this moral landscape that the study described in this chapter is situated.

During the 1990s, young people displaying those varieties of socially unacceptable behaviour that attract a diagnosis of what is now known as 'first-episode psychosis' were served by generic mental health services. By the turn of the century it was recognized that people were encountering delays of up to two years between the 'onset' of psychosis and the provision of 'treatment' (DoH, 2000). This delay was considered problematic in the light of research that claimed an association between the 'duration of untreated psychosis' and poorer long-term outcomes (McGorry et al., 1996). In consequence a new area of service provision, Early Intervention in Psychosis (EIP), emerged (NIMHE, 2009). A key feature of national guidance in this area is an emphasis on working with the families of people who use EIP services. This approach is exemplified by the identification of families as a specific 'focus of intervention' for EIP teams, who are encouraged to engage with the client's family at the time of referral, involve the family in ongoing reviews, and provide the family with 'psychoeducation', and 'psychoeducational family intervention' (DoH, 2003: 3). This chapter examines parents' experience of that focus.

Parents and the 'psy' professions

While central government is abundantly clear about parents' moral and legal responsibility 'for the actions of their children', since Freud's abandonment of the 'seduction hypothesis' (Masson, 1984) the 'official' psy view of parents' responsibility for the madness of their children has been inconsistent, one might even say schizoid. Paradoxically, whereas the laity views the actions of parents as being instrumental in the emotional development of their children, some commentators suggest that it is, for the psy professions, now a prohibited topic: 'Few people doubt that our emotional well-being as adults has a lot to do with how we were raised as children. However, the possible role of families in the causation of "schizophrenia" has become a taboo subject.' (Read et al., 2004b: 253). A brief history of the varying conceptions that psy has had of this issue may help in understanding this paradox.

Although Freud's theories of the aetiology of schizophrenia went through a number of changes, which Masson (1984) suggests were motivated by political, social and financial motives rather than scientific ones, a consistent feature was that pressures from *both* the internal and external world lead to intrapsychic conflict (Lemma, 2003).[1] This view was expanded by object–relations theorists such as Klein, Fairbairn and Winnicott who suggested, to varying degrees, that problems such as schizophrenia have their genesis in the interplay between phantasy and the real actions of parents, particularly mothers. However, what unites the psychodynamic theories of schizophrenia is the basic premise that the conflict that gives rise to madness is the result of the failure by *the child* to successfully negotiate a particular stage of psychical development. That is to say, the primary focus is directed *away* from factors in the child's upbringing, which may have a role in the production of distress, onto the putative failure, one might say vulnerability, of the child.

By the late 1940s the notion that mothers play a significant role in the aetiology of schizophrenia began to receive more attention, and the phrase 'schizophrenogenic mother' was coined to denote the impact of maternal rejection on the developing child (Fromm-Reichmann, 1948). However, other contemporaneous research suggested that schizophrenia was not solely caused by *maternal* actions, but rather was the result of a severely disrupted *family* environment: 'the parental home was usually markedly unstable, torn by family schisms and constant emotional turmoil, and frequently patterned according to the whims of grossly eccentric and abnormal personalities' (Lidz & Lidz, 1949: 332). Yet it was not until the flourishing of the antipsychiatry movement that the role of families in 'causing schizophrenia' really began to take centre stage.

In a number of publications throughout the 1960s Laing wrote extensively on the subject of schizophrenia, and particularly the families of those people labelled as schizophrenic (Laing 1960, 1969; Laing & Esterson, 1964). Laing did not view schizophrenia as a mental illness, but rather saw the unwanted (Sarbin, 1990) and socially unacceptable conduct taken to be 'symptomatic' of schizophrenia to be an understandable response to family conflict; and therefore to be 'socially intelligible' (Laing & Esterson, 1964: viii). Thus, in contrast to Lidz and the object relations theorists, where family dysfunction was seen to lead to individual intrapsychic pathology, Laing suggested that whatever 'pathology' there was resided in relationships between family members: what was held by mainstream psychiatry to be schizophrenia was, actually, an existentially meaningful reply to extremely problematic interpersonal dilemmas. As is well known, the reaction of the public, media, and the majority of the psychiatric profession was to accuse Laing of *blaming the family* for causing schizophrenia (Johnstone, 1999).[2]

Perhaps in an effort to modulate the presumed moral condemnation of parents that Laing's existential account of schizophrenia was seen to be handing down, the vulnerability–stress model was proposed, whereby 'stressful' events are held to trigger a pre-existing 'vulnerability'. Whereas in its original conception 'family experiences' could, theoretically, act as either an 'acquired vulnerability', or as an 'environmental stressor' (Zubin & Spring, 1977: 109), over time the model has become synonymous with the notion of an underlying *biogenetic* vulnerability, again *in the child*, being 'triggered' by a precipitating environmental event. It is this version which the psy disciplines have, since the late 1970s, attempted to 'sell to parents' (Read et al., 2004b: 254) as the truth about schizophrenia and, in more recent years, to account for the onset of first-episode psychosis (Spencer et al., 2001).

In concert with the selling of the vulnerability–stress model, has been the promotion of the concept of familial Expressed Emotion (EE) as crucial to, variously, the development of both first-episode psychosis (McNab et al., 2007; Raune et al., 2004) and the maintenance of, or relapse into, schizophrenia (Ivanovic et al., 1994). Originally introduced by Brown et al. (1962), EE is a term used to describe the hostility, criticism, and emotional overinvolvement that relatives of people said to have schizophrenia may show towards the 'patient'. What exactly EE is said to cause, and in which direction causality is said to flow, is a matter of debate: some researchers have concluded EE is associated with relapse (Bebbington & Kuipers, 1994), others that it is not a causal factor for schizophrenia (Kuipers et al., 1992) and yet others that EE does not precede the onset of schizophrenia, but rather is a response to it (King, 2000). That EE is responsible for relapse but not cause, a product but not a precursor is, suggest critics, a rather unlikely specification for the direction of causality, which is perhaps more accurately conceptualized as a covert ideological effort to avoid being seen to blame the family (Johnstone, 1993; Read et al., 2004b).

In contrast, and recapitulating the early Freud, over the last two decades the strong relationship between trauma, childhood sexual and physical abuse, and madness has, to a very limited extent, been 'rediscovered' in the psy literatures (Dillon, this volume; Johnstone, this volume; Read et al., 2004a; Read, Rudegeair et al., 2006; Vetere, this volume). Some researchers have been prepared to name the relationship as more than just an association; for example, Read, van Os et al. (2005: 330) straightforwardly state that 'child abuse is a causal factor for psychosis and "schizophrenia"'. The implication of this, then, for parents of those who receive a diagnosis such as schizophrenia, is that at best they may have failed to protect their children from such abuse or, at worst, they are the perpetrators of the abuse itself. This has been cited as the reason this type of research has taken so long to appear; a (professional) fear that it would be received as a return to the family blaming of the 1960s: 'it cannot be published without levelling accusations at the parents. And that is something that is still prohibited in our society, in fact to an increasing degree' (Miller, 2005: 30).

In contrast to the delicacy surrounding the publication of 'family blaming' research, in recent years, the term 'mental health literacy' has been used to describe the strenuous efforts psy has made to 'educate' the public about what mental disorders 'really' are, how to identify them, and how they should be treated. This campaign explicitly suggests that 'there is a continuum of mental health literacy running from lay *beliefs* to professional *knowledge* ... professionals have *expert knowledge* which is to a large extent based on *scientific evidence* and *expert consensus*, while the public have a range of *beliefs* based on *personal experience, anecdotes* [and] *media reports'* (Jorm, 2000: 398, our emphasis). It is apparent then, that psy is clear: while holding anecdotal 'beliefs', when it comes to 'mental health' the 'illiterate' public do not *know*, do not necessarily know that they do not know, need to know that they do not know, and need to know there are there are those who do.

So what *do* ordinary ('illiterate') members of society know? In 1970 Sarbin and Mancuso concluded that despite their best efforts, the psy professions had failed to persuade the public that mental illness should be viewed in the same way as physical illness. Almost two decades later Wahl (1987) found that members of the public cited environmental factors most frequently as the cause of schizophrenia, and considered parenting to be a causal factor. Rogers and Pilgrim's (1997) lay participants were also found to favour environmental explanations, including family conflict, and more recently Read and Haslam (2004) have suggested that the layperson still favours nonbiological accounts of mental illness. Thus, despite some contrary findings (e.g. Angermeyer et al., 2010), most studies suggest that the 'uninformed' favour psychosocial over biological explanations of madness.

It could, however, be suggested that members of the public are naive due to an absence of familiarity with the lives of people who are diagnosed with 'serious mental illness', and that those who receive a diagnosis such as schizophrenia, and indeed their families, have far greater insight into the true (biological) nature of such 'illness' by virtue of their personal experience. However, existing research does not support this proposition. Holzinger et al. (2003) report that individuals who have themselves been diagnosed with schizophrenia cite psychosocial causes twice as often as biological causes (increasing to three times as often for relatives), with the type of problems cited often being difficulties in early life, including being repeatedly placed in care, not having a relationship with either parent, or being physically, or sexually, abused by a parent. Perhaps unsurprisingly, while Ferriter and Huband (2003: 553) suggest that, in the abstract, parents rate biological theories of causation most frequently, and theories implicating parents least frequently, in conversation parents frequently blamed themselves, and expressed their guilt, despite their apparent endorsement of biological causation.

So, there we have it. The professional prohibition against suggesting parents might be responsible for the madness of their children is the twist in the present paradox: a society obsessed with naming and shaming any and (almost) all forms of 'antisocial' behaviour, a political class entirely comfortable with 'levelling accusations at ... parents', and a professional elite that not only dare not do so but, currently, vociferously denies what appears to be, *pace* Larkin (1974), prevailing cultural commonsense. What then, do parents of 'psychotic' children make of all of this?

What do parents say about first-episode psychosis?

Using the 'hybrid' EM/CA-informed discursive psychological analysis of McHoul & Rapley (2005)[3] we describe the ways in which parents talk about, and make sense of, the conduct and 'illness' of their children. Based on eight extended interviews, our analysis focuses on the ways in which the parents attend to the work of *moral accounting* in talking about their children, and their parenting of them.[4]

I'm just, you know, Joe Bloggs, I'm not, I'm not a professional

Throughout the interviews, all parents explicitly oriented to the interviewer's professional occupation (trainee clinical psychologist) and engaged in a concerted effort to work up their own identities in contrast to this. That is, all interviewee's positioned themselves as 'non-experts', as being unqualified to make 'psychological remarks' (cf. Sacks, 1992). For example, in the first extract Sue works up her identity as an 'average person'.

Extract 1

1728	Carlton:	Do you think you can recover from schizophrenia?
1729	Sue:	(.) I didn't think you could, no.
1730	Carlton:	Okay.
1731	Sue:	Whether you can or not, I don't know. I, as I say, I don't know, but
1732		obviously that's why you're asking me these questions, because I'm,
1733		I'm just, you know, [Joe] Bloggs, I'm not, (.)
1734	Carlton:	[Mmm.]
1735	Sue:	I'm not a professional (.)

Sue makes it clear, three times, (lines 1729 to 1732) that she doesn't know whether recovery from schizophrenia is possible, which she then justifies by explaining that her understanding is based on lay knowledge. She is 'not a professional'; she is just 'Joe Bloggs', 'everyman', rather than an expert. Sue, in common with all parents interviewed, thus makes an explicit contrast between her knowledge and (pre-eminent) ratified professional knowledge, and displays deference to the knowledge of experts in the field of mental health. Notably the interviewees did *not* present themselves as having a *different* knowledge, as being 'experts by experience', but rather (*pace* Jorm, 2000) as not having any worthwhile knowledge of such matters at all.

Orienting to parental responsibility

Despite invariably constructing themselves as lacking the necessary expertise to understand their children's first-episode psychosis, parents routinely demonstrated that they *did* know that the mental health professional to whom they were talking may hold them responsible for its genesis. In a pertinent absence, no parent explicitly said, 'I know you probably think it is my fault' but all, rather, tacitly declined acceptance of any responsibility. That is to say, in dealing with this *unspoken but omnirelevant* accusation, parents used a variety of rhetorical strategies to defuse their potential culpability. The extracts below show some of these strategies.

In extract 2, Sue orients to the possibility that making her daughter, Kate, attend her grandmother's funeral may have been the decisive factor that led to Kate's madness. However, Sue then goes on to undermine this claim, and to suggest that, actually, her decision was not critical.

Extract 2

```
0556  Sue:      Oh yeah. (.) And, and cos I wouldn't let her go to see my mum, (.)
0557            [I, I    ] just didn't think it
0558  Carlton:  [Mmm.]
0559  Sue:      was right, you know, a young girl, (.) with, (.) well it, (.) it, it's, (.) an
0560            adult (.) it's bad enough, but (.) I didn't want to go and see my mum,
0561            (.)      [and   ] I, I just think I'd rather
0562  Carlton:           [Right.]
0563  Sue:      she'd remembered my mum (.) as she was, not, (.) ((cries)) not dead
0564  Carlton:  Mmm.
0565  Sue:      ((sniffs)) (.) ((cries)) But, er, (.) ((sniffs)) anyway, I didn't think much
0566            of it, I just (.) ((sniffs)) said, "No, no.". I thought she'd had a dream.
0567            But then after that, ((sniffs)) after the funeral, she said to me, "I
0568            don't want to go the funeral", (.) and I made her go. ((cries)) I made
0569            her go ((cries)). And I don't know (.) whether that tipped her over
0570            the edge, or (.) I don't know. But, ((sniffs)) (.) erm, after that, (.) erm,
0571            (.) she just seemed to (.) have lots of conversations with herself.
0572  Carlton:  Right.
0573  Sue:      Erm, (.) but it was like (.) not nasty,
0574  Carlton:  Uh      [hmm.]
0575  Sue:              [she   ] was laughing. (.) She was giggling, (.) and, (.) but
0576            then, when I, in hindsight I think perhaps that had been going on
0577            before we realised it. Perhaps that's what these (.) you know this (.)
0578            phoning people or (.)
0579  Carlton:  Okay.
0580  Sue:      because she seemed to, (.) she was, she seemed to be having (.)
0581            conversations with (.) people she knew, (.) but (.) erm, (.) they
0582            weren't there.
```

Sue initially works up a justification for not letting her daughter Kate see her grandmother after she had died (lines 556–63). Then, in line 566, Sue uses direct reported speech to construct her response to a question that Kate was said to have asked, regarding whether it is possible to hear the voice of someone who is dead.

Sue then begins to describe what happened 'after that' and after the funeral' (line 567), but shifts timeframes, and uses further direct reported speech to construct what Kate said prior to the funeral; specifically that she did not 'want to go' (lines 567–8). Holt (1996) suggests that direct reported speech often functions within narrative sequences both to dramatize interactions between people and to make them more vivid, and is commonly used when it is particularly important to provide *evidence* of what a person said on a given occasion. In this instance the device serves to accentuate Kate's wish not to attend the funeral, which is critical in working up the causal implications of Sue's subsequent actions.

Sue's statement that she made her daughter attend her grandmother's funeral is given particular prominence by the fact that it is repeated twice in succession (lines 568 and 569), which helps to emphasize the contrast with Kate's wishes. Then, in lines 569–70, Sue orients to the possibility that her decision to make Kate go to the funeral may have been what 'tipped her over the edge'. Via this idiom, Sue invokes the commonsensical causal explanation that traumatic events can precipitate madness (lines 570–1). This type of pivotal event is, of course, also a feature of a number of *professional* explanations of 'psychopathology', such as vulnerability–stress models of schizophrenia, and cognitive formulations of psychosis. However, rather than claiming a factual causal link, Sue's initial orientation to the possibility serves as a preface to an account directly undermining any such relationship.

In lines 569–71 Sue bookends the idiom that suggests a causal link with markers of uncertainty, stating, 'I don't know' before and after. Beach & Metzger (1997) suggest that insufficient knowledge claims serve to mark uncertainty about the next positioned statement, such that it can be heard as a guess or opinion, rather than as a fact. In this instance, Sue's repeated statement that she does not 'know', works to present her orientation to the causal status of her decision as personal conjecture, and not certainty. Furthermore, Sue can also be seen to mark the consequences of her decision with additional uncertainty by stating not that Kate *had* 'conversations with herself', but that this is what '*seemed*' to happen (line 571).

The way Sue constructs Kate's behaviour also downplays any distress associated with her experiences. Thus, Kate's conversations with herself are described as 'not nasty', and are said to have involved both 'laughing' and 'giggling' (lines 573–75). By describing her daughter in this way, Sue formulates Kate's behaviour in essentially positive terms, minimizing the potentially negative emotional consequences of her decision, and reducing the potential for her actions to be seen as worthy of censure.

Following Sue's favourable construction of Kate's behaviour, she also makes the claim that 'in hindsight' she thinks Kate may have been having such experiences before she and her family were aware of them, on the basis that Kate previously appeared to be having conversations with acquaintances that were not with her at the time (lines 576–82). However, this statement creates a paradox, since what Sue is claiming is that she observed Kate having conversations with people who 'weren't there' (line 582), before she 'realised' (line 577) that Kate was having 'conversations with herself' (line 571). Thus, although hindsight allows Sue to introduce new information to undermine the causal status of her funeral decision, it does so at the expense of her account following a coherent narrative sequence.

The contradiction introduced by hindsight is managed by Sue once again marking her claims with uncertainty, on this occasion by the repeated use of the word 'perhaps' in lines 576 and 577. However, possibly of even more note is the self-repair that occurs in line 580, where Sue corrects her statement that Kate '*was*' having conversations with acquaintances, with the much less definite '*seemed to*'. This repair manages the hindsight paradox by producing Sue's observation of her daughter's behaviour as speculative.

Sue thus orients to the possibility that she may have precipitated her daughter's madness, but then immediately works up a case to undermine this. Of the eight interviews that were conducted, this was the nearest that any parent came, on the face of it, to acknowledging the possibility that they may have played a part in causing their child's first-episode psychosis. Analysis of the narrative structure suggests, however, that Sue's funeral story is not in fact an admission but rather the first part of an 'at first I thought *x*, then I realised *y*' account structure (Jefferson, 2004): that is to say the power of Sue's repudiation of blame is heightened by her prior admission of possible culpability.

Refuting parental responsibility

Like Sue, Derek also orients to the possibility that parents can cause their children to experience mental health problems. However, Derek makes this claim in reference to his son's friend and, from this springboard, works up a far more positive version of the upbringing that he provided for his own child.

Extract 3

0813	Carlton:	You mentioned with, erm, Dexter's friend that his (.) parents
0814		hadn't treated his friend very well, and yo [u]
0815	Derek:	[B]ut I found that
0816		out after, yeah.
0817	Carlton:	you wondered whether that was one of the (.) erm, reasons why he
0818		had, (.) [had]
0819	Derek:	[He,] he was abused as a young (.) boy. He told us. They
0820		didn't tell us what it was, (.) but ( ) and things like that.
0821	Carlton:	Okay.
0822	Derek:	And I suppose that, with him, (.) it was with his step-dad, and his
0823		step-dad hits him and everything, [like,] he's seventeen,
0824		like, you
0825	Carlton:	[Mmm.]
0826	Derek:	know. I think you know, I suppose ( ) ((*mobile phone rings*)), right
0827		and I suppose that is the reason (.) he's gone like that.
0828	Carlton:	Ye [ah.]
0829	Derek:	[You] know because he was abused as a little boy.
0830	Carlton:	Right.
0831	Derek:	(.) Erm,
0832	Carlton:	Whereas Dexter y [ou]
0833	Derek:	[He]'s had the best life and, you know, I
0834		mean, what we give him, he's (.) had everything, like you know and
0835		he's, you could give him.
0836	Carlton:	Mmm.

As soon as the issue of parental conduct, and by implication responsibility, is raised at the beginning of the extract, Derek interrupts the interviewer, stating that he only 'found that out after' (line 816). By claiming to have only known about Dexter's friend's mistreatment 'after', Derek deflects any responsibility accruing from such knowledge: clearly he could not have intervened in any way to stop it. In lines 819–27, Derek goes on to state explicitly that Dexter's friend was 'abused' when he was younger, and then begins to construct a link between this abuse and the mental health problem that he has described earlier in the interview.

As discussed previously in this chapter, child abuse has been associated with the occurrence of madness in the psychological literature. However, rather than stating the link in terms of a definite causal relationship, Derek claims insufficient knowledge by displaying uncertainty with the phrase 'I suppose' on three occasions (lines 822, 826 and 827) to construct a connection as personal supposition rather than as fact. In falling short of making an explicit claim that Dexter's friend's parental abuse caused his mental health problem, Derek skilfully manages the possible implications for himself, as a father of a child diagnosed with first-episode psychosis.

This project is furthered in line 827, with Derek's stress on the word 'he's' in his statement 'that is the reason (.) he's gone like that', emphasizing the specificity of Dexter's friend's situation, and implicitly excluding Dexter from such circumstances. However, in line 832 the interviewer forces the comparison to become explicit by initiating a direct contrast with Derek's own son, which is immediately interrupted by Derek, allowing him to seize control of any comparison that is to be made, and thus demonstrating the magnitude of what is at stake. That is to say, like Sue, Derek orients immediately to the unspoken possibility of personal responsibility for Dexter's madness.

Derek continues to work up the contrast between his son's upbringing, and that of his son's friend, through his statements that Dexter has not just had a good life, but the 'best life' (line 833), and not just that he has provided Dexter with whatever he could, but rather he has given him 'everything' (line 834). In constructing Dexter's upbringing in these extreme terms Derek maximizes the contrast between Dexter's childhood, and that of his friend, which again works to negate the possibility that he is in any way responsible for Dexter's first-episode psychosis. However, what is of crucial importance to note here is that, in the final lines of this extract, Derek manages the issue of responsibility for his son's psychosis by direct recourse to his own moral credentials as a 'good parent'. Thus, rather than relying on claims of insufficient knowledge to undermine parental responsibility for the madness of a child, this strategy utilizes the moral character of the parent to make such responsibility seem incongruent and, thus, implausible.

Being a 'good parent'

A pervasive feature of all the interviews was the assiduous attention parents paid to working up the 'goodness' of their parenting. It would seem that the category 'good parent', and its predicates, have wide common-sense currency within Western culture. Aside from the plethora of legislation and policies mentioned earlier, there is a multitude of commercially available self-help books, many featuring the term 'good parent' in their title, dedicated to specifying in explicit detail how one should go about the business of parenting.[5]

In the following extract Bob works up his membership of the good parent category by describing the activities that he and his wife, Shirley, have undertaken for the benefit of their son, Luke; particularly in respect of Luke's pre-existing physical disability.

Extract 4

1510	Bob:	But yeah, I mean, ((*blows air through lips*)) (.) er, we, we don't treat
1511		Luke any, we don't wrap Luke up; we'll help him, but we don't wrap
1512		him up. I mean, (.) er, er, nobody's mentioned that Luke's got a, (.) a
1513		dodgy side if you like. (.)
1514	Carlton:	Yeah.
1515	Bob:	Erm, (.) she knows the posh name for it, I don't know.
1516	Carlton:	I think Shirley said earlier right-sided weakness.
1517	Shirley:	Hemiplegic.
1518	Bob:	Yeah, [well] done Shirl. Erm, (.) I, huh, Luke
1519	Carlton:	[Mmm.]
1520	Bob:	had a rotten, I mean, (.) a bit of a hard time really. Erm, (.) we used
1521		to do a lot of swimming, (.) erm, (.) and from, and a very early age
1522		we encouraged him to use that side,
1523	Carlton:	Uh hmm.
1524	Bob:	to the stage, that if he didn't u-, lose it, he'd get a little slap. (.) Erm,
1525		when he was older enough to understand we bought him multi-
1526		gyms; we've done this for him, we've done that for him, he's got a
1527		running machine upstairs. ( ) fit bloke, he's got fat since he's been
1528		on this lark, but he has.
1529	Carlton:	Uh hmm.
1530	Bob:	But he's true, if he, he's never smoked, as, I don't think he's ever,
		((*lines 1531 and 1532 omitted as Bob addressed Luke directly and Luke replied*))
1533	Bob:	Erm, (.) ((*tuts*)) (.) we, we have encouraged him, yeah,
1534	Carlton:	Uh hmm.
1535	Bob:	yeah. Erm, (.) obviously we've never encouraged him to drive, ((*very*
1536		*short laugh*))
1537	Carlton:	Su [re.]
1538	Bob:	[for] obvious reasons. But, (.) yeah, I mean er, I like to think
1539		we've treated Luke (.) as, as best as we could possibly treat a child.

At the opening of the extract Bob heads off any possible suspicion that he and Shirley may have overprotected Luke, that they may have demonstrated, in the terms of the EE literature, 'emotional over-involvement', by qualifying the support they have offered: they did not 'wrap him up' (lines 1511 to 1512). Then, in line 1513 Bob states that Luke has a 'dodgy side', which he implies contributed to what he begins to describe as a 'rotten' [childhood?], and then self-corrects by the use of 'I mean', to 'a bit of a hard time' (line 1520). This self-correction serves to downplay the difficulty of Luke's early life experiences, and presents his childhood in a more favourable light, which works to limit the parental responsibility that might otherwise have been expected to accrue, if Bob's description of Luke's childhood had remained 'rotten'.

Bob then continues his account of Luke's upbringing by constructing how he and his wife supported Luke with his hemiparesis. In line 1524, Bob works up an account of the ways in which they 'encouraged' Luke to use his weaker side, which Bob states took the form of a 'little slap', when the family went swimming (line 1524). By describing their actions in this way, Bob minimizes the physical nature of this 'encouragement': it is both 'little' and a 'slap', rather than, for example, a 'sharp smack' or a 'good whack'.

In contrast to their actions when Luke was younger, Bob also provides a list of measures that he and his wife took to help Luke to improve his physical abilities when he was 'older enough to understand' (lines 1525 to 1528). In a widely used rhetorical device, a three-part list, Bob itemizes this family support: he and Shirley have provided multigyms and done 'this' and 'that'. The generalized list completers, and the running machine appended as an afterthought, do not just identify items on their own, but present them as representative exemplars of a much bigger project. In effect, then, Bob suggests that, as Luke's parents, they took every possible course of action that they could to support him with his disability. Bob validates the efficacy of this support by citing as evidence that, despite the fact that 'since he's been on this lark' (his neuroleptic medication) Luke has become fat, he is 'a fit bloke' (lines 1527–30), who has 'never smoked' (line 1536).

In lines 1538–9 Bob concludes his description of how he and Shirley have performed as parents with the assessment that he likes to 'think' that they have treated Luke 'as best' as they could have possibly treated a child. One of the interactional advantages of claiming to 'think' is that it is a class of claim that cannot be directly refuted. However, in addition to its irrefutability, Bob's assessment of his own, and his wife's, parenting abilities serves to summarize the numerous parenting activities that he described earlier in the interview, including protecting, encouraging, and purchasing items for Luke, thus cementing their credentials as 'good' parents.

Discussion and conclusions

Analysis of these interviews permits some tentative observations on the professional project of psy and, in particular, on the reception by parents of the 'psychoeducational' agenda of EIP services which seek to 'engage' them. Parents were observed to deploy two key strategies to defuse the unspoken, omnirelevant, but professionally denied, accusation that their conduct, as parents, was responsible for the first-episode psychosis of their children.

The first strategy, in a neat turning of the 'mental health literacy' tables, was to claim insufficient knowledge. Parents took great pains to stress their ignorance of professional understandings of madness and to defer to the 'expertise' of their interviewer: a ratified psy-professional. By working themselves up as just 'Joe Bloggs', as the cultural dopes that psy considers them to be, as lay people not possessed of expert knowledge, parents rendered incoherent the idea that they could possibly be responsible for outcomes of which they know nothing about the cause.

The second strategy employed by the parents was to use their own moral character to render any accusation of responsibility for the first-episode psychosis of their children as wholly implausible. This was achieved by parents working up their membership of the 'good parent' category via descriptions of the parenting activities they engaged in for the benefit of their children, including itemizing the many ways they supported their children, offered them advice and encouragement, bought them the physical goods they needed, and loved and cared for them. In so doing, parents demonstrated that they had fulfilled their moral duties towards their offspring, absolving themselves from any responsibility that might otherwise have been expected to accrue. Thus, via both strategies, parents clearly demonstrated that, whatever the squeamishness about 'parent blaming' of the psy professions, they understood all too clearly that recent legislation *is* a direct political expression of the commonsense cultural understanding that parents *are* responsible for the moral development, well-being, behaviour ('psychotic' or otherwise), and life outcomes of their offspring. So where does this analysis leave the issue of parental blame that has been the bane of psy for over a century?

In instances of unequivocal and deliberate abuse (see Dillon, this volume), where their conduct self-evidently contravenes commonsense understandings of the 'moral duties' that parents have towards their children, professional blaming of parents appears unproblematic. Yet in circumstances without apparent gross violation, where the moral status of parents' actions is not obvious, and where it is difficult to discern malign intentionality it is clear that, while psy may be incoherent about parental culpability, parents are not. Perhaps theorizing *parental involvement* in the genesis of madness in a way that recognizes that 'being in some way responsible for' an outcome does not, inevitably and necessarily, imply the *intent* to cause it (and hence attract the moral opprobrium that is 'blame'), may offer a way out of the current reliance on either 'a simplistic illness-blaming model that says it's *not at all* their fault, or an equally simplistic family-blaming model that says it's *all* their fault' (Read, Seymour et al., 2004b: 264, italics in the original).

Of further, and final, note is the observation that none of the parents explained first-episode psychosis as a biological phenomenon, despite the fact that this would have immediately exonerated them from the responsibility they consistently oriented to. In contrast, the mobilization of moral credibility as leverage adds yet further weight to the argument that what is held by psy to be medical diagnosis is actually an assessment of, and verdict upon, moral conduct (Sarbin & Mancuso, 1980).[6] Thus, it would seem that it is *still* the case that 'the general public has not been persuaded that illness is an appropriate metaphor for deviant behaviour'. (Sarbin & Mancuso, 1970: 159). Parents are rather, it would appear, only too well aware that, whatever the blandishments of psy, they are (cf. David Blunkett) 'accountable for the actions of their children and set the standards they are to live by'. In so doing they again demonstrate that what passes as 'professional knowledge' of, and 'expert consensus' on, matters pertaining to mental health is, in practice, parasitic upon mundane commonsense.

13
The Myth of the Antidepressant: An Historical Analysis

Joanna Moncrieff

What are 'antidepressants' and where have they come from?

Intense marketing of antidepressants over recent decades has resulted in a dramatic rise in their use, and in the widespread social acceptance of the idea that depression is caused by a 'chemical imbalance' that can be rectified by drugs. In 2002 eleven per cent of women and over 5 per cent of men in the United States were taking antidepressants (Stagnitti, 2005). This situation led Nikolas Rose to conclude that a large proportion of people have come to 'recode their moods and their ills in terms of their brain chemicals' (Rose, 2004: 28). Although there has been some criticism of levels of prescribing of antidepressants, and recent guidelines recommend that their use is restricted to people with more severe conditions (NICE, 2004), the idea that an antidepressant drug can reverse depression has not seriously been challenged. In this chapter I describe evidence that suggests that the very concept of 'an antidepressant', rather than emerging from scientific data, was constructed to fulfil the pre-existing desire of the psychiatric profession, allied with the pharmaceutical industry, to present psychiatric interventions as specific treatments. At the time the concept was invented there was little evidence to support the idea that drugs could exert a specific 'antidepressant' action, and there remains little such evidence to this day.

Certain drugs have been known as 'antidepressants' since the 1950s. Since that time they have been thought to act as specific treatments for depression according to what can be called a 'disease centred' theory of drug action (Moncrieff & Cohen, 2006). This suggests that drugs exert their effects by reversing the particular brain abnormalities that give rise to symptoms, or, in more colloquial terms, by rectifying a biochemical imbalance. This contrasts with an earlier understanding of the action of drugs in psychiatric conditions, which can be called a 'drug centred' theory. This is the idea that psychiatric drugs are psychoactive substances, which induce abnormal or altered states, in just the same way as more familiar psychoactive drugs like alcohol, ecstasy and heroin. The only difference between psychiatric drugs and recreational drugs is that the altered states produced by most psychiatric drugs are usually disliked, whereas those induced by recreational drugs are usually experienced as pleasant. According to this model, psychiatric drugs *can* be helpful, not because they reverse an underlying brain abnormality, but because the psychoactive state they induce may suppress or mask the manifestations of emotional or behavioural problems. Alcohol, for example, was once thought to be useful for people with social phobia, because one of the behavioural effects of alcohol intoxication is disinhibition. Similarly, the drug-induced effects of benazodiazepines like Valium and Librium include feelings of calmness, relaxation and sedation, which can be useful in many psychiatric situations. The point about the drug-centred model is that psychiatric drugs do *not* work by returning the brain to normal, they work, or appear to work, when they do, by putting people into a drug-induced state which is preferable (often to relatives and professionals, if not the person themselves) to whatever state they are in when drug-free.

Views about how psychiatric drugs worked changed during the 1950s. Prior to this drugs were understood as acting in a drug-centred fashion, usually acting as chemical restraints through their sedative properties. However, the new range of psychiatric drugs introduced from the 1950s onwards came to be seen as having disease-specific actions. Although at first drugs like chlorpromazine, first referred to as 'neuroleptics', were believed to act through inducing an abnormal neurological state, akin to Parkinson's disease,[1] they soon came to be seen as treating the underlying basis of psychotic symptoms and even of schizophrenia itself (NIMH Psychopharmacology Service Center Collaborative Study Group, 1964; Whitaker, 2002). In line with this view they became known as 'antipsychotics'. Drugs that became known as 'antidepressants' were also introduced in the late 1950s.

Michel Foucault suggests that modern disease theory started to emerge at the beginning of the nineteenth century when diseases came to be seen as discrete processes that could be located within particular parts of the body (Foucault, 1973). This view contrasted with the older 'humoral' notion of disease as a general state of bodily imbalance. However, historians Edmund Pellegrino and Charles Rosenberg suggest that it was only during the late-nineteenth and early-twentieth centuries that the new outlook was widely accepted. The idea that substances might have specific actions on disease processes was first clearly articulated at the end of the nineteenth century by Paul Erlich the discoverer of tetanus antitoxin and arsenic treatment of syphilis. He described the new drug therapies as 'magic bullets' that could chemically target the infective agent without affecting the rest of the body (Mann, 1999). At first these ideas were greeted by scepticism among medical practitioners and their patients and much medical practice continued along humoral lines. However, over the first decades of the twentieth century confidence in science and scientific medicine grew. There was an acceptance of the disease theory of medicine and therapeutics among professionals and the public even before many effective medical treatments were available. Medicine became strongly associated with specialism and 'cure by specific therapy became the 'only really proper sphere for the physician' (Pellegrino, 1979: 255).

The new ideas brought with them a change in the nature and status of the medical profession and its relation to science. Prior to modern conceptions of disease and treatment, drug taking and prescribing were part of a 'fundamental cultural ritual' based on the shared humoral model of bodily health and disease (Rosenberg, 1977). In this context, patients and doctors had a more equal relationship than today. People took home remedies to produce purging, frequented quacks as well as regular physicians and all treatments were based on the same principles. By contrast, modern ideas about disease and its treatment require a detailed technical understanding of the specific mechanisms of disease that is not available to the layman. Through the exclusive possession of this technical knowledge, the medical profession acquired 'enormous social power' (Rosenberg, 1986: 25). And as we have seen in the opening chapter, the acquisition of such social power has been a key goal of the psychological professions since at least the days of Freud. In return doctors were expected to deliver more potent therapies.

Therefore, from the late-nineteenth century on, the whole of medicine was seeking disease specific treatments, a process that resulted in some very effective drugs being developed starting with antibacterials like sulphonamides and hormones including thyroxin and insulin. Thus, in developing disease-specific models of treatment, psychiatry was following a general trend within medicine, one that offered the hope of more effective therapies and promised to empower medical professionals. Most research on the history of psychiatry has accepted the portrayal of modern psychiatric drugs as specific or disease-centred agents. Hence drugs are often credited with revolutionizing psychiatry by bringing it in line with medical science and breaking the influence of psychoanalysis and social psychiatry (Shorter, 1997).

However, there is little evidence to support the assumption that psychiatric drugs act in a specific, disease-centred manner (Moncrieff & Cohen, 2005, 2006). In the case of antidepressants, recent meta-analyses suggest that their advantage over a placebo is small, and possibly clinically meaningless (Kirsch et al., 2002; Kirsch, this volume; NICE, 2004), and it has never been demonstrated that they have consistently superior effects to other drugs with psychoactive properties. Contrary to popular belief, it has *not* been demonstrated that depression is associated with an abnormality or imbalance of serotonin, or *any other* brain chemical, or that drugs act by reversing such a problem (Moncrieff & Cohen, 2006).

The rest of this chapter describes an historical study, using a range of sources, of how drugs now classed as antidepressants came to be seen as disease-specific treatments for depression. I trace the development of the concept of the antidepressant during the 1950s and 1960s as portrayed in major textbooks of psychiatry, psychiatric and medical journals and more specialist publications on psychopharmacology. I also examine early advertisements for antidepressants and statements produced by professional bodies such as the Royal College of Psychiatrists (in the United Kingdom) and the American Psychiatric Association to determine what extra-scientific forces may have influenced the adoption of a particular view of the nature of unhappiness and the (licit) drugs that could be used to 'treat' it.

Treatment of depression prior to the 1950s

Although melancholia is a longstanding psychiatric diagnosis, there was little coverage of depression in textbooks or journals prior to the 1940s, apart from in the context of manic depression. It was generally felt that there was 'no specific form of therapy' for depression or for mania (Henderson & Gillespie, 1927: 154). However, patient notes demonstrate that sedative drugs were commonly prescribed to people with features that would now be classified as depression, and from the 1930s on amphetamines and other stimulants were also used. In other research Nicolas Rasmussen has shown that stimulants were marketed as antidepressants from the 1940s onwards and helped to define a market for the drug treatment of neurosis with depressive features largely based in primary care (Rasmussen, 2006). Rasmussen's research shows how stimulants were identified with a particular profile of depressive symptoms characterized by anhedonia above all, suggesting the beginnings of the idea of the specificity of action. Pharmaceutical advertisements examined for this study in the *American Journal of Psychiatry* in the 1940s and 1950s confirmed that stimulants were marketed for depressive conditions. However, there was little coverage of stimulants, or any other drugs, in the British textbooks examined or in the academic articles in both the British and American Journals of psychiatry. In fact not a single paper covering stimulants was identified in any of the issues examined in either journal. The only discussion of stimulants was found in *An Introduction to Physical Methods of Treatment in Psychiatry* in which it was suggested that not only were they not a specific treatment, but also that they were not particularly helpful in depression (Sargant & Slater, 1944).

Convulsive therapy was introduced in the 1930s and by the 1940s electro-convulsive therapy (ECT) was in widespread use in psychiatric hospitals. It was initially viewed as a treatment for schizophrenia but gradually came to be seen as having its best effects in depression, particularly in involutional melancholia (Mayer-Gross, Slater & Roth, 1954). Although there is still no agreement about how ECT induces its effects, it was generally regarded as acting to rectify a putative neuropathological basis of depression, according to various speculative theories (Paterson, 1963; Sadler, 1953). For involutional melancholia it was described as a 'specific and adequate means to relieve this common illness' (Moss, Thigpen & Robinson, 1953: 896). With the arrival of ECT depression came to be seen as a treatable condition that made up an important part of psychiatric practice. In 1944 the authors of the leading British psychiatric textbook claimed that 'the immediate outlook in depressions, whether manic depressive or involutional, has been transformed by the introduction of "shock" treatment, first by the cardiazol method and now by electricity' (Henderson & Gillespie, 1944: 261). By the 1950s, when the modern idea of an antidepressant drug first emerged, psychiatrists already believed that depression might respond to a specific physical intervention, namely ECT, and that there was a precedent for the use of drugs alone for milder cases.

From stimulants to 'psychic energisers'

The introduction of chlorpromazine transformed the way drug treatment was regarded. Even before the disease-centred theory of its action crystallized, chlorpromazine was received with great enthusiasm. It was viewed as being superior to previous drug treatments and it inspired extensive research and publicity (Moncrieff, 1999). It immediately stimulated a search for similar compounds and for possible drug treatments for depression (Lehmann & Kline, 1983).

The antituberculous drugs that were used for the treatment of depression were initially regarded as stimulants and were known to produce serious psychiatric side effects similar in nature to those associated with amphetamine. Given that amphetamine was being widely used to treat psychological problems in general and psychiatric practice, the suggestion that other stimulants might be useful could be expected. In a paper published in 1956, George Crane likened the effects of iproniazid to amphetamine and pointed out the frequent occurrence of 'overactivity, insomnia, agitation and paranoid trends' (Crane, 1956: 330). Hans Lehmann referred to it as a 'drug with stimulant properties' (Lehmann, Cahn & deVerteuil, 1958). French researchers Jean Delay and Jean-Francis Buisson described the immediate subjective effects of isoniazid as 'a sensation approaching euphoric dynamism' (Delay & Buisson, 1985: 52) and he noted the occurrence of 'psychomotor subexcitation', insomnia and anxiety (Delay & Buisson, 1958).

However, within a short space of time a change in the conception of the effects of these drugs can be detected. There came to be less emphasis on the nature of the effects the drugs produced, and more stress on their effects on the patient's mental condition. In particular, efforts were made to distinguish them from stimulant drugs. Thus in a paper published in 1957 Crane divided the effects of iproniazid into 'therapeutic effects', which were presented first, and 'toxic effects' including 'psychological side effects', presented later. This is in contrast to the earlier paper in which an overall profile of the drugs' effects was presented. In the second paper the therapeutic response was described as 'marked psychological improvement' with no reference to stimulant effects or hyperactivity. However, in the section on side effects it was briefly mentioned that three of the 20 subjects developed psychotic reactions and a further 15 had 'behavioural disorders' or 'overstimulation' (Crane, 1957).

1957 was also the year that the idea of the 'psychic energiser' was first elucidated by American psychiatrist Nathan Kline and colleagues. The concept of a psychic energizer was designed to differentiate the antituberculous drugs from other stimulants. It was suggested that a 'psychic energiser' was a drug that stimulated the psyche without stimulating the body thus exerting a 'general rather than a specific action' (Loomer, Saunders & Kline, 1957: 130). The authors argued that 'it has heretofore been impossible to increase psychic energy without simultaneously increasing motor, alerting and cerebral activity – without resulting undesirable side effects when a certain level is reached'. But, they continued, 'it is our conviction that the present preparation, iproniazid, acts more selectively than any of the others' (Loomer, Saunders & Kline, 1957: 130). Kline and colleagues attributed the effects of psychic energizers to monoamine oxidase inhibition, which they linked to all stimulant drug activity. However, they did not explain how the difference between general stimulants and psychic ones was mediated.

'Antidepressants'

The other 'antidepressant' drug that emerged around this time was imipramine. Unlike the tuberculostatic drugs, imipramine is not a stimulant. It is chemically similar to chlorpromazine. In volunteer studies, this type of 'tricyclic' antidepressant is found to be strongly sedating, to impair intellectual functioning, to slow reaction times and generally are found to be unpleasant. Therefore, in contrast to stimulant drugs with their activating and euphoric effects, it was difficult to construct a drug centred rationale for the usefulness of imipramine in depression. In other words it was difficult to see that any of the physiological and subjective effects it induced would be particularly useful in someone who was depressed, especially as there were other sedatives available to address insomnia and agitation. Its use could only be rationalized on the basis that it exerted its effects by acting on the pathological basis of a depressive illness.

Imipramine was first used by Swiss psychiatrist Roland Kuhn, who subsequently described how his experience with ECT had produced a 'conviction that it must be possible to find a drug effective in endogenous depressions' (Lehmann & Kline, 1983: 234). Kuhn is said to have tried imipramine first in patients with chronic schizophrenia who were withdrawn from chlorpromazine (Healy, 1997). Many of the patients became agitated and some became euphoric, which was attributed to imipramine, although in retrospect it seems possible that it was due to the sudden withdrawal of chlorpromazine. However, Kuhn took this as evidence that imipramine might be useful in depression. Kuhn's reports of imipramines' effects in patients with depression contained no quantitative data and consisted of personal impressions and opinions (Kuhn, 1957, 1958). Kuhn claimed that imipramine had 'markedly antidepressive properties' (1958: 459) and 'potent antidepressant action' (Kuhn, 1958: 464). He reported that people who had been depressed for years were suddenly cured, usually in two to three days and that patients and their relatives claimed 'they had not been so well for a long time' (Kuhn, 1958: 460). He described how a homosexual man had been transformed back to heterosexuality through treatment and another man had been cured of impotence.

Kuhn admitted that imipramine's mode of action was uncertain, but he was at pains to deny that imipramine had euphoriant effects. Although Kuhn did not explicitly propose a mechanism of action, one can be inferred from his remarks. Kuhn said that if imipramine was discontinued 'the illness breaks out again, usually with undiminished severity' (Kuhn, 1958: 60). He also believed that imipramine could induce mania in susceptible individuals, a belief that has persisted ever since in psychiatric folklore, despite the fact that controlled studies show no evidence that this occurs (Visser & Van der Mast, 2005). Kuhn's report conveys, implicitly, idea that imipramine reverses the biochemical or physical substrate of depression: if the drug is stopped the abnormalities resurface and use of the drug may tip the patient into the opposite state of mania. Kuhn was also the first to claim that imipramine's effects were most pronounced in people with 'endogenous depression', a syndrome he described as consisting of 'general retardation in thinking and action, associated with fatigue, heaviness, feeling of oppression and a melancholic or even despairing mood' (1958: 459). This claim also suggests a disease-specific notion of the effects of imipramine. It implies that the drugs' effects are not universal, but confined to people with a certain sort of neuropathology, manifested in a particular behavioural syndrome.

Dissemination of the concept of an 'antidepressant'

The term 'antidepressant' quickly caught on. Figure 13.1 shows the number of papers published using the term 'antidepressant' somewhere in the text between 1957 and 1965, as retrieved from a search of Medline. By 1959 the term was being used routinely in over 100 papers. Many papers repeated the assertion that imipramine's effects were strongest in endogenous depression. Often there was no reference to Kuhn's paper or to anything else, suggesting that the association between the benefits of imipramine and endogenous type depression was regarded as established beyond doubt (Ayd, Jr, 1961a; Dally & Rohde, 1961). However subsequent reviews have not confirmed this association (Joyce & Paykel, 1989).

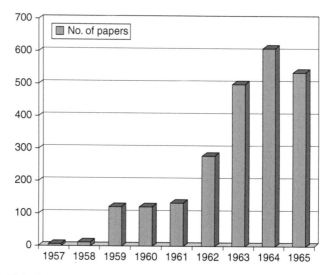

Figure 13.1 Papers using term 'antidepressant' on Medline 1957–65

As early as 1959 the idea that the new drugs for depression were disease-specific treatments was explicitly endorsed by prominent psychiatrists. At a conference on depression held in 1959 Professor Erik Jacobsen, referring to the antituberculous drugs, expressed the belief that '[T]he mono-amine oxidase inhibitors seem, in theory, to be closer to the ideal psychotropic drugs, with strong and clear-cut effects on pathological states and almost no effect on normals' (Jacobsen, 1964: 210). Jacobsen suggested that the effects of these drugs were clearly distinguishable from effects of stimulant drugs. At the same conference Pierre Deniker, a French psychiatrist who was involved in the first studies of chlorpromazine, and his colleague declared that '[T]he action of imipramine, and to a lesser extent iproniazid, is not merely sedative and symptomatic, like that of the neuroleptics, but is curative' (Deniker & Lemperiere, 1964: 230).

However some researchers questioned the view that antidepressants were disease-specific. Authors of an early study of imipramine noted that 'similar results may have been obtained with other drugs' (Lehmann, Cahn & de Verteuil, 1958: 161). Authors of a trial comparing 'Drinamyl', a widely used preparation containing barbiturates and amphetamine, with imipramine, which found no difference between the two treatments concluded 'that imipramine has no specific antidepressive action' (Hare, McCance & McCormick, 1964: 819). Referring to tricyclic antidepressants such as imipramine, they also suggested that 'in so far as antidepressive drugs are effective in the treatment of depressive illness, this is in virtue of a sedative action' (Hare et al., 1964: 819) and recommended that they should be compared with other 'purely sedative' drugs (Hare et al., 1964: 820). Authors of another study comparing imipramine and the neuroleptic thioridazine concluded that they could not confirm 'the specificity of action ordinarily attributed to antipsychotic and antidepressant drugs' (Overall, Hollister, Meyer, Kimbell, Jr & Shelton, 1964: 608).

However, these were already exceptional views by the 1960s. The overwhelming majority of research and other 'official' information such as textbooks and formularies implicitly accepted the notion of a specific drug for depression. As early as 1960 textbooks referred to iproniazid and imipramine as 'antidepressants' and distinguished them from stimulant drugs (Mayer-Gross, Slater & Roth, 1960). Participants at a psychopharmacology conference held in 1962 also contrasted the specificity of antidepressants to the implied non-specificity of stimulants thus:

> The earliest reports of the use of antidepressant medication seemed to indicate that the purpose of the medication was simply some special kind of stimulation which was useful in relieving lethargy and withdrawal. It was soon evident, however, to good clinical observers, that the action of antidepressant substances was much more specific.
>
> (Goldman, 1966: 526)

The British National Formulary first included a category of 'antidepressants' in 1963, noting that 'the treatment and prognosis of mental depression has been considerably enhanced by the use of antidepressant drugs' (British Medical Association and Pharmaceutical Society of Great Britain, 1963: 85). The formerly used category of 'stimulants' was abandoned in this edition and amphetamines and other stimulants were included in the category of antidepressants along with imipramine and iproniazid.

Antidepressants and the concept of depression

By the 1950s the use of amphetamines had already carved out a niche for the use of drugs with people considered to have 'neurotic depression' in both general and out patient practice (Rasmussen, 2006). The use of ECT had also helped to establish the idea that depression was an important and, crucially, a *treatable* psychiatric condition. The idea of an antidepressant strengthened the notion that depression was an important and independent category of psychiatric disorder. By 1961 leading psychiatrist Frank Ayd characterized depression as the most common psychiatric condition (Ayd, Jr, 1961b). However, many psychiatrists, including Kuhn, proposed that drug treatment was only specific in cases of 'endogenous depression' which was seen as equivalent to a physical disease caused by a biological disturbance. According to this view 'milder' conditions were seen as a reaction to life events and not thought to be particularly amenable to drug treatment. In contrast, others proposed that depression was a single entity, differing only in terms of severity. The debate about whether depression was categorical or dimensional raged throughout the 1970s (Healy, 1997). However, the notion that any sort of depression might be amenable to a specific type of drug treatment helped to cement the existence of a generic category of depression. The idea that depression was a single condition won the day with the publication of DSM III in 1980 – which did away with the concept of neurotic or 'reactive' depression altogether (Healy, 1997). The generic category brought together severe depressive psychosis and endogenous depression with neurotic or reactive depression and formed a rationale for the use of antidepressants in primary care and outpatient practice along clear disease-centred lines. The notion of 'depression' as a single and clear-cut entity also formed the basis for the pharmaceutical industry to develop an extensive market for the new antidepressants such as Prozac that emerged in 1990s. In turn, the widespread use of antidepressants helped to strengthen the concept of depression as a common biological disorder and the idea that personal problems could be attributed to a chemical imbalance. That is, the very concept of the antidepressant helped to fashion our modern notion of depression.

The influence of the psychiatric profession

The idea of an antidepressant was, then, embraced long before there were any placebo-controlled trials of antidepressants, and in the absence of any evidence that might support the idea that the drugs had a disease-specific action in depressive states. This situation begs the question as to what functions the concept of an antidepressant fulfilled, and whose interests it served?

Throughout the first half of the twentieth century the psychiatric profession was concerned to integrate with general medicine, to establish its scientific credentials and improve its status, along with that of its patients (Bond, 1915; Moncrieff & Crawford, 2001; Petrie, 1945). The physical treatments of the twentieth century, especially ECT and insulin coma therapy, were embraced for their ability to confirm the medical nature of institutional psychiatry. The authors of a *Manual of Shock Treatment in Psychiatry* argued that, with ECT, 'the psychiatrist takes on, in the patients mind, the characteristics of a "real doctor" in that he is able to apply and utilise a physical method of treatment' (Jessner & Ryan, 1943). Subsequently, the new drugs introduced from the 1950s also assumed this role (Shepherd, 1994). In a California Senate investigation, drugs were credited with making 'the mental hospital a medical institution in the minds of the public' and producing a 'profound intensification of medical orientation'. They were also used as an argument for increasing numbers of psychiatrists (California State Senate, 1956; Swazey, 1974: 209).

The psychiatric profession's other concern throughout the twentieth century was to disengage itself from its former power base in the asylum. The county mental hospitals of the nineteenth century were overcrowded with people with chronic and severe conditions, and were perceived as a source of stigma and embarrassment for both the psychiatric profession as well as their patients. By 1915, the president of the Medico-Psychological Association had identified the asylum as the cause of the unpopularity of psychiatry, and recommended the establishment of 'psychiatric clinics' in general hospitals. As David Armstrong has documented, the whole of medicine during the twentieth century was developing a greater focus on milder conditions and their overlap with normality (Armstrong, 1983). Psychiatry's increasing preoccupation with neurosis, outpatient practice, community psychiatry and the psychological health of the general population were expressions of this general trend. However, it was impossible to attract people with milder conditions to have cumbersome and dangerous procedures such as ECT and insulin coma therapy and, anyway, these could not be conducted in an office-based practice. Psychoanalysis and psychotherapy were more suitable, which may partly explain their increasing popularity in this period. So was drug treatment, and drugs had the added advantage of seeming to be a 'proper' medical treatment.

Subsequently, during the 1970s, when psychiatry was under attack from antipsychiatrists and was hit by funding cuts in the United States, there was a concerted attempt to reinforce biological psychiatry and purge American psychiatry of the influence of psychoanalysis and social psychiatry (Wilson, 1993). The resultant publication of DSM III saw the deliberate restitution of medical diagnosis to the heart of psychiatric practice and research. Drugs, and their presumed specific effects, formed an essential part of the justification for this reorientation. In a response to the Rosenhan experiment, which had cast doubt on the validity of psychiatric diagnosis (Rosenhan, 1973), leading American psychiatrist Robert Spitzer, the engineer of DSM III, defended psychiatric diagnosis by referring to the specificity of treatment. He argued that evidence for the 'superiority of the major tranquillisers (neuroleptics or antipsychotics) in schizophrenia, of electro convulsive therapy in psychotic depression and more recently of lithium carbonate for the treatment of mania' justified the application of a medical process of diagnosis (Spitzer, 1975: 450).

The influence of the pharmaceutical industry

The pharmaceutical industry played a significant part in establishing the role of the new psychiatric drugs in the 1950s and beyond. In 1961 the industry was described as 'launching an aggressive search for more antidepressant compounds' (Ayd, Jr, 1961a: 32). The *British Medical Journal* published one or two page adverts for antidepressants, involving seven different drugs or drug combinations, placed by eight different companies, in the first two months of 1962 alone.

Merck, who finally won the patent for amitriptyline, is often credited with establishing the common use of the tricyclic antidepressants. According to David Healy, Merck distributed 50,000 copies of Frank Ayd's book, *Recognising the Depressed Patient* (Ayd, Jr, 1961b; Healy, 1997), which suggested that depression was commoner than was generally realized and that it often went undiagnosed. Indeed, Ayd suggested that one in ten people required some sort of psychiatric treatment in their lifetime, most commonly for depression. He suggested that depression was most commonly encountered in general practice, where it could be satisfactorily treated by the general practitioner. Like more recent marketing campaigns, Merck sought to establish the concept of depression as a *common medical condition*, amenable to drug treatment.

Early antidepressant marketing reflected the commercial opportunities that the pharmaceutical industry saw in promoting antidepressants as disease-specific drugs, and in distinguishing them from non-specific drugs on the market. Imipramine, marketed by Geigy as Tofranil, was described as a 'specific therapeutic measure in the treatment of depression' (Tofranil advertisement, 1961). Nialamide (Niamid, a MAOI) was described as a 'specific treatment' for 'depressive illness' (Niamid advertisement, 1962). Phenelzine (Nardil) was claimed to be a 'true antidepressant which acts selectively on the brain' (Nardil advertisement, 1961). A North American advertisement emphasized that it 'removes the depression rather than merely masking the symptoms as do tranquillisers, CNS stimulants or sedatives' (Nardil advertisement, 1960). Amitriptyline was recommended for its broad profile of action, including its 'intrinsic tranquillising properties' (Tryptizol advertisement, 1964). However, it was also described as having a 'pronounced antidepressant effect' (Saroten advertisement, 1962a) and as being a 'specific treatment for depression and anxiety' (Saroten advertisement, 1962b). In contrast, benzodiazepines, stimulants and occasionally neuroleptics were advertised for their non-specific drug-induced effects in a range of situations, including 'emotional fatigue' (Parstellin advertisement, 1962), 'the menopause' (Ritalin advertisement, 1964) and the 'querulousness of old age' (Largactil advertisement, 1964).

The history of psychiatry

This chapter has charted the rapidity with which drugs that are now currently regarded as 'antidepressants' came to be seen as specific treatments for depressive disorders. The earliest drugs – that are retrospectively regarded as antidepressants – the antituberculous drugs, were clearly similar in nature to stimulants. Although stimulants had been successfully promoted as 'antidepressants' in the 1940s, by the 1950s and 60s a distinction started to be drawn between stimulants, which were regarded as non-specific, and drugs that were thought to target depression specifically. The antituberculous drugs metamorphosed into antidepressants through the concept of the psychic energizer. However it was imipramine that finally established the modern notion of an 'antidepressant'. Imipramine *had to be* regarded as acting on a 'disease', because it was difficult to see how any of the effects that imipramine was known to induce could be at all useful in depression. The idea that imipramine was an 'antidepressant' caught on despite the lack of any quantitative data to support its benefits and before there were any controlled trials to establish its efficacy compared with placebo. In addition, there was, and remains, no evidence to suggest that imipramine and other antidepressant drugs act in a disease-centred fashion on the biological basis of depressive symptoms.

This challenges the conventional view of the recent history of psychiatry, which suggests that modern day drugs helped to transform psychiatry into a genuine scientific activity. This view is premised on the idea that modern drugs are disease- or symptom-specific treatments; that they work by reversing some or all of an underlying physical pathology. It is the idea of the *specificity of action* that makes drug treatment *appear* to be a therapeutic, medical enterprise. If, in contrast, modern psychiatric treatments are not specific, if they act merely by inducing psychoactive effects that suppress or contain psychiatric distress and problematic behaviours, then psychiatry has not moved far from its historical roots as a superficially, or metaphorically medicalized form of social control.

The evidence suggests that extra-scientific interests have played a crucial role in shaping our current understanding of the nature of depression and the drugs that are used to treat it, illustrating Rosenberg's thesis of the symbiosis between treatment specificity and professional prestige (Rosenberg, 1977). Over the course of the twentieth century there were various reasons why the psychiatric profession wished to embrace the idea of disease specific drugs. During the early part of the century, the profession was actively seeking to improve its status through a closer association with general medicine. In addition, psychiatry was moving away from the asylum and seeking to build up outpatient and community-based practice. The antidepressants provided a medical-seeming treatment for a common problem that could be managed outside hospitals. The claimed specificity of drug treatments also helped the profession to weather the storms provoked by the antipsychiatry critiques and economic challenges of the 1960s and 1970s. The pharmaceutical industry also helped to establish the market for antidepressants and disseminate the disease-specific view of antidepressants, providing an early example of the power of the pharmaceutical industry to shape scientific 'facts' in the area of psychiatry (Busfield, 2006).

Over the last 20 years, many millions of people around the world have been persuaded that their difficulties arise from a brain disorder that can be called 'depression' and corrected by drug treatment. The ideas of 'depression' and 'antidepressants' have been marketed, as 'diseases', to a general audience as never before. Few people are aware that these concepts have their origins, not in robust scientific research, but rather in the interests of a psychiatric profession desperate to cement its professional position, and in the marketing tactics of the pharmaceutical industry. Antidepressants have transformed a myriad of social and personal problems into a source of corporate profit and professional prestige.

14
Antidepressants and the Placebo Response

Irving Kirsch

Introduction

I used to think that antidepressants worked. As a clinical psychologist, I had for years referred some of my clients to psychiatric colleagues who could prescribe antidepressants for them. Sometimes the antidepressants did not seem to help, but when they did, I assumed that the benefit derived from the chemical properties of the drug. In this chapter, I describe the process by which I came first to doubt and then to disbelieve the hypothesis that antidepressants had a biochemical affect on depression, a process more fully documented in *The Emperor's New Drugs: Exploding the Antidepressant Myth* (Kirsch, 2010).

My entry into the world of antidepressant research was serendipitous. I was not particularly interested in evaluating the effects of antidepressants. Instead, I began looking at antidepressant clinical trials because of my long-standing interest in a psychological construct called response expectancy (Kirsch, 1985). Response expectancies are anticipations of automatic subjective reactions, like changes in depression, anxiety, pain and so on. I have argued that response expectancies are self-confirming. The world in which we live is ambiguous, and one of the functions of the brain is to disambiguate it rapidly enough to respond quickly. We do this, in part, by forming expectations. So what we experience at any given time is a joint function of the stimuli to which we are exposed and our beliefs and expectations about those stimuli (Kirsch, 1999).

When I first began researching antidepressants, the response expectancy hypothesis was the focus of most of my research. The particular topic areas (hypnosis, psychotherapy, placebo effects, etc.) were chosen merely because they provided a convenient opportunity for examining expectancy effects. It seemed to me that depression ought to be particularly responsive to expectancy effects because hopelessness is a central feature of depression (Abramson, Seligman, & Teasdale, 1978), and hopelessness is an expectancy. Specifically, it is the expectancy that a negative state of affairs will not get better, no matter what one does to alleviate it.

If you ask depressed people what the worst thing in their lives is, many will tell you that it is their depression. They believe that their depression will continue, no matter what they do – a very depressing thought indeed. As John Teasdale (1985) noted, these people are depressed about their depression. If this is the case, then the expectancy of improvement should produce improvement. That is, the belief that one will improve is the opposite of the hopelessness that may be maintaining the depression, or at the very least is an important component of it. In other words, theoretically there ought to be a substantial placebo effect associated with the treatment of depression.

Listening to Prozac™ but hearing placebo

In 1998, Guy Sapirstein and I undertook a meta-analysis to evaluate the placebo effect in depression (Kirsch & Sapirstein, 1998). We searched the literature for studies in which depressed patients had been randomized to receive antidepressant medication, an inert placebo, psychotherapy, or no treatment at all. We included studies of psychotherapy, because those were the only ones in which patients had been randomized to a no-treatment control condition, and we needed that condition to evaluate the placebo effect. The *response* to a placebo is not the same as the *effect* of the placebo. The placebo response (as opposed to the placebo effect) may at least in part be due to the passage of time, spontaneous remission, the natural history of the disorder, and regression to the mean. Just as the difference between the drug response and the placebo response is deemed to be the drug effect, so the difference between the placebo response and improvement in a no-treatment control group can be interpreted as the placebo effect.

The results of our meta-analysis indicated equal and substantial improvement among patients given medication or psychotherapy. However, patients given placebos also got better, whereas those in no-treatment control groups showed relatively little improvement. We found that approximately 25 per cent of the improvement in the drug group would have occurred without any treatment whatsoever, 50 per cent was a placebo effect, and only 25 per cent was a true drug effect. In other words, the placebo effect (which is the difference between the response to being given a placebo and what would have happened had no treatment been given at all) was twice as large as the drug effect (the response to the drug minus the response to the placebo). This was indeed surprising. After all, antidepressants have been hailed as miracle drugs that produced a revolution in the treatment of depression (see Double, this volume; Moncrieff, this volume).

Our surprise at the outcome of our analysis led us to wonder whether it may have been due to the diversity of antidepressants in the clinical trials we had analyzed. Perhaps some of the medications were very effective and others not, leading us to underestimate the drug effect? To assess this possibility, we returned to our data set and classified the various studies in terms of the type of medication evaluated. We categorized them into four types: tricyclic medications, SSRIs, miscellaneous other antidepressants and other medications. The consistency was remarkable: regardless of the type of medication studied, 75 per cent of the response to the active drugs was duplicated by placebo, leaving a true drug effect of only 25 per cent in each case. What makes this particularly surprising is the response to what we labelled 'other medication'. These were active drugs that are not regarded as antidepressants (e.g., lithium, barbiturates and thyroid medication given to depressed patients who were not suffering from depression). They too produced substantial improvement in depression, as that as great as that produced by tricyclics, SSRIs, and other antidepressants. Joanna Moncrieff has described similar data concerning an even wider range of medications that all surpass placebo in the treatment of depression (Moncrieff, 2008a), and the same 'antidepressant' effect can be produced by drugs that are supposed to decrease, rather than increase, serotonin levels (Kirsch, 2010). What do you call a substance, the effects of which are independent of its physical properties? A placebo.

The finding of equivalent antidepressant effects of all of these different drugs led us to search for their commonality. One thing they have in common is that they all produce side effects. Placebos can also produce side effects, but they do so to a much lesser degree than active medications (Philipp, Kohnen, & Hiller, 1999). Why is this important? Imagine that you are recruited to a clinical trial for an antidepressant medication. As this is a double-blind trial, you are told that you may receive medication or you may receive placebo. You are also told that the active medication has been reported to produce a number of side effects, such as dry mouth and drowsiness, and you are told that the therapeutic effect may not become evident for some weeks. You are likely to wonder to which group you have been assigned, the active-drug group or the placebo-control group. You notice that your mouth has become dry and that your feel drowsy. At this point, you are likely to conclude that you have been assigned to the drug condition. Indeed, data indicate that about 80 per cent of patients assigned to the active drug condition in clinical trials of antidepressants break the blind and conclude that they are in the active drug condition (Rabkin et al., 1986). Being more certain that you have been assigned to the drug group, you will have a stronger *expectancy* for improvement, which according to the response expectancy hypothesis should *produce* greater improvement. In other words, it is possible that the superiority of active antidepressant to inert placebo is due to the breaking of blind by patients in the active drug condition. Rather than being a true drug effect, it is an enhanced placebo effect.

The emperor's new drugs

Needless to say, our first meta-analysis proved to be quite controversial. Its publication led to heated exchanges. The response from critics was that these data could not be accurate. Perhaps our search had led us to analyse an unrepresentative subset of clinical trials? Antidepressants had been evaluated in many trials and their effectiveness had been well established.

In an effort to respond to these critics, we replicated our study with a different set of clinical trials (Kirsch, Moore, Scoboria, & Nicholls, 2002). We used the Freedom of Information Act to request that the Food and Drug Administration (FDA) send us the data that pharmaceutical companies had sent to it in the process of obtaining approval for six new-generation antidepressants that accounted for the bulk of antidepressant prescriptions being written at the time. There are a number of advantages to the FDA data set. First, the FDA requires that pharmaceutical companies provide information on *all* of the clinical trials that they have sponsored. Thus, we had data on unpublished trials as well as published trials. Second, the same primary outcome measure – the Hamilton depression scale (HAM-D) – was used in all of the trials. That made it easy to understand the clinical significance of the drug–placebo differences. Third, these were the data on the basis of which the medications were approved. In that sense they have a privileged status. If there is anything wrong with them, the decision to approve the medications in the first place can, and must, be called into question.

In the data sent by the FDA, only 43 per cent of the trials showed a statistically significant benefit of drug over placebo. The results of our analysis indicated that the placebo response was 82 per cent of the response to these antidepressants. Subsequently, my colleagues and I replicated our meta-analysis on a larger number of trials that had been submitted to the FDA (Kirsch et al., 2008). With this expanded data set, we again found that 82 per cent of the drug response was duplicated by placebo. More important, in both analyses, the mean difference between drug and placebo was less than two points on the HAM-D. The National Institute for Clinical Excellence (NICE), which drafts treatment guidelines for the National Health Service in the United Kingdom, has established a three point difference between drug and placebo on the HAM-D as a criterion of clinical significance (NICE, 2004). Thus, when published and unpublished data are combined, they show no clinically significant advantage for antidepressant medication over inert placebos.

At roughly the same time as our second meta-analysis of the FDA data set was done, Corrado Barbui and his colleagues (Barbui, Furukawa, & Cipriani, 2008) analysed the data on paroxetine that had been reported on the GlaxoSmithKline (GSK) website. As part of the settlement of a lawsuit brought against GSK by the State of New York for withholding data showing negative results, the company was required to post summary data from all of its clinical trials of antidepressants, including those that had not been published (Spitzer, 2004). Unlike the FDA data, which are limited to pre-approval trials, the GSK website includes postmarking trials as well. Barbui et al. (2008) found 40 placebo-controlled studies of *Seroxat*™ for the treatment of major depression, including the 16 that had been sent to the FDA. Although they analysed response rates rather than mean symptom change, the results of their analysis of these 40 studies were virtually identical to the results of our analysis of the studies that had been sent to the FDA. In their analysis, the placebo was 83 per cent as effective as the real drug. Thus the failure to find a clinically significant difference between drug and placebo holds for post-marketing as well as pre-marketing trials.

There are two types of design in the clinical trials submitted to the FDA. The most common involved allowing prescribing physicians to adjust the dose as needed during the course of the trial. In addition, approximately one quarter of the trials used a fixed dose design, in which patients were randomized to receive particular doses of the medication. Thus we were concerned that the data we had analysed might have included patients who were assigned to receive an inadequate or sub-clinical dose of the medication. If this were the case, then we might have underestimated the drug effect.

To eliminate this possibility, we performed an additional analysis on the fixed-dose clinical trials. Specifically, we compared improvement among patients given the lowest dose in the trial with those with improvement among patients given the highest dose. We found that improvement at the lowest dose (9.57 points on the HAM-D) was virtually identical to improvement at the highest dose (9.97 on the HAM-D). Nor was there any apparent advantage for mid range doses. In fact, of approximately 40 comparisons of different doses of the same antidepressant, only one significant difference was reported. In a study of fluoxetine in moderately to severely depressed patients, the two lower doses were significantly more effective than the high dose, which was not significantly more effective than placebo.

The 'dirty little secret'

The response to our earlier meta-analysis was incredulity. However, in an invited commentary on our paper, the response to our analysis of the FDA data was unanimous acceptance by 12 groups of independent scholars, some of them participants in clinical evaluations of antidepressants for pharmaceutical companies. As one group of commentators put it: 'many have long been unimpressed by the magnitude of the differences observed between treatments and controls, what some of our colleagues refer to as "the dirty little secret" in the pharmaceutical literature' (Hollon, DeRubeis, Shelton, & Weiss, 2002).

Perhaps the most disturbing aspect of the keeping of this secret is the role of the FDA. Among the data we received using our Freedom of Information request were copies of internal memos. One of these, written by the Director of the Division of Neuropharmacological Drug Products, includes the following revealing information:

> The Clinical Efficacy Trials subsection within the Clinical Pharmacology section not only describes the clinical trials providing evidence of citalopram's antidepressant effects, but make[s] mention of adequate and well controlled clinical studies that failed to do so. I am mindful, based on prior discussions of the issue, that the Office Director is inclined toward the view that the provision of such information is of no practical value to either the patient or prescriber. I disagree. I believe it is useful for the prescriber, patient, and 3rd party payer to know, without having to gain access to official FDA review documents, that citalopram's antidepressants effects were not detected in every controlled clinical trial intended to demonstrate those effects. I am aware that

clinical studies often fail to document the efficacy of effective drugs, but I doubt the public, or even the majority of medical community, are aware of this fact. I am persuaded they not only have a right to know, but should know. Moreover, I believe that labeling that selectively describes positive studies and excludes mention of negative ones can be viewed as potentially 'false and misleading'.

(Leber, 1998, p. 11)

How did these drugs get approved?

How is it that medications with such weak efficacy data were approved by the FDA? The answer lies in an understanding of the approval criteria used by the FDA. The FDA requires two adequately conducted clinical trials showing a significant difference between drug and placebo. But there is a loophole: there is no limit to the number of trials that can be conducted in search of these two significant trials. Trials showing negative results simply do not count. Furthermore, the *clinical* significance of the findings is not considered: all that matters is that the results are *statistically* significant.

A typical example of the implementation of this criterion is provided by the FDA file on citalopram. Seven controlled efficacy trials were conducted. Two showed small but significant drug–placebo differences. Two were deemed too small to count. Three failing to show any significant benefit for the drug were deemed 'adequate' and 'well controlled', but were 'not counted against citalopram' because there was a 'substantial placebo response' (internal memo by T. P. Laughren, FDA Team Leader for Psychiatric Drug Products). Thus, citalopram was approved on the basis of two clinical trials despite negative results in five other trials.

Conclusions

There is a strong therapeutic response to antidepressant medication. But the response to placebo is almost as strong. This presents a therapeutic dilemma. While the *drug effect* of antidepressants is not clinically significant, the *placebo effect* is. What should be done, clinically, in light of these findings?

One possibility would be to prescribe placebos, but this entails deception. Besides being ethically questionable, it runs the risk of undermining trust, which may be one of the most important clinical tools that clinicians have at their disposal. Another possibility that has been proposed is to use antidepressants as active placebos (Hollon et al.,

2002; Moerman, 2002), but the risks of side effects, suicide, withdrawal symptoms and drug interactions render this alternative problematic. A third possibility is the use of alternative treatments. Physical exercise, for example, has been shown to produce clinical benefit in moderately depressed people (Kirsch, 2010). This might also be a function of the placebo effect, but the difference in the side effect profile can be considered. Side effects of antidepressants include sexual dysfunction, insomnia, diarrhoea, nausea, anorexia, bleeding, forgetfulness, seizures, and an increased risk of suicide. Side effects of physical exercise include enhanced libido, better sleep, decreased body fat, improved muscle tone, longer life, increased strength and endurance, and improved cholesterol levels.

Finally, the social and economic causes of depression need to be addressed. Depression is associated with unemployment, poverty, poor education, and unaffordable housing, and the people who benefit most from antidepressant or psychotherapeutic interventions tend to be white, well paid, and well educated (Kirsch, 2010). Treating depression is not enough. We also need to prevent it by changing the social conditions that increase the increased risk of becoming depressed.

15
Why Were Doctors So Slow to Recognize Antidepressant Discontinuation Problems?

Duncan Double

The recognition of antidepressant discontinuation problems

The *Defeat Depression* campaign was a five-year-national programme launched in January 1992 by the Royal College of Psychiatrists in association with the Royal College of General Practitioners. The aim of the campaign was to educate health professionals and the public about depression and to reduce the stigma of mental illness.

A door-to-door survey of public opinion was undertaken to obtain baseline data before the campaign started (Priest et al., 1996). Most of the people questioned in the sample, that is 78 per cent, thought that antidepressants were addictive. This finding caused some consternation among those running the campaign, because, as far as they were concerned, the public was misinformed on this issue. Part of the education programme, therefore, was to teach doctors that patients should be told clearly when antidepressants are prescribed for the first time, that discontinuing treatment in due course will not be a problem.

In retrospect, this guidance may seem surprising. The *British National Formulary*, which doctors use for reference about medication, has given a warning since 1990 that symptoms may occur if an antidepressant is stopped suddenly after regular administration for eight weeks or more. In fact, case reports of discontinuation reactions have appeared since antidepressants were first introduced (Mann & MacPherson, 1959).

Tricyclic antidepressants began to be prescribed in the mid-1950s. A new class of antidepressants called serotonin specific reuptake inhibitors (SSRIs) were introduced onto the UK market in 1987. Discontinuation symptoms were only recognized in this new group of drugs after the SSRIs had been in widespread clinical use for several years.

The drug companies were concerned about these discontinuation problems and a consensus meeting of experts, sponsored by Eli Lilly, the manufacturers of fluoxetine, or Prozac™, as it is known by its trade name, was held in Phoenix, Arizona, at the end of 1996. This led to an editorial in the *British Medical Journal* in 1998 acknowledging that antidepressant discontinuation problems existed (Haddad et al., 1998). It suggested, though, that they were both preventable and simple to treat.

The *BMJ* editorial seems to have understated the seriousness of the problem. The same authors only two years later acknowledged that discontinuation symptoms are common in a letter to the *Lancet* (Young & Haddad, 2000). There was also confusion about the meaning of terms like dependence and addiction. Eventually, the pharmaceutical company GlaxoSmithKline dropped its insistence that paroxetine, its SSRI drug, is not addictive (Boseley, 2003). Even though there may be little evidence of physical addiction, in the sense that the body gets addicted to SSRIs, commonsense understanding of the word also includes psychological dependence, and despite what the *Defeat Depression* campaign said, the public knew, even if doctors did not, that taking antidepressants could become a habit.

Modern guidelines, therefore, such as the one for depression from the National Institute for Health and Clinical Excellence (NICE, 2004), actually state the opposite of what was recommended by the *Defeat Depression* campaign. This is that all patients prescribed antidepressants should be informed that discontinuation/withdrawal symptoms may occur on stopping, missing doses or, occasionally, on reducing the dose of the drug.

Antidepressant discontinuation reactions are now established. However, there is still no accepted definition of an antidepressant discontinuation syndrome. Many of the reported symptoms associated with SSRI withdrawal are physical rather than psychological. Schatzberg et al. (1997) divided the somatic symptoms into five clusters: (1) disequilibrium (e.g. dizziness, vertigo, ataxia) (2) gastrointestinal symptoms (e.g. nausea, vomiting) (3) flu-like symptoms (e.g. fatigue, lethargy, myalgia, chills) (4) sensory disturbances (e.g. paraesthesias, sensations of electric shock), and (5) sleep disturbances (e.g. insomnia, vivid dreams). As well as the somatic symptoms, several core psychological symptoms – anxiety/agitation, crying spells, and irritability – are associated with SSRI discontinuation.

Antidepressant discontinuation problems are commonly seen as being related to reregulation of brain receptors and transporters. The theory is that as antidepressants prevent the reuptake of serotonin and other monoamines, when they are discontinued, the brain has to reregulate its balance of receptors (Blier & Trimblay, 2006).

However, I want to concentrate on wider aspects of antidepressant discontinuation and, in particular, psychological dependence. In its broadest sense, dependence means a negative affect experienced in the absence of the drug (Russell, 1976). Taking antidepressants can become a habit. People may form attachments to their medications more because of what they mean to them than because of what they do. Patients often stay on medications, maybe several at once, even though the actual benefit is questionable. It can be more of a problem than it is worth to stop medication. Any change threatens an equilibrium related to a complex set of meanings that the medications have acquired. For example, patients may think, or may be unsure, that the drug is preventing relapse, so they do not want to take the risk of stopping it.

Deciding when to withdraw antidepressant treatment, especially maintenance treatment, can be difficult and requires careful discussion of the potential benefits and disadvantages (*Drugs and Therapeutic Bulletin*, 1999). If treatment is discontinued, the doctor and the patient need to be alert to the risk of discontinuation effects and the re-emergence of depressive symptoms, which can occur on cessation of any antidepressant. Antidepressants should not be stopped abruptly, nor treatment courses interrupted, unless there is a good clinical reason, for example a serious adverse effect or patient request.

So, in summary, doctors do not always know best. It took some time for them to recognize the nature of antidepressant discontinuation problems. They did not use their common sense to realize that discontinuing a drug that is thought to improve mood may cause problems. Antidepressants are likely to be habit forming, so however much the medical profession may declare that they are not primarily reinforcing like psycho stimulants, the public has always understood that there may be difficulties in discontinuing antidepressants. The general public might reasonably have expected that psychiatrists, who are supposed to be specialists in disorders of the mind, would recognize psychological dependence, base their advice on clinical experience, and use their common sense.

I want to suggest that there are at least three reasons for doctors' neglect of the significance of antidepressant discontinuation problems:

(1) Doctors concentrate on short-term rather than long-term treatment,
(2) Doctors focus on neurobiological rather than psychosocial factors,
(3) Doctors are biased about the effectiveness of medication.

These factors help to explain why there was so much delay in doctors recognizing that antidepressants can cause discontinuation problems. In general, doctors are advocates of antidepressant treatment and this has led to them overlooking what should have been obvious about the risk of discontinuation problems. I will consider each of the reasons I have listed in turn.

Doctors concentrate on short-term rather than long-term treatment

Medication is often prescribed in life crises and serves to reinforce defensive mechanisms against overwhelming anxiety. When people are desperate they will accept almost anything that is proposed to help them. The power of the placebo needs to be recognized (Shapiro & Shapiro, 1997; Kirsch, this volume). Medicines may provide relief just because patients and their doctors believe in them.

It is not just doctors that hope for a 'quick fix'. Ideally, we may all want a simple, quick, cheap, painless and complete cure. In fact, in the real situation, motives may be more complex than this. In surveys, people express a reluctance to take drugs, but an inability to be free of them (Townsend et al., 2003). Nonetheless the wish-fulfilling nature of both patient and doctor expectations is a driving factor in outcome.

There can be disastrous consequences for patients investing their faith in the omnipotence of doctors. The combination of impressionable patients and misinformed doctors is a particularly powerful mix. As noted by Oliver Wendell Holmes as long ago as 1871:

> There is nothing men will not do ... to recover their health and save their lives. They have submitted to be half drowned in water, ... half choked with gases, ... buried up to their chins in earth, ... seared with hot irons like galley slaves, ... have needles thrust into their flesh, and bonfires kindled on their skin, to swallow all sorts of abominations, and to pay for all this, as if blisters were a blessing and leeches were luxury. What more can be asked to prove their honesty and sincerity?
> (Oliver Wendell Holmes, 1871: 427)

Modern medicine likes to think it has moved on from such quackery. It may believe itself to be ethically beyond reproach, glossing over, for example, how practitioners still accept considerable amounts of hospitality, gifts and other freebies from the pharmaceutical industry and commercial medical device manufacturers. Rather than just going along with any intervention that may seem to make a difference, it tries to assess the evidence for treatments scientifically by performing randomized controlled trials. It, therefore, attempts to justify its interventions as evidence-based.

However, clinical trials tend to be tests of short-term interventions. The results do not always generalize to real-life clinical practice. For example, the average duration of trials in the NICE analysis of SSRIs versus placebo is only $6^3/_4$ weeks (National Institute for Clinical Excellence, 2004). This emphasis on the short-term and the episodic nature of depression helps to create the impression that occurrences of depression are easy to treat.

The resources required for longer-term studies can be prohibitive. Moreover, there are methodological problems due to attrition of subjects, leading to potential bias in the results. When longer-term treatment is studied, this tends to be done by looking at what happens when medication is withdrawn, rather than comparing outcome from the start of treatment. Patients do not do well when antidepressants are stopped. Discontinuation trials of antidepressants have a substantial relapse rate, with estimates from 36 per cent (Klerman et al., 1974) to as high as 92 per cent (Prien et al., 1974).

At face value, the evidence of discontinuation studies is that people should maintain their antidepressant treatment. But then why, if people should continue antidepressants, is the outcome for the treatment of depression over the long-term so poor? The introduction of antidepressants onto the market should have been expected to improve the long-term prognosis for depression. However, only $1/_5$th of people make a complete recovery over a period of 15 years (Andrews, 2001). Such poor long-term results contrast with the impression created over the short-term that antidepressants are effective.

Withdrawal studies may also not be the best way to assess the value of antidepressants over the long-term. In clinical practice, distinguishing discontinuation reactions from true relapse is not always clear-cut. Maybe what is being detected in withdrawal trials is more due to discontinuation effects than true relapse. After all, we recognize the placebo effect of antidepressants when they are started. Expectations are as likely to play a role in discontinuing medication, producing a negative placebo effect, known as a nocebo reaction.

Discontinuation reactions may be particularly likely to bias the results of withdrawal studies if patients are unblinded in the clinical trials. To try and eliminate the effect of expectancies, both patients and doctors are masked from knowing whether active or placebo medication is prescribed. However, 'double-blind' designs are not truly double-blind (Oxtoby et al., 1989). Both patients and raters are cued into whether active or placebo medication is being prescribed by a variety of means, including the recognition of the side effects of the active medication.

Although not specifically examined for withdrawal studies, there is evidence from short-term antidepressant trials that blindness can be breached. When patients are asked whether they have been put onto a placebo or an active antidepressant, it is found that they can guess correctly better than would be predicted by chance (Even et al., 2000). This 'unblinding' effect is likely to be at least as strong in withdrawal studies, as patients become accustomed to the effect of taking their antidepressant and will notice when it has been discontinued.

There is also evidence of a loss of benefit emerging with long-term treatment and also on re-treatment after discontinuation of antidepressants (Baldessarini et al., 2002). In clinical practice, it is not uncommon to find that the effect that a patient obtains from medication may seem to reduce over time. Similarly, medication may not work as well after the first time if it needs to be reintroduced. These findings reinforce the notion that the original reaction was a placebo effect.

In fact, there is some naturalistic evidence that people treated without antidepressants may do better over the long term. Using antidepressants may actually increase recurrences (Fava, 2003). The possibility that taking antidepressants may, therefore, create a vulnerability to relapse needs to be taken seriously. Maybe people who work through their problems without medication actually do better (Whitaker, 2010). This may require hard work, not a quick fix.

Evidence to support this view comes from the finding – in trials comparing psychotherapy and medication – that psychotherapy shows a significant advantage over medication at follow-up (Imel et al., 2008). The longer the follow-up the greater the difference between drug and psychotherapy. Furthermore, patients previously exposed to cognitive therapy are significantly less likely to relapse following treatment termination than patients withdrawn from medication (Dobson et al., 2008). This indicates that antidepressant discontinuation could well be hindering patients doing better over the long-term.

Whether antidepressants actually create a vulnerability to relapse should be a major research question. However, besides the methodological difficulties of testing this hypothesis, there is also an ideological barrier to considering it, as doctors want to believe in their prescriptions. However, proper learning from the lesson of the history of the resistance to the recognition of antidepressant discontinuation reactions should help to create a more open attitude to examination of this important issue.

Doctors focus on neurobiological rather than psychosocial factors

It is commonly believed that mental illness is due to a chemical imbalance in the brain. In fact, doctors frequently tell patients that their problems are due to a 'chemical imbalance'. However, there is no rigorous corroboration of any chemical-imbalance theory, such as the serotonin theory of depression (Lacasse & Leo, 2005). In fact, there is a significant body of contrary evidence to the simple notion that depression is due to a deficiency of serotonin in the brain. The serotonin theory of depression is no more than a theory, and most of the evidence is against it.

Psychopharmacologists trying to understand the mechanism of action of antidepressants long ago abandoned the theory. It is practising doctors who continue the myth in their everyday work. They have faith in the theory and influence their patients to believe as well. Doctors generally assume there is widespread evidence for mental illnesses being proven biological diseases of the brain. To question this presumption is almost heretical.

This conviction extends to professional medical bodies that represent doctors. For example, the American Psychiatric Association (2003), in a statement on the diagnosis and treatment of mental disorders, properly acknowledged that there are: 'no discernible pathological lesions ... that in or of themselves serve as reliable or predictive markers of mental disorder'. However, it then went on to say that 'mental disorders will eventually be proven to represent disorders of intercellular communication or disrupted neural circuitry'. Psychiatry has always had the belief that the answer to mental illness will eventually be found in the brain. It will not give up this wishful thinking, even if the evidence is against it. To be a psychiatrist seems almost to demand this step of faith.

However, my experience is that patients are able to understand that the 'chemical-imbalance theory' is only a theory. After all, people believe all sorts of things. What patients find more difficult to appreciate is why they are told that this theory has been proven, when this is not the case. Their doctors rarely tell them, for example, that there is evidence against the serotonin theory of depression.

So why does the myth persist? One reason is that the chemical-imbalance theory is used as a means of persuading patients to take their medication. Doctors do not want to give up the theory, because they want patients to take their prescriptions. If people believe that medication corrects a chemical imbalance, this provides a rationale that they can understand and follow by complying with doctors' orders.

Actually, modern medicine is supposed to be a partnership between doctors and patients (Stewart et al., 2003). Patients require the expertise of doctors to make sense of health information available to them. They need details to be given to them correctly. They expect psychiatrists not to be biased by interests other than those that are directed to the welfare of patients. However, medicine can be more doctor-centred than it should be, tilting the balance away from properly patient-centred practice.

The way doctors think about illness and treatment may satisfy a variety of needs, including their own professional security needs. The chemical-imbalance theory helps to protect doctors' roles and their income, prestige, and power. Modern psychiatry is no different in this respect to its nineteenth-century origins in society's acceptance of the need to 'care for' the mentally ill by building the asylums. The chemical-imbalance theory is just a modern variant of the belief that mental illness is due to brain pathology.

For example, John Haslam (1817), at the turn of the nineteenth century, noted that 'insanity is "a corporeal disease"'. He elaborated his reason for this belief by saying, 'I have never been able to conceive ... *a disease of the mind*' [his emphasis] (Haslam, 1798: 104). It was just too complicated for Haslam to believe anything other than that mental disorder is a brain disease. To quote from him again: '[T]he various and discordant opinions, which have prevailed in this department of knowledge, have led me to disentangle myself as quickly as possible from the perplexity of metaphysical mazes' (Haslam 1798: ix). A biological psychiatrist hopes to be relieved of having to deal with complicated philosophical issues about the connection between mind and matter and how it impinges on the relationship between facts and values.

Reductionistic beliefs, reducing mind to brain, have always been dominant in psychiatry and still persist. It is obviously attractive to believe that the phenomena of human experience can be understood in exclusively biological terms. This viewpoint seems to give some certainty, perhaps particularly in the field of madness and mental illness, which may be difficult to understand. However, it is legitimate to question whether an explanation of human nature can take the same form as the laws of natural science. Human beings do not behave like machines.

However much we may wish it were the case, the laws of cause and effect that are derived from the study of material objects, cannot be used to understand human phenomena (Dilthey, 1976). Due accord needs to be given to matter and still allow a meaningful worldview. The way to preserve nature as a meaningful entity is to integrate mind and body. An interpretative approach needs to be used that looks at human beings as whole persons and the study of persons should not be dominated by concepts related to the physical. This perspective acknowledges the importance of development, history and the potential for the continual reconceptualization of human understanding. There is an inevitable uncertainty and lack of finality in the description of human behaviour.

The implication of taking the step of faith and accepting the biomedical hypothesis is that psychosocial approaches tend to be disparaged (Clark, 1981). The insistence on somatic explanations of madness produces a resistance to psychological and social interpretations. For example, Henry Maudsley, in the latter half of the nineteenth century, broadened psychiatry by promoting treatment and research rather than just confinement and 'asylum'. As editor of the *Journal of Mental Science*, he expanded its scope to include psychology and philosophy. However, he still believed that, 'the explanation, when it comes, will not come from the mental, but from the physical side' (Maudsley, 1874). Maudsley's position was that the only sound psychological science was founded on physiology.

The biomedical hypothesis is so fundamental to the edifice of psychiatry that the 'chemical-imbalance theory' is still believed despite contrary evidence. However, psychodynamic thinking and attempting to integrate such understanding should not be avoided because it seems difficult and requires effort to make sense of people's feelings and actions. Honest assessment should prevail rather than professional security needs taking precedence.

To summarize, the problem for biomedical psychiatry is that, at its most extreme, it reduces people to brains that need their biology cured. There is insufficient focus on the person. Objectification of people by reducing them to abnormalities of their brains may have ethical implications for the doctor–patient relationship in assessment and treatment. Psychiatric assessment needs to be explicit that it is about understanding of the person. Shared decision-making with patients needs to be encouraged in treatment.

Furthermore, suggesting that mental illness has a physical basis serves as the justification for psychiatric interventions and institutions. The biomedical hypothesis functions as an apologia for psychiatric practice. It needs to be defended and promoted because it appears to provide the foundation for and legitimizes psychiatric intervention, such as antidepressant prescribing. To deny that mental illness is a physical disease may therefore be seen as hazardous as it seems to undermine orthodox practice.

As an illustration, in the Osheroff case, an argument was made for the right to effective treatment for depression with medication (Klerman, 1990). In this example, a patient, Dr Osheroff, sued the Chestnut Lodge for negligence. This renowned private hospital in Maryland specialized in intensive individual psychoanalytically orientated psychotherapy. Osheroff's claim was based on the failure to administer what was regarded as appropriate antidepressant medication for his condition. The hospital's management policy was seen as being unreasonable in view of the apparent lack of research evidence for the effectiveness of psychotherapy.

However, the apparent consensus about psychiatric conditions and their treatments, as, for example, expressed in clinical guidelines and other apparently authoritative sources, may merely represent the opinion of a dominant group (Stone, 1990; Moncrieff & Timimi, 2010). The inadequate scientific basis of psychiatry allows for widely varying interpretations and the inevitable clash of different opinions. The current authoritarian control of practice by biomedical psychiatry, based on its alleged firmer foundation, needs to be rebuffed.

Over recent years mainstream psychiatry, in fact, has become more biomedical in emphasis. There was a time when it was more pluralistic. For example, Karl Menninger's (1963) *The Vital Balance* represented a broadly conceived psychosocial theory of psychopathology. The perceived need to create explicit diagnostic criteria, as in DSM-III (American Psychiatric Association, 1980), ushered in a new emphasis on biomedical aspects of psychiatry. This approach has been called neo-Kraepelinian (Klerman, 1978), as it promotes many of the ideas associated with the views of Emil Kraepelin, often considered to be the founder of modern psychiatry.

Symptom checklists and formal decision-making rules for diagnoses are now established in diagnostic manuals, following the original call for such standardization by Feighner et al. (1972). This operationalization of diagnostic criteria was developed specifically to respond to criticisms of the basis of psychiatric classification. The attempt to make psychiatric diagnosis more reliable, combined with a return to a biomedical model of mental illness, promotes psychiatry as a scientific, medical speciality. Mentally ill patients, who require treatment, are seen as clearly demarcated from normal people. Belittling of the value of psychiatric diagnosis is discouraged.

Biological models of mental illness have been further encouraged by neuroimaging studies of the brain, genetic linkage studies and evidenced-based evaluations of the effectiveness of psychiatric treatment (Bullmore et al., 2009). Although psychosocial approaches have always been a minority paradigm within psychiatry, biomedical attitudes are now even more dominant. This encourages an emphasis on physical treatments, such as psychotropic medication.

The increase in antidepressant prescribing that has occurred over the last two decades illustrates this point clearly. Numbers of prescriptions in the UK for antidepressants increased more than twofold in the period 1975–98 (Middleton et al., 2001) and continued to rise by another 36 per cent between 2000–5 (Moore et al., 2009). The latest figures from the Prescription Cost Analysis, on the DoH website, show prescribing has gone up from around 10 million prescriptions in 1992 to 36 million in 2008, up from 22 million in 2000 (DOH, 2010). The reason for this rise may not necessarily be due so much to an increase in new cases, but because people are staying on antidepressants long-term (Moore et al., 2009). It only needs a small number of people to stay on antidepressants long-term to increase the total number of prescriptions dramatically. This finding emphasizes that it may well be fear of discontinuation problems that is the predominant explanation for the increase in antidepressant prescribing over recent years.

It is true that patients may want an antidepressant prescription, but the problem is that doctors do not always appreciate how much they may not, and doctors find it easier to continue repeat prescribing. Doctors need to be truthful about the evidence for the chemical-imbalance theory of depression, and to help people make up their minds about medication, such as antidepressants. It may be obvious, but doctors should not deceive their patients. They should be interested in helping patients decide how long they need to stay on medication.

Doctors are biased about the effectiveness of medication

It is generally claimed that antidepressants have been proven to be effective. In fact the results of thousands of studies of antidepressants are not nearly as conclusive as they are often claimed to be. For example, about a third of the earlier published studies showed no difference between antidepressants and placebo (Morris & Beck, 1974).

These are only the studies that have been published. Negative studies of antidepressants are much less likely to be published if only because the medical journals are more interested in publishing positive findings. Even in the trials that are published, outcomes are not always reported, particularly if the findings are negative (Chan & Altman, 2005). Trials are written up – and not necessarily by the researchers who conducted them – to emphasize the positive findings.

There are other ways in which bias is introduced. For example, conclusions in trials funded by drug companies tend to be more positive than those in which a more neutral experimenter has been involved (Als-Nielson et al., 2003). The quality of the study is also important. Better quality studies tend to find less treatment effect than the less methodically sound studies (Juni et al., 2001).

Putting these factors to one side, when the actual difference between antidepressant and placebo is measured, it is much smaller than most people realize. The mean drug-placebo difference in improvement scores has been found to be only 1.8 points on the Hamilton Rating Scale of Depression in data submitted to the Food and Drug Administration by drug companies to obtain a licence for their antidepressant drugs (Kirsch, this volume; Kirsch et al., 2002).

The Hamilton depression rating scale is a 17-item scale (in the most frequently used version) for assessing depression symptoms that is completed by a clinician. It is the most common rating scale used in clinical trials of depression. Items are scored from 0–4 or 0–2, giving a total score range of 0–51 on the 17-item version. 1.8 points may not be very clinically significant on a scale of 51. The National Institute for Health and Clinical Excellence (NICE) discriminated between statistical and clinical significance in this way and suggested that the small difference between antidepressants and placebo found in its own meta-analysis was too small to be clinically relevant (NICE, 2004).

Even though the small difference is statistically significant, could this finding still be biased? Controlled clinical trials have been introduced because the very expectation that medication will produce improvement may itself produce apparent benefit. As has already been noted, there is a large placebo effect with antidepressants and trials are not always conducted double-blind.

The breaking of the double blind on occasions has been interpreted as the explanation for a positive trial result. For example, Karlowski et al. (1975) found that ascorbic acid seemed to reduce the duration of the common cold, but these differences were eliminated when taking into account correct guesses about medication. Doctors may tend to be sceptical about the scientific value of vitamin C in the treatment of the common cold, so are happy to explain away a positive trial outcome in this situation as the result of faulty methodology. However, unblinding in clinical trials is commonplace and the problem will not be solved merely by pleas for improved study design and execution.

Some early trials of antidepressants reported more sceptical findings about their value. For example, Porter (1970) found no difference between imipramine and placebo. Interestingly, Porter did not pretend his trial was double blind, because he recognized that no trial of this kind can be conducted under completely blind conditions. In fact, he openly declared his bias that tricyclic antidepressants probably had no specific action in depressive illness, although they may suppress anxiety and agitation by their sedative effect. He actually argued that his attitude towards the effectiveness of the drug might neutralize the influence of the breaking of the blind.

The unblinding of antidepressant trials should not be ignored, but the dilemma is to know what to do about it. Nonetheless, there should be no pretence that objective, sound evaluation of antidepressants has confirmed their effectiveness. A misleading self-deception is encouraged that trials can be conducted double-blind, and the role of expectancies is underestimated. The wish for a scientific basis for psychiatric treatment is understandable, but professional status should not mean that the challenge to double-blind methodology goes unnoticed.

Furthermore, the degree of unblinding correlates with treatment effect size (Even et al., 2000). Unblinding, therefore, seems to be introducing expectancies that affect the results. Raters' expectations and patients' suggestibility could entirely explain the small effect sizes found. In other words, antidepressants may be merely amplified placebos.

Side effects may be the most common way in which the blind is broken (Thomson, 1982). Effect sizes also correlate with the proportion of patients having side effects. Furthermore, controlling for the difference in side effects means that drug-placebo differences become nonsignificant (Kirsch, 2010). Although this evidence may not be absolute proof, it strongly implies that the small difference between antidepressants and placebos, although statistically significant, is an artefact.

Doctors should at least tell patients about the small effect size and substantial nonresponse rate of antidepressants. At least part of the reason that they do not do so is because of fear of undermining their effectiveness. We do need to be clear that the issue of whether antidepressants work has not yet been decided in a scientific sense. Questioning the effectiveness of antidepressants is still legitimate. In fact, we should be more confident in stating that antidepressants are merely placebos with side effects.

Conclusion

It is perhaps not that surprising that doctors were slow to recognize antidepressant discontinuation reactions, as they focus on short-term fixes, they are not psychologically minded and they are too quick to peddle medication. I do not want to be accused of overstatement. I do recognize that not all doctors fit this stereotype.

The root problem is the belief that mental illness is a brain disorder. It needs to be recognized that psychiatry can be practised without postulating brain pathology as the basis for mental illness. Again, I do not want to be misunderstood. I am not saying that the brain and mind are separate. Perhaps a way to express what I am saying is that mental disorders must show *through* the brain but not always *in* the brain (Double, 2006).

Psychiatry has been found out on the issue of antidepressant discontinuation problems. Therapeutic zeal has led to the justification of all sorts of groundless medical interventions. Antidepressants may turn out to be yet another example. We need to be reminded of Plato's view that appearances on the surface may be different to the way things really are. The limits of the effectiveness of antidepressants need to be recognized. More attention should be given to the fact that doctors have made so many people dependent on them.

16
Toxic Psychology

Craig Newnes

For some, especially those claiming benefit from counselling or others who have found clinical psychologists less harmful than medication-wielding psychiatrists, the idea that psychology might be toxic will seem odd. After all, is it not clinical psychology that has done its utmost to supplant and undermine the ubiquitous 'medical model' in psychiatry? Is it not to counselling that so many turn, either as directed by their General Practitioners or via the expert advice of a newspaper columnist with suitable letters after her name? Surely modern day psychology is the new alchemy, turning all it touches to gold and laughing at the physically constrained treatments of medicine and its offspring, psychiatry? I want to explore a less benign discourse of psychology, particularly clinical psychology, by examining some of the ways the discipline has embraced the post-industrial language of progress and the gloss of science in order to position its practitioners as, almost by definition, noble seekers after both truth and the general good.

Any history of a given profession, as any historiographer will tell you, will reveal the nature of the prism through which it is glimpsed, something of the agenda of the historian and something of the context in which the historian works. Histories tend, in addition, to be written by the winners and lean toward a glorification of those winners. There are many histories of clinical psychology and psychiatry from the simple personal accounts of retired practitioners through to archival records held in various public or professional collections and numerous published volumes regularly updated through new editions or replaced by fresh accounts of our professional background. Perhaps the best place to find a condensed, though typically thorough, history of the psy professions is Roy Porter's (1997) *The Greatest Benefit to Mankind* wherein the author nails his subject in 30 (out of 716) pages of lucid text.[1] Many of the usual suspects are in place in those 30 pages; treatment, legislation, famous names, trends and fashion, the patient's perspective, professionalization and institutions. Less evident, but with entire canons of their own elsewhere, can be found histories seen through the prisms of gender, power relations, progress and protest.

Critical histories are increasingly common and it is through a critical frame that I shall present something of a history of clinical psychology. The frame here leans heavily on Wolf Wolfensberger's (1987) concept of *deathmaking*, but for those of a post-modernist and political bent there are traces of a Foucault-inspired philosophical analysis and a hint of Marxism.[2]

It is necessary to start, I think, with something of a caveat, almost an apology for what is to follow. For reasons that will hopefully become clear, I cannot claim that the harm revealed by a more critical view of Psy has been, and continues to be, perpetuated deliberately, maliciously or knowingly by the perpetrators. Indeed, it appears, to me at least, that one of the fundamental flaws of modernist psychological theory – the belief that we can somehow control what we think and do – absolves (if the belief *is* utterly flawed) psychologists from blame. After all, if they, like the rest of us, just do things because they do – with no control over their conduct – then how can we blame professionals for their actions?

Following from the above, the essence of the – admittedly fairly Anglocentric – history presented here is the repeated attempts by individuals, often designated experts, to help others either by alleviating their distress or enabling them to better fit with society's demands. The fact that such efforts can be seen to have led repeatedly to harm, even to death, is not an indictment – though perhaps it should be.

Reading history

Certain principles can be deduced (some might say invented) from a reading of a profession's history, principles that, of course, only emerge if the historian sets out on their elucidation. Since the nineteenth century one common principle – or thread – in any given historical path, has been the idea of progress. Science inexorably improves through better, faster, technologies and better explanatory theories. Space here precludes debating the possibility (or, indeed, knowability) of 'progress' but it is a common perspective to be found in histories of technology-based endeavour. Here, I wish to highlight some rather different threads in the history of our attempts to help each other via 'professional' intervention.

Early attempts to heal and help have something of the 'kill or cure' mentality, a mentality that dramatically reappeared in the twentieth century with the use of Psycho-surgery and Electro-convulsive therapy (ECT). Trepanning, for example, was a procedure (still very occasionally used today, though for different reasons) whereby holes were drilled into a person's skull in order to (we are told) release evil spirits. The procedure frequently ended in the patient's (victim's) death and many thousands of trepanned skulls have been found in excavations of Ancient Egyptian burial sites. It is not possible to conclude that the perpetrators of what would now be regarded as a barbaric treatment *hoped* their patients would die, but it might be possible to speculate that possession by spirits was seen as serious enough to *take the risk* that death would immediately follow their expulsion.

Such risk assessments remain commonplace in various physical treatments by psychiatrists (aided and abetted by clinical psychologists) where the dangers of the supposed illness (diagnosed as depression, schizophrenia, etc) are exaggerated in order to justify 'life-saving' but potentially lethal physical treatments such as ECT or experimental doses of powerful medication. ECT itself has Egyptian antecedents in the ancient use of electric eels to ameliorate melancholy. The lethal nature of modern treatments might offer some validity to the concept of deathmaking – the idea that treatment of distressed and 'marked' individuals is *designed* to kill either the body or spirit (or both) under the guise of aid. The disciplines of psychotherapy and counselling can be seen to play their part here. From a critical perspective, both professions are, at best, bystanders in a medically dominated psychiatric world where experimentation (e.g., via the lack of acknowledgement that *all* drugs effect people in different ways and thus need to be systematically monitored) is the norm and, at worst, active accomplices in a deathmaking enterprise (for more on psychotherapy-as-bystander see Jeffery Masson's (1988) chapter on Carl Rogers in *Against Therapy*).

Active killing of the spirit is everyday practice for many Psy-professionals. Imagine you have little spare money, live in a frequently frightening part of town and regret having the three young children that now live alone with you since their father left. You see a counsellor who reassures you that Cognitive Behaviour Therapy (CBT) or a close relation is the answer. Better still, it won't take long. But, of course, although the counsellor is patient and kind, the office warm and the buses not too inconvenient in terms of dropping the kids off at your mum's, you don't feel a lot different after a dozen visits. After five more you are told that your time is almost up and you seem to be 'resisting'. Your spirit dies a little.

This is not the fault of the counsellor, nor a particular limitation of the counselling brought on by the material context of the patient's life. Talking treatments are *bound* to kill a little of the spirit *despite* the best intentions of patient and therapist.

A second thread appears in the continuous promotion of humoral theory (or updated variants thereof) derived from the Hippocratic Corpus in around 250 BCE. In essence, sickness was seen to result from imbalances in the humours (*chymoi*). Vomiting, melancholy and mania were directly linked to bile and a healer's task was to effect rest or diet in order to increase or decrease the patient's bile relative to the other main humors. Porter (1997: 57) further suggests that the natural evacuation of blood (via nose bleeds and menstruation) led to the practice of blood-letting: 'systematized by Galen, and serving for centuries as a therapeutic mainstay'. Again, we find an attempt to restore humoral balance. It is this conception of the essential balance of the healthy body (or 'mind') that influences much psychiatric and psychological discourse today – whether in the wholly untested (and, indeed, untestable) theory of brain biochemical imbalance used to promote the necessity for corrective psychopharmacology – or in the glib assertions of 'life coaches' who advocate a 'work–life balance'.

A third thread is that of 'distantiation' examined by Foucault (1961) in relation to a combination of confinement and banishment (see, for example, his discussion of the 'ship of fools' and, later, the work of Pinel). Distantiation is a term used by Wolfensberger to capture one aspect of deathmaking – the removal of a person (invariably for that person's 'best interests') from socially valued sources of support (family, neighbours, friends, familiar local environments and so on). Such removal may actually be life-saving (as when a car accident victim is taken to a specialist intensive care unit miles from where she lives) but is more often in the case of the Psy professions *justified* as being life-saving when the removal (distantiation) is actually for the sake of persons distressed by the patient's conduct (as when a person labelled 'psychotic' is placed in a psychiatric unit against his will or a woman diagnosed with a so-called eating disorder is moved hundreds of miles from home to a specialist centre for eating disorders). This loss of the familiar and the – hopefully – supportive care available from local friends leads to disorientation and a loss of spirit. This particular aspect of deathmaking is probably one in which clinical psychology presents more as a collaborator than bystander as numerous clinical psychologists are actively involved in assessment protocols that are said to determine whether any given person merits psychiatric incarceration. Indeed, the bedrock of the profession, as first established in England and France, was the provision of intelligence testing to determine whether children could benefit from mainstream schooling or would need to be excluded (thus saving on the State education budget).

Positioning clinical psychology

In this section I want to provide some background from which to develop the theme of harm perpetrated by clinical psychology and psychotherapy both in the shadow of the overarching discipline of psychiatry and in their own right as disciplines offering deathmaking rather than healing. Again, I am not suggesting that this professional course has, in the main, been a deliberate attempt to hurt the people we are meant to help, though some examples will be given that offer little leeway for alternative conclusions.

A useful map for tracing the history of the profession of clinical psychology in Great Britain is provided – albeit for different purposes – by Goldie (1977). He describes three possible positions which can be taken up by non-medical professions in a context where medicine is the dominant discourse. Life-coaches and people offering therapy sessions for 'personal growth' would be excluded from Goldie's schema – though it is quite possible to argue that they and their clients have been seduced by an altogether more invidious Zeitgeist, the world of psychobabble. In Goldie's schema professions and individual professionals can move between the three positions depending on context and the point in their professional development. Non-medical professions, relative to medicine, can be positioned as *compliant, eclectic* or *radically opposed*.

To offer an example of how difficult it is for *anyone*, professional or not, to escape the discourse of medicine, take the simple word 'anxiety'. Newspaper columnists, reporters, ordinary people on the bus, even politicians, tend to talk of a person, whether the person is a well-known media idol or a close friend, as being 'anxious' – about money, a job interview, their child's health – rather than frightened, alarmed, ill-at-ease or a host of other similes. People are described as 'depressed' rather than overwhelmed, crushed, dispirited and the rest and journalists shunt so-called celebrities the way of the public as illustrations of 'bi-polar disorder' rather than personifications of being up-and-down or at-sixes-and-sevens. It is not hard to see how these medically derived words come to replace the far richer vocabulary of colloquial English; they are promoted by drug-company sponsored press releases, all-too-willing 'expert' psychologist-columnists, and press agents of the media-savvy seeking headlines. Ironically, as specific terms, these labels – anxiety, depression, bipolar disorder – have no validity and little enough reliability (it is a commonplace that any three psychiatrists will offer three different diagnoses of the *same* conduct in any given individual). The *impact* of such terminology from a psy-professional, however, is very different and can have devastating results.

Thus, if my neighbour calls me 'crazy, a nut, even (pause) schizophrenic' not much is going to happen. If my neighbour happens to be a Senior House Officer in Psychiatry called out by another neighbour alarmed by strange sounds coming from my house and I am described as 'Schizophrenic' a variety of State-supported interventions are likely to follow, from possible incarceration to forcible injection of medication and assessment by a clinical psychologist. Goldie's framework thus makes sense; in language, as in much else in society, a medical discourse prevails and it is reasonable to examine non-medical professions in relation to that discourse.

Compliance

Goldie's first position – *compliance* – is best summarized as taking care not to rock the medical boat. In the United Kingdom since clinical psychology's establishment as a profession under the 1948 National Assistance Act, compliance has been a persistently held position. An example is the use of psychometric assessment procedures for a host of assumed ills – from the tests for Schizophrenogenic Thought Disorder of the 1960s to many different tests for so-called Attention Deficit Hyperactivity Disorder of today. In the United States, where the majority of health care is paid for via private insurance, it has long been the case that insurance companies *insist* on psychometric assessment and subsequent psychiatric labelling before agreeing to fund treatment. Though not constrained by such institutional demands in the UK, clinical psychologists in the *compliant* position still perform psychometric assessment and, by implication, support the diagnostic system upheld by such procedures. This can range from agreeing that someone 'has' post-traumatic stress to confirming that a person's IQ is less than 70.

Eclecticism

The second position – *eclecticism* – has all the signs of a collaborative endeavour with sufficient hint of offering an alternative to the diagnostic and physical excesses of psychiatry to appeal to those clinical psychologists unwilling to be seen as bystanders. An example of practice that fits the eclectic schema is psychotherapy offered as an adjunct to medication for a host of diagnosed individuals. In such cases the clinical psychologist neither directly challenges the diagnosis ('What on earth do you *mean* by the term schizophrenia?') nor the use of medication ('Have you tested for the brain–biochemical imbalance you say is producing this person's feelings of overwhelm?') Instead, the clinical psychologist offers a variety of psychotherapy to the patient and reports progress to the referring physician or psychiatrist. Such practice has been a regular feature of clinical psychology in the UK for over 50 years from the Behavioural Therapies of the Maudsley Hospital under Eysenck, via the psychoanalytic approach of the Tavistock Clinic through to the modern obsession with Cognitive Behaviour Therapy and post-modern narrative approaches. There is – an admittedly flagging – drive in Britain to promote Cognitive Behaviour Therapy as the latest panacea. CBT holds that mood and emotions can be directly influenced by thoughts despite the reality that thoughts, feelings and behaviour are entirely different – rather than mutually influencing – modalities. Further, the therapy is based on the assumption of an internal world that can be accurately conveyed to others through speech.

It might be argued that Clinical Psychology in the UK rather missed the boat when it came to truly embracing a psycho-therapeutic discourse: though some practitioners dabbled with so-called humanist therapies (e.g., Gestalt therapy) and others took up a body-centred praxis (e.g. Bio-energetics) public debates within the profession tended in the 1970s to focus on a Psycho-dynamic versus Behaviourist discourse, and more recent debates revolve around CBT versus community psychology approaches. Along the way, clinical psychology in the UK seems to have neglected hundreds of other therapies that it might have embraced. The profession is, however, constrained in the UK in a way not familiar to practitioners from countries where health care is based on private insurance or direct payment such as the USA. Public funding and the much heralded public accountability in the UK limits clinical psychology training courses and their graduates to certain approved therapeutic modalities of which CBT is, presently, the mandatory market leader.

Radical opposition

The third position – *radical opposition* – Goldie identifies as a polarized fight or flight modality. Here, non-medical professions and individual professionals might take up a public opposition to the dominant medical discourse or attempt to leave the conflict zone. There are many variants of the latter ranging from early retirement to specializing in areas of psychology only tangential to a medical discourse, for example, conversation analysis – though it might be added that a number of exponents of CA use it to demonstrate the vacuity of much medical discourse and thus find themselves in the 'fight' position. Clearer examples of the fight pole are to be found in the work of some critical clinical psychologists, for example, those authors who actively challenge the medical paradigm frequently by sharing a platform with service survivors (see, e.g. Coleman, 1999) or offer alternative, normative means of – frequently – local and community rather than professional aid (see Cromby et al., 2006).

Individual practitioners, depending on context, might *claim* a position not easily identifiable to an observer, for example, a newly qualified practitioner might well screw up the courage in a case conference to challenge a consultant psychiatrist's proposed diagnosis or treatment. The psychologist may well assume herself to be in at the fight pole of the fight-or-flight position. From a critical perspective, however, that psychologist is still attending the case conference as a professional and implicitly supporting a medical discourse wherein complete strangers are designated 'cases' by powerful others. As such, the majority of the profession is positioned as either compliant or eclectic. Certainly, as a professional body, the Division of Clinical Psychology of the British Psychological Society adopts a public stance which consistently fails to challenge a medical discourse and academic journals like *The Journal of Clinical Psychology* or *Clinical Psychology and Psychotherapy* have a long history of support for psychiatric diagnostic nosologies and professional/ patient dichotomies. In terms of Goldie's nosology the profession of clinical psychology in Great Britain can be seen as moving – broadly – between a primarily compliant position and a – broadly – eclectic one, with fluctuations between the two.

In general then, the discipline of psychology has, since the first edition of *The British Journal of Psychology*, positioned itself as representing a value neutral science. Psychological science, however, differs from genuine science in at least two key respects. First, psychology employs un-testable hypotheses, which can neither be proven nor refuted (cf. Popper, 1963). In claiming, for example, that unwanted or upsetting conduct is due to childhood trauma, unconscious drives, the economic climate or whatever psychologists fail to explain why the conduct is inevitable nor – in the case of drive theory for example – can they prove the existence of such drives.

The second key departure from science in clinical psychology – arising directly from the failure to deal in refutable explanation – is the inability to say, 'We were wrong. We shall drop that theory.' Instead, people are treated as if the underlying theory is correct but the evidence not quite available yet. Thus some forms of psychological practice involve interminable searches for evidence of, say, hostility towards one's parents, faulty thinking, repressed desires or behavioural reinforcers when such evidence is not to be found.

Clinical psychology has been a major contributor to, and benefactor from, the modernist smoke screen concerning distress, diagnosis and the alleviation of distress. Combining physical causal explanation with an equally obscurantist 'psychological model' has proven profitable for the profession. The gloss of science is provided by a fixation with classification that shores up and expands psychiatry's own endeavours. Thus, a person's conduct will be classified and coded via observation and testing and, if required, explanations will then be proffered which might combine any number of physical, personal and environmental causes. A typical example could be the use of the Beck Depression Inventory, which marks a person as 'depressed'. Suggested reasons for the diagnosis can include genetic pre-disposition, 'faulty' cognitions, brain-biochemical imbalance, unconscious drives, early childhood experience, recent trauma, unemployment and so on. No effort is made to reason that millions of people would not receive such a diagnosis after experiencing similar life events and – of course – no physical evidence is forthcoming to substantiate the genetic or bio-chemical hypotheses. Psychologists might appeal to the idea that a 'combination' of factors is necessary to produce conduct that is classifiable as deviant or abnormal. Such analyses are coded ways of saying, 'All sorts of things make us who we are and I'll keep throwing factors into the pot until you ask me to stop.' These multi-factorial analyses cloud the whole endeavour in more expert-led obfuscation and give no verifiable weighting to any particular stated 'cause'.

Foucault termed the way in which professionals discipline themselves and others through coding conduct as 'the gaze' (1963). Through observation of those less powerful than themselves, professionals – particularly those in the so-called mental health professions – define abnormality and, by default, normality. As willing servants of psychiatry, clinical and educational psychologists thus perform a powerful social function. They are the guardians of what is to be considered normal. Clinical psychologists have thus contributed both to the labelling as deviant of numberless persons over the last century and, in many cases, their destruction at the hands of so-called mental health services. The so-called mental health services do not serve people, at least not those they claim to serve – rather, they observe, label and persecute in the name of a normality governed by those with power.

Clinical psychology, as a normalizing profession, is the tip of a vast psychological iceberg. Educational psychologists run tests on perfectly ordinary, if annoying, children and diagnose them with Attention Deficit Hyperactivity Disorder, military psychologists are involved in devising interrogation techniques (as if it takes an expert to understand that isolating and blindfolding someone, not to mention half drowning, will frighten them) and occupational psychologists make all sorts of claims which justify exploitation of workers by management looking for 'efficiency savings'.

In summary, clinical psychology and its allied psy-disciplines are positioned, for the most part, as a more-or-less-knowing accomplice to the medical profession of psychiatry in developing nosologies of human conduct that categorize our thoughts, deeds and whole persons as deviant. Claims that such an endeavour is 'scientific' are made to maintain psychology's position in the labour force and market place rather than as a genuine reflection of psychology praxis. At one level, psychology operates as part of the gaze, defining normality by default and maintaining a societal status quo through the observation and assessment of supposed 'abnormality'.

Thus summarized, clinical psychology might be seen as a relatively benign, indeed normal profession – no more, in Bernard Shaw's (1908) terms, than an everyday 'conspiracy against the laity'. In the next section, through the prism of deathmaking, I explore the ways in which this particular conspiracy appears malign.

Toxic (clinical) psychology?

From the very early days of professional clinical psychology in the UK, clinical psychologists have been involved in *incarcerating* members of the public. This may be as part of so-called risk assessment protocols given to people under the auspices of either the criminal justice or psychiatric systems. Clinical psychologists have consistently offered assessment or therapy within institutional settings where citizens are held against their will from psychiatric units utilizing holding powers under the Mental Health Act to prisons and specialist centres for the criminally insane or learning disabled, for example, Broadmoor, Ashworth and Rampton hospitals. *Incarceration* is but one potential feature of *distantiation* and clinical and educational psychologists have a long history of involvement (or, indeed, *encouragement*) in the removal of individuals – 'in their best interests' – to specialist centres where unwanted or challenging members of society are clustered together away from public view.

Physical invasion without consent is one way in which psychiatric and similar systems add to the destruction of the spirit. It is a rare clinical psychologist who speaks publicly about forced injections in psychiatric units (equally, it is a rare psychiatric nurse who feels able to voice concerns). In 40 years of publication the monthly in-house journal of the Division of Clinical Psychology, *Clinical Psychology Forum*, has not published *one* article about forced injection of patients. In this way clinical psychologists can be seen to condone such practices without being put in the position of injecting patients themselves.

It is a commonplace that people receiving so-called mental health services, children and those with learning disabilities receive *little or no relevant and understandable information* about the reasons for their referral to a clinical psychologist. Patients are thus not treated with respect and frequently the much promoted option of choice is neglected altogether. How can you choose if you don't know what you have been referred to and have little or no information about your diagnosis and the likely approach of the professional you are to see?

Until recently in the UK state system patients attending clinical psychology appointments were not routinely given *access to personal files*. Thus, incorrect factual information could easily remain unchecked for as long as files were held (even this is a grey area: various rules exist for the destruction of psychiatric and similar records but I am unaware of *anywhere* which has a system in place for acting on the destruction policy). Ironically, the collection of files on deviant individuals is one area where the gaze is at its most inefficient – records are kept, but rarely read and frequently lost; rather like CCTV cameras, it only *appears* that Big Brother is watching.

As noted above, clinical psychologists are actively involved in *assessing* and *labelling* people. In the UK, psychometric assessment was one of the main branches of the profession (alongside behavioural therapy and psychodynamic therapy) in the early 1950s; John Raven led the way at the Crighton Royal Hospital near Dumfries. Assessment invariably leads to a label, rarely the kind of 'mark' esteemed by the general public. Thus people can be described as deviant in a huge number of ways. It has been argued that describing a child as suffering from Attention Deficit Hyperactivity Disorder brings necessary services to the child in the form of medication and other 'help'. Equally, much needed financial benefits (in the form of Disability Living Allowance), may follow a diagnosis, parents will be excused blame for their child's conduct on the basis that the child is 'ill', teachers may receive additional classroom support and so on.

In such a well-balanced – and apparently mutually beneficial – system it can be difficult to remember that the child is being given toxic and experimental drugs that 'work' by effectively overdosing his metabolism. There are increasing claims that children who are difficult to manage have a neuro-developmental disorder. The phrase 'neuro-developmental disorder' is one aspect of a lexicon designed to simultaneously obscure meaning and give power to 'those that know' – in this case so-called child experts. In fact we have no idea how any given individual is meant to develop neurologically, nor can we readily know that a person is neurologically disordered from casual behavioural observation. Yet ADHD is solely diagnosed through such observation and clinical psychologists then *infer* a neurological problem. This is perfectly in step with child psychiatrists who then prescribe medication in order to suppress the conduct. Moreover drugs such as Ritalin become access drugs for illegal and very similar stimulants like speed (amphetamine) and cocaine and, of course, the very existence of that first diagnosis points to a future 'career' in human services for the growing child. In an age of ferocious drug company marketing it is no accident that the diagnosis of ADHD has risen a hundred fold in the UK in the last 20 years (McHoul & Rapley, 2005; Timimi, this volume; Timimi & Radcliffe, 2005).

This last example of the *physical harm* meted out to recipients of services is one which illustrates the bystander mentality of many professions allied to medicine or its sub-discipline, psychiatry. No doubt many clinical psychologists would be appalled by the charge that they are implicated in a system which harms individuals: a cursory glance through clinical psychology journals would, however, indicate few examples of clinical psychologists speaking out against complicity in harmful services (Newnes, 2001) and numberless examples of authors supporting the status quo of assessment and treatment in the context of such services.

What of clinical psychologists who work in services for older people? Older people are – by far – the largest group receiving ECT in the world today, a procedure described as an 'electrical lobotomy' (Breggin, 1998). Clinical psychologists working in services for older people frequently offer therapeutic alternatives (the eclectic position) to electrocution but the Zeitgeist is such that the majority of persons over the age of 65 'marked' as depressed will receive drug treatment or ECT rather than kindly comfort from a middle-class psy-professional. Again, clinical psychologists are hesitant to take up a position of active and public conflict with medical colleagues pursuing physically damaging ends for their patients. Indeed, like many journalists and members of the public, there are many qualifying clinical psychologists unaware that ECT – as a treatment option – even still *exists* and are horrified to discover that it is the *treatment of choice* for many older people diagnosed as depressed. Again, this ignorance has not been ameliorated – nor should it be excused – by the fact that only *one* article in the last 30 years in the in-house journal for UK clinical psychologists has addressed the issue (Newnes, 1991).

As a profession clinical psychology and indeed educational psychology and their parent discipline, psychology, sit firmly near the top of the income hierarchy. It should not be surprising that the vested interest in supporting that hierarchy is – in the main – glossed over by the profession (Smail, 2005). The profession nests in a cultural context wherein sexism, racism and ageism are endemic – various protocols promulgated by clinical psychologists reflect all three positions for example, the use of the Wechsler Adult Intelligence Scale for measuring IQ; a scale that explicitly includes norms for men *and* women as if they are a different species when in fact Wechsler introduced the different norms as soon as he – rapidly – realized that women scored *higher* than men. One aspect of the profession – those accepted for clinical psychology training – reveals a gender and race bias wholly different from many other professions. The overwhelming majority of psychology graduates are women in their early-twenties. As – for no demonstrably useful reason – an upper second degree in psychology remains the basis for potential acceptance on a state funded Doctorate in Clinical Psychology it should be no surprise that in excess of 90 per cent of newly qualified clinical psychologists are women, the majority white and in their mid-twenties. As a psycho-*technology* the profession thus continues an erosion of the role of men as foreseen by Engels – who predicted 170 years ago that the family would be undermined as men in work were replaced by women who were cheaper, more malleable and more efficient at operating machinery (Engels, 1845). But what if you happen to be an elderly Jamaican man who has waited 30 minutes for a delayed bus to get to a therapy session with a well-paid, car-owning white, female, doctoral professional in her mid-twenties? Would you want to tell her anything that might lead to her offering genuine assistance – like the truth about your lack of money or the state of your council house?

Clinical psychologists should not be seen as operating in bad faith. Many take for granted that there is an internal world that can be accurately described and assume that links between our conduct and various brain functions have been proven. Similarly, many work in multi-disciplinary teams where the expression of doubt in any shared model of conduct – be it the idea of madness, brain–biochemical imbalance or the parlous condition of modern housing estates – is socially undesirable and a slight on colleagues. All will have been inducted into the modern obsession with the importance of the brain and numerous psychological theories based on so-called human attributes like personality, cognitive schemas and the like. There are exceptions to this rule and a small cadre of professional psychologists takes very seriously indeed, notions of social construction. But it hardly matters – they still take an income from a social framework which declares them experts and, by comparison with the numbers in the majority (there are more than 100,000 clinical psychologists trained in the individualistic modernist framework in the United States alone), their constituency barely raises a voice.

In this respect clinical psychology remains firmly embedded in the professional hierarchy that enacts death making in its many guises. Failure to speak out at multi-disciplinary meetings is only part of the sorry story. Though trained in research methodology clinical psychologists tend to research subjects who have already been psychiatrically diagnosed or psychologically labelled and apply a myriad of therapies that are wholly individualistic at their core – 'Think this and you'll feel different', 'Keep a stress diary and it will help', 'Tell me your dreams and I'll explain them', and so on. In this way psychologists maintain their position of privilege and deny individuals the right to protest collectively.

A final irony

A few years back a colleague and I conducted a series of seminars for clinical psychologists entitled 'Prescribing Rights'. We were interested in seeing what proportion of psychologists – supposedly against physical interventions – would not wish to pursue the trend in the US whereby clinical psychologists are gaining the right to prescribe medication. Despite a full day exercise outlining the physical harm *inherent in any psychotropic drug*, a quarter of participants ended the training by saying they wanted the right to prescribe; some even said they wanted the drug companies on their side so they would receive, like psychiatric colleagues, free lunches and computer equipment. Their rationale was familiar – somehow, unlike their psychiatric colleagues, they would know better and therefore prescribe lower doses of medication to patients. (In the US, these prescribing rights have been claimed in a number of states and thus far there are no clear data demonstrating any overall reduction in prescribing; common sense, however, would suggest that drug companies would only promote prescribing by non-medical personnel if prescriptions increase.)

These seminars illuminate a final irony in the world of professional clinical psychology. Despite the profession-generated myth that clinical psychologists are determinedly anti-psychiatric, many not only ape medical colleagues in the use of diagnosis or so-called treatment but also are silent when it comes to opposing medically defined ills and aid. Clinical psychologists barely come over the parapet in their anti-psychiatric credentials. Breggin, Healy, Jackson, the Critical Psychiatry Network, even Laing have been outspoken critics of psychiatry – all of them psychiatrists. Instead of speaking out, clinical psychology has played a politically astute game of alternating between *compliance* and *eclecticism* to ensure the profession's survival. That it has contributed to the spiritual and physical deaths of thousands might be regarded as an unfortunate necessity.

17
Psychotherapy: Illusion with No Future?

David Smail

Having spent the past 50 years involved in, and thinking about therapeutic psychology I find myself, with some embarrassment, coming to the inescapable view that for much of that time I, along with so many others, have been pursuing an illusion. Therapeutic psychology may just prove to be the great red herring of the twentieth century, a masterstroke of ideology which has managed to obscure from our view the full significance for our emotional suffering of the workings of material reality. Instead of seeing with absolute clarity that what makes people happy or sad, triumphant or despairing, lucid or confused, is a function of what happens to them in the real, material world which lies beyond their skin, our view has become clouded by a haze congealing all too easily into a mirage of personal responsibility and control. We are deceived into believing that mastery of our fate follows from the deployment of our psychological resources as private individuals.

Not everyone, of course, has succumbed to this illusion, and it may have been much more dominant in the capitalist West than in the – until fairly recently – communist East. It is striking that, despite the cultural breadth of his view, Eric Hobsbawm makes absolutely no mention of psychology and psychotherapy in his absorbing account of the 'short twentieth century' (Hobsbawm, 1994). Freud doesn't appear in the index to *Age of Extremes*, nor do any of the other psychological architects of our notions of self. In some ways this must be regarded as an oversight on Hobsbawm's part, but in another it is an excellent indication of the importance of psychological ideas for the actual events of the time. The century which Isaiah Berlin characterized as the 'most terrible in Western history' unrolled at the behest of powers scarcely glanced at by the likes of Freud and Jung, Rogers, Perls or Berne.

And yet if psychological notions have been largely irrelevant to the actual course of events of the last 100 years or so, and have failed to have any significant impact on the suffering that they have occasioned, in some ways this could still be called the Century of Psychology. Certainly in the so-called liberal democracies, there can be hardly anyone who hasn't derived their view of self, and ideas about the scope of personal responsibility, from the kind of 'dynamic' psychological approach whose origins are attributed to Sigmund Freud.

Freudianism has enjoyed a remarkable revival in Britain over the past 30 years, and even within academic psychology, traditionally most suspicious of Freud's ideas, psychoanalysis has enjoyed a surprising rehabilitation. In the United States, of course, Freud has had a strong following right from the early years of the twentieth century. If one regarded Freud's contribution as being simply about founding a system of therapy for the relief of psychological distress, his success would be hard to explain, because the evidence for the effectiveness of psychoanalysis as a therapeutic medium is slender, if not non-existent. Rather, Freud has to be regarded as the great ideologue of the Western World (Marx, of course, being – for a considerable period, anyway – his counterpart in the East). I don't suppose Freud would have been terribly happy to think that he might come to be seen in this role, but there is something about his ability as a psychological sophist; his genius for performing the conceptual conjuring tricks which can turn black into white, reality into imagination (and vice-versa); his literary skill in fudging arguments and obscuring the stuffy bourgeois morality underlying them, which makes him the ideal person to provide an intellectual backing for the capitalist world. For this world depends for its survival on a huge, docile consumership instantly internalizing manufactured needs and exquisitely vulnerable to endless cycles of changing fashion, and psychoanalysis is a marvellous medium for making 'all that is solid melt into air' – while convincing those driven to distraction by the process that somehow it is all their own fault.

This is not to suggest that Freud was some kind of evil genius deliberately weaving woolly notions to pull over the eyes of the masses, but rather that, inevitably caught up himself in the inescapable net of capitalist socio-economic relations, he was drawn quite without noticing into constructing some of the most influential conceptual foundations for it. And if I seem to be giving particular prominence in what follows to Freud's writing, it is not because psychoanalysis is necessarily the most widespread psychotherapeutic system in operation today, but because Freud, in constructing the philosophical and moral framework of therapeutic psychology, was intellectually streets ahead of his professional successors who, though they have quarrelled endlessly over details of therapeutic practice, have hardly questioned the fundamental tenets of the therapeutic enterprise.

Freud's achievement, then, was to detach the person from the noxious influences of a real, material world, and render the causes of their suffering imaginary and, simultaneously, to remove from people the right to judge the significance of their own actions, while at the same time affirming their personal moral responsibility for the ills befalling them. These two processes combine to establish a comprehensive psychological privatism that all but destroys the possibility for credible political understanding and action. Let me try to give some substance to these allegations.

The claim that Freud rendered the causes of suffering imaginary might seem to be refuted by his oft-quoted view that 'hysterical misery' is but a perverted form of 'common unhappiness'. What he actually wrote was as follows:

> "Why, you tell me yourself that my illness is probably connected with my circumstances and the events of my life. You cannot alter these in any way. How do you propose to help me, then?" And I have been able to make this reply: "No doubt fate would find it easier than I do to relieve you of your illness. But you will be able to convince yourself that much will be gained if we succeed in transforming your hysterical misery into common unhappiness. With a mental life that has been restored to health you will be better armed against that unhappiness."
>
> (Freud, 1974: 393)

For me, the most significant aspect of the view Freud articulates here – a view with which I have some sympathy – is that, it was one he shortly afterwards abandoned. It was in fact written in 1895, very much towards the beginning of the development of Freud's ideas, and reflected his experience that the so-called neurotic symptoms of his mainly young, female patients seemed surprisingly often to be related to sexual traumata that had befallen them in childhood (that sexual abuse, especially by members of their family, happens to children disturbingly frequently is something that we have of course rediscovered in much more recent times (see Johnstone, Vetere, Dillon, this volume)).

At this stage, then, Freud seemed to have embarked upon the thesis that psychological disturbance in later life was likely to be the consequence of actual injuries sustained earlier on in infancy and childhood. He quickly discovered, however, that this was not a popular view, and, as has been persuasively documented by Jeffrey Masson in *The Assault on Truth* (Masson 1984), Freud very soon revised his view fundamentally, suggesting instead that the sexual assaults and seductions which seemed to lurk behind his patients' distress were in fact the products of their own wishful fantasy. Far from being the result of painful and damaging abuses of power, his patients' symptoms were thus transformed into events that they guiltily wished to have happened.

One can see that this revision of his theory must have brought Freud considerable relief: quite apart from mitigating some of the odium in which he had found himself with colleagues, it no doubt made it easier for him to make a living. Freud himself never seems seriously to have considered as psychologically important the kinds of material necessities which form such a prominent part of the motivation of the great mass of humanity, but there is no doubt that he was at this time of his life greatly preoccupied with the need to make ends meet, and it must have been easier for him to persuade the senior male members of his patients' households to pay his bills if they were not at the same time being accused of incestuously assaulting their offspring. It is particularly relevant at this point to quote a passage written by Freud in a letter to his friend Wilhelm Fliess around this time, as it demonstrates how acutely aware Freud was of material necessity in his personal circumstances while insisting in his writings on the primacy of fantasy for everyone else.

> A patient of mine with whom I have been negotiating, a 'goldfish', has just announced herself – I do not know whether to decline or accept. My mood also depends very strongly on my earnings. Money is laughing gas for me. I know from my youth that once the wild horses of the pampas have been lassoed, they retain a certain anxiousness for life. Thus I have come to know the helplessness of poverty and continually fear it. You will see that my style will improve and my ideas will be more correct if this city provides me with an ample livelihood.
>
> (Freud, quoted in Masson, 1984: Letter of 21.9.1899, 374)

So there was nothing very reflexive about Freud's psychology: goose and gander had distinctly different diets, and while Freud himself constantly worried about money, power and influence, the world for those who were the objects of his study was collapsed into the contents of their 'psyches'. What made *them* tick was the (largely) morally repugnant contents of their 'Unconscious', which for the sake of their psychological health had to be 'interpreted' by a psychoanalyst such that 'Id' was 'transformed' into 'Ego'. What was actually going on in the world around people, together with what had actually taken place in their past, were explicitly ruled irrelevant to their mental state by psychoanalysis, which insisted instead on the fundamental significance of the individual's psychic apparatus, which in turn could be understood and influenced solely through the carefully guarded and esoteric arts of psychoanalysis itself.

Not the least important aspect of this process was the morality it espoused. Responsibility for their predicament lay squarely with patients themselves. True, they would not be considered by most psychoanalysts to be exactly in control of their own fate (that privilege would depend on how far they were able to make use of the benefits of analysis), but they would certainly be held responsible for it, and somewhere buried in the middle of the technical verbiage is, as in all brands of psychotherapy which have been concocted since, an extremely naive view of 'will power'. Essentially, this encompasses the view that once someone sees the reasons for their conduct (as revealed, in the case of psychoanalysis, by 'insight' gained from the interpretations of the analyst) they may be expected to adjust their previously 'neurotic' conduct by means of an act of will.

Freud was of course always at pains to invoke the authority of 'science' for his position and it was doubtless his scientific aspirations which led him to develop the notion of 'psychic determinism' as a means of rendering human conduct amenable to the technical operations of psychoanalysis. But the result seems to be merely cosmetic. In fact 'psychic determinism' seems to mean little more than the shifting of everyday cultural ideas about blame and responsibility and the operation of will power from one mental sphere (the conscious) to another (the unconscious). For example, modestly claiming a triumph for the interpretative art of psychoanalysis in revealing the origin of 'parapraxes' such as slips of the tongue, Freud wrote that such events were strictly determined and revealed as an expression of the subject's suppressed intentions or a clash between two intentions, one of which was permanently or temporarily unconscious (Freud 1986). All that seems to have happened here is that Freud has transferred the processes of will from the conscious to the unconscious mind; unconscious mental acts come about in exactly the same way as conscious ones, apart, of course, from the individual's not knowing about them.

That Freud was unable to free himself from a very mundane – one might be tempted to say *petit bourgeois* – conception of morality is demonstrated particularly clearly in his treatment of the Oedipus legend. In a fascinating passage in one of his *Introductory Lectures*, written, interestingly, only a year or two before the outbreak of World War I (Freud 1973), Freud chides Sophocles for the 'amorality' of his treatment of the Oedipus legend. How Freud managed to derive his version of the Oedipus Complex (in which the male child wishfully fantasizes the sexual conquest of his mother and the destruction of his father) from Sophocles' tragedy (in which Oedipus is fated to fulfill the oracle's prediction that he will murder his father and marry his mother) is a mystery. But this passage makes it plain: Freud simply dismisses the tragedian's concern with the relation between Oedipus and powers greater than and outside himself (the Gods), and wrenches the structure of the work into a form which will support his own, entirely contrary notion of internalized will and unconscious morality. Completely disregarding the fact that Oedipus is overtaken by fate despite the best efforts of all to avoid its coming to pass, and tries, desperately and unsuccessfully, to discharge his duty by obeying the dictates of superior power, Freud maintains instead that there is a 'secret sense and content of the legend' to which the auditor reacts.

> He reacts as though by self-analysis he had recognized the Oedipus complex in himself and had unveiled the will of the gods and the oracle as exalted disguises of his own unconscious. It is as though he was obliged to remember the two wishes – to do away with his father and in place of him to take his mother to wife – and to be horrified at them. And he understands the dramatist's voice as though it were saying to him: 'You are struggling in vain against your responsibility and are protesting in vain of what you have done in opposition to these criminal intentions. You are guilty, for you have not been able to destroy them; they still persist in you unconsciously.' And there is psychological truth in this. Even if a man has repressed his evil impulses into the unconscious and would like to tell himself afterwards that he is not responsible for them, he is nevertheless bound to be aware of this responsibility as a sense of guilt whose basis is unknown to him.
>
> (Freud, 1973: 374)

To arrive at this interpretation, Freud has to mutilate Sophocles' play in order, like a cuckoo, to install within it his own brainchild. The tragic inevitability of Oedipus's innocent fulfilment of the Oracle's prophecy, and his horror at the discovery that it has indeed come to pass, are turned by Freud, as of course were the violations of his patients by their male relatives, into matters of personal responsibility. Instead of the kind of objective analysis of the working on individuals of powers beyond their control which might lead to a compassionate solidarity with them (much more Sophocles's intention, of course), we are offered an account in terms of 'evil impulses' for which 'we like to tell [our]selves afterwards that [we] are not responsible' an account typical of the kind of moral bigotry which makes rape victims complicit in the crime which has been perpetrated upon them. Indeed, this is moralism with knobs on: the individual is placed in a moral double-Nelson. Not only are we to be held responsible for our conduct, but we are also guilty of repressing our knowledge of that responsibility so that it has to be elucidated for us by a professional expert (the analyst) before we have an opportunity for atonement.

In fact, the kind of social philosophy underlying Freud's moralism is all too clear, and expressed quite unashamedly in his *The Future of an Illusion*. It's all a question of ignorant masses and enlightened leaders. The masses, he writes,

> are lazy and unintelligent; they have no love for instinctual renunciation, and they are not to be convinced by argument of its inevitability; and the individuals composing them support one another in giving free reign to their indiscipline. It is only through the influence of individuals who can set an example and whom masses recognize as their leaders that they can be induced to perform the work and undergo the renunciations on which the existence of civilization depends. All is well if these leaders are persons who possess superior insight into the necessities of life and who have risen to the height of mastering their own instinctual wishes. There is a danger that in order not to lose their influence they may give way to the mass more than it gives way to them, and it therefore seems necessary that they shall be independent of the mass by having means to power at their disposal. To put it briefly, there are two widespread human characteristics which are responsible for the fact that the regulations of civilization can only be maintained by a certain degree of coercion – namely, that men are not spontaneously fond of work and that arguments are of no avail against their passions.
>
> (Freud, 1985: 186)

Freud goes on to pour scorn on religion as a means of containing and disciplining the masses, but certainly does not notice that in proffering psychoanalysis as the (scientific) answer he is simply replacing one opiate with another. Rather than criticizing religion, he was competing with it. In fact, over the first three decades of this century what Freud did was to lay the foundations of a psychotherapeutic ideology that, whether explicitly or not, underpins all subsequent approaches in the field. To summarize the psychotherapeutic credo, then, the fundamental propositions of the therapeutic state would seem to be as follows:

- Psychological distress arises not from the *injuries inflicted by a material social environment*, but from the *desires and fantasies* (and more recently, from the *faulty cognitions*) of individuals themselves.
- Although desires, fantasies and cognitions are largely unconscious and/or 'automatic', the rules of conventional morality still apply: people are 'responsible' for their distress, and guilt over its causes is not inappropriate, even if the way to expiation is only to be found through engagement in the formal process of psychoanalysis/ psychotherapy.
- The functioning of society requires that for the mass of ordinary people some kind of disciplinary procedure is necessary if their natural inclination to indolence and anti-social conduct is to be contained. In contrast to the illusory and increasingly discredited rules and dogmas of religion, psychology offers the scientific means of achieving this discipline.

We do not of course have to be aware of the conceptual underpinnings of our practice, and the fact that many psychotherapists today would dissent emphatically from so blunt a statement of this basic therapeutic creed does not invalidate it. The whole manner and context of the practice of psychotherapy betrays its most basic assumptions, that is, that people are responsible for their suffering and that in the final analysis its up to them to will the appropriate changes to their lives. The fact that these assumptions are clearly false, and that, moreover, there is not a shred of evidence for the effectiveness of the therapeutic practices which are based upon them further betrays the fundamental rationale of psychotherapy: to represent social damage as personal failure and to transmute potential political dissent into an anxious concern with individual adjustment.

The only way we can explain the continued existence – indeed the positive flourishing – of psychotherapy since the serious doubts which were raised about its efficacy in the middle of the last century (particularly by H. J. Eysenck), is through the recognition that it serves some purpose other than the therapeutic. Psychotherapy has of course had its scientific apologists, and there is a truly vast literature on the supposedly objective measurement of its apparent benefits, but even these justify no more sanguine a conclusion than that psychotherapy, in the safest and most experienced hands, is only marginally more effective than the healing passage of time. However, Epstein has more recently launched several spanners into the psychotherapeutic works that could prove even more destructive than Eysenck's efforts in the 1950s.

In *The Illusion of Psychotherapy* (Epstein, 1995) and *Psychotherapy as Religion* (Epstein 2006), he systematically demolishes the propsycho-therapy research literature in a way which, though it scarcely disguises his own partiality, leaves very little comfort to anyone wishing to claim that, on any conventional understanding of 'evidence', the practice of psychotherapy can be justified by its demonstrable results. Epstein contends that the reason for the continued thriving of psychotherapy – despite its ineffectiveness – is precisely its political expediency. He suggests that psychotherapy is

> an immensely attractive strategy for a society that is reluctant to allocate substantial funds to address its problems. If it were effec-tive, then psychotherapy would offer efficient, low-cost remedies. Yet, even apart from the issue of its effectiveness, psychotherapy still provides a useful vehicle to proselytise the ideology of social efficiency in evading more productive and expensive approaches to social problems ... [T]he ideology of therapeutics is ... consistent with a conservative social ideology that is unwilling to accept broad-based social expenditures to provide greater social equality through government action.
>
> (Epstein, 1995: 6)

Epstein's achievement is to hoist psychotherapy researchers by their own petard – including devotees of currently fashionable cognitive behavioural therapy – and leave the official apologetics of psychotherapy in tatters. Even if the profession treats Epstein's thesis with disdainful silence, his books nevertheless demonstrate that the future of an essentially illusory psychotherapy industry is vulnerable to exactly the kind of analysis by means of which it has sought to justify itself.

But there are other, personally more compelling, reasons for questioning the efficacy of psychotherapy, not least of which is that, in my case anyway, a lifetime's practice as a clinical psychologist reveals precisely the opposite of what is usually theoretically claimed for it: people are not responsible for their distress, cannot 'change' themselves from the inside, but are, so to speak, fixed in place by the social powers enveloping them.

Working in a publicly funded health service with people whose resources – or rather lack of them – leave them very few options when it comes to deciding how to order their lives makes it obvious how 'choice' and 'will power' are epiphenomena of material advantage, rather than the innate moral potentialities which, explicitly or not, psychotherapy suggests they are. I have too often come across people with perfect insight into the reasons for their distress, who are absolutely desperate to change things, who struggle with enormous courage against all the odds, and who in the end succumb to the overwhelming influences which have damaged them in the past or oppress them in the present, too often, to believe any more in the potency of psychotherapeutic magic.

Certainly, well-educated, relatively affluent, relatively socially well-connected people may make use of the opportunity for reflection on their situation afforded by psychotherapy to redeploy their assets or formulate strategies to better their lot. The richest may buy a five-times-a-week psychoanalyst to act as a kind of personal confidant, providing solidarity in their troubles for as long as they can afford to pay. But for ordinary people, that which shapes their lives and, too often, causes them pain, is a combination of powers and influences well beyond their own or any therapist's ability to control. Epstein is absolutely right to point out that the ideology of psychotherapy serves principally to divert our gaze from the real causes of our troubles in the outside environment. Instead, we are offered a moralistic appraisal of our so-called inner worlds, the provision of which (we are assured) will fuel feats of will power, flashes of insight and engineerings of attitudes that will 'adjust' us better to a reality taken as given and immutable.

A psychological analysis of personal distress must, in my view, diagnose not individuals, but their environments. What we need is not the moral crusade of psychotherapy, in which our ills are made a matter of 'responsibility', but the patient laying-bare of the social and material structures through which oppressive power is transmitted and which ends up impinging on the individual's body as the sensation of pain. What we then do about these structures is not a matter for psychology, but inescapably, for politics.

As it is, most people, conditioned by over a century of dynamic psychology and its offshoots, have very little understanding of the origins of their own distress and are profoundly mystified as to its nature and significance. The commonest reactions to distress are probably panic and guilt, at once a terror of 'abnormality' and an intimation of responsibility for it. Let me give as an example a description of a predicament widespread among younger people who grew up in the Regan/Thatcher years, and particularly noticeable in the student population with whom I was working around the turn of this century.

The subjective experience was primarily one of anxiety, but not about anything specific. Rather, young people described experiencing a *pervasive uncertainty* about whether what they were feeling and thinking were appropriate, whether they were 'like' other people or seemed strange to them, and this uncertainty flared from time to time into seemingly uncontainable panic – 'freaking-out', as it was often put. The degree of subjective suffering attached to this state seemed out of all proportion to the person's actual ability to cope. Sufferers were often intelligent, competent students able to cope well with the intellectual demands made on them (though exams could become a serious obstacle) and even functioning socially quite effectively – they had friends, social networks, active lives and seemed outwardly well-adapted to student life. And yet under the surface were profound doubts and anxiety about the validity of their own experience – which at its worst looked very like the uncontrolled terror and distress of an abandoned baby.

Another interesting feature was an *impairment of desire*. Young people often said that they had absolutely no idea of what they really wanted. Whether courses of study, prospective jobs, choices of girl- or boy-friend, outside-work activities or even food, they seemed devoid of an internalized arbiter of taste, no flash of lust, no gut feeling to guide their conduct. Choices had to be arrived at by some kind of, prosthetic device. I asked one young man to imagine being really hungry in a wonderful restaurant, money no object – what would he choose from the limitless menu? He wrestled with this for some time. 'I really don't know', he said. 'I suppose I'd have to choose the most expensive.'[1]

The things which particularly 'freaked out' young people suffering in this way were very often experiences which are simply the unavoidable lot of human beings as they grow up. One of the most frequent was, put at its simplest, love. I encountered several students, young men and women, who were panicked to the point of incapacity by meeting someone whom they were seriously attracted to. Casual relationships were unproblematic (and taken or left), but the experience which used to be referred to as 'falling in love' seemed often to be simply unmanageable. The bodily feelings that overwhelmed them were experienced as alien, utterly confusing, frightening; the obsession with the beloved was felt as an intolerable form of derangement. It was if they had never come across any understanding of this condition in our culture, had read no novel nor seen any film which made intelligible the experience of falling in love. The beloved was not experienced as *desired*, but as dangerous, even terrifying.

It was extremely difficult to shift people who found themselves in this condition from a view of themselves as personally and morally defective, to seeing that they were perfectly intact individuals whose lack of understanding about the nature and origins of their experience was the result of deprived environments ('I'm such a sad git; why can't I get a grip on myself?' was typical). To give a full account of the nature of this deprivation, one would have to go beyond immediate factors such as parental influence (or, perhaps better, a *lack* of parental influence) to the socio-economic settings shaping those factors.

Just to hint at what some of these influences might be, many of the students were brought up in homes where their parents (often, but not always, professional people from working-class backgrounds) were struggling with the aspirations of upward mobility, the insecurity consequent upon threats to their jobs, an almost irresistible belief in the importance of 'image', or 'appearances', and the consumerist philosophy underpinning it. Preoccupied by their own struggles for survival, difficulties in relationships generated by profound changes in the job market and, consequently, male and female roles, their parents did not realize that their children needed instruction in *what it is to be a human being*. In particular, the closest thing to a meaningful relationship some of the boys had, was with the computer their parents were so keen to provide them with. You can pick up a good sense of binary logic, what passes for human intimacy in massively available pornography, or quick draw techniques for destroying aliens by spending hours with computers, but not much of an idea of *human desire* and what to do with it. A significant proportion of this generation, it seems, were brought up with a kind of crude, bottom-line instrumentality, a basic survival kit for a 'real world' consisting of a disorientating combination of hostile competition and consumerist fantasy, but very little appreciation of the warm flesh and blood of embodied humanity.

When it comes to the conduct of our lives in the present, the cultural message we are given, heavily endorsed by the psychotherapy industry, is that our survival and success depend on our personal initiative and our ability to exercise responsibility (precisely the attributes so stifled, we are led to believe, by the 'outmoded' welfare state). This view, in fact, entirely fails to recognize that what enables us to live reasonably comfortably in the social world is the kind of exoskeleton provided by its institutions – we cannot hold ourselves together psychologically *just* by our own internal structures.

There needs to be a world of which any young person can become part, and by 'world' I mean, among other things, the provision of a range of valued social roles. As it is, the young, as increasingly the old, find themselves an impediment to social worth. Far from being beckoned into a society which has need of them, even the relatively advantaged young are grudgingly loaned the means of an education which is seen as a personal privilege of dubious value rather than a social need, and at the end of their period of study they are left to cobble together the means of their livelihood with very little in the way of social approbation – unless, that is, they have a vocation for banking, finance or business administration. Understandable enough, in circumstances such as these, to feel lost and panicky.

There is in fact no form of psychological distress not best understood as damage done to people by the world they inhabit, past and present. We will make no impact on distress by holding ourselves responsible for it and/or trying to tinker with the psychological processes through which the world is experienced. We need to detach ourselves from the illusory promises of psychological therapy and turn our attention to making the world a more comfortable place for people to live in. It is hard to judge how much longer the hotchpotch of 'postmodern' make-believe and crude business pragmatism, which constitute present-day culture, can maintain their symbiotic relationship with the ideology of psychotherapy. The sooner reality intrudes, the better.

18
The Psychologization of Torture

Nimisha Patel

> The whole world should see what they did – but even
> when they see they don't care ... we are being crushed
> like ants, like we are nothing, nothing ... so tell me, what
> are my human rights if I am not even human to others?
>
> A survivor of torture

Introduction

Torture, one of the absolute prohibitions in international humanitarian, human rights and criminal law, has fallen victim to psychology, and in ways which have obscured the essentially moral (and, since 1948, the legal) position that torture, as deliberate, state-sanctioned violence towards another human being is wrong, should be stopped and should be remedied. How we use psychology to address torture, largely by an unquestioning reliance on dominant discourses of 'trauma', as well as some of the possibilities beyond the psychologization of gross human-rights violations, is the focus of this chapter. Underlying my argument is the dilemma that I wrestle with: in the face of unimaginable brutality and profound distress, why shouldn't we do all we can, even if it means disguising the limitations of psychology and the masquerade of a professional identity, when we are engaged in the politicization of distress? The risk is that, whether we draw on psychology or human-rights law, when we talk of justice, redress and well-being we forget we are talking about people, and what it means to be human.

The psychologization of torture

Dehumanizing persons, through various means, is arguably the precursor to systematic marginalization, persecution and torture. Torture is an extreme form of discrimination, deliberate violence, State-endorsed,

239

often used against marginalized people, on grounds of gender, sexuality, religion, political beliefs, ethnicity – for a purpose: to silence, terrorize, oppress and eliminate dissenting voices, individuals and communities. Its aims include the destruction of agency, and severance of trust, and hence social bonds within communities. In this sense, torture is an exertion of institutional power, 'a ritual display of the infinite power to punish' (Foucault, 2003: 85) and control. Torture is currently systematically used in over 159 countries by both State organs and non-State actors (Amnesty International, 2010), despite being an absolute prohibition in international law. Torture is a crime, a human rights violation. Needless to say, torture is not an illness, disease or syndrome.

For laypersons and psychologists alike, it should not be surprising that torture causes suffering and pain. As one torture survivor explains:

> They did things you cannot even imagine how they thought of this – they forced drugs by pushing injections in me when I was tied and blindfolded, they pulled my toe nails, one by one, they burnt me with cigarettes – all over my body, they pulled out chunks of my hair, they hung me upside down until I lost consciousness, they raped me, many of them, again and again ... they forced a baton and broken glass inside me, beating me, saying disgusting things to me ... you become aware of every part of your body, like you never knew what pain it could give you. I do not want this body anymore – every mark, every scar, every pain – all remind me what happened, what I am ... a person inside this marred body, when people look at me, do they see me or my scars? Do they see the emptiness in my eyes? Do they see my suffering, my nightmares, the things I saw in prison – things I will never forget? What do you see? Do you see me?

Feeling stripped of his humanness, he asks repeatedly 'Do you see me ... did they take that away from me?' While psychologists among others have sought to convey the horror of torture by describing in technical language what torture does to people, simply put, what torture does is to break moral codes and taboos, degrading and dehumanizing people, often causing unimaginable pain, anguish, suffering and misery. It intentionally targets not just the individual, but their family and communities in the service of oppression and social control.

How then have psychologists and other health professionals so successfully transformed torture into a psychological phenomenon, obscuring its political nature? Not by describing acts of torture, or examining its anatomy and socio-political context, but by examining the tortured individual and meticulously describing their 'symptoms' and 'disorders', arguably to highlight the harm inflicted. Torture survivors often do describe their suffering and 'symptoms' in detail, but not necessarily in forms psychologists would be familiar with. One man who had experienced brutal torture over several years in solitary confinement described his pain, and memories related to injuries to his spinal column, sustained as a result of torture thus:

> The pain is my friend, like my comrade. Every pain in every vertebra of my spine has a memory ... often I cannot sleep, or even stand up straight or walk because of the pain. The pain wakes me at night, then I fall asleep and wake up again after a nightmare, and the pain is still there, always there. The memories are terrible, they are like a library in my body – for each pain I can tell you a memory – of what I saw in prison, how they executed people, what torture they did to others, the screams from the other prisoners in the cells, seeing my father being blindfolded, pushed against the wall in the yard and then shot, the sound of the lorries coming before dawn to carry out the bodies of those killed ... hundreds of them ... I can tell you dates, images, smells, the time of day. These memories I never want to forget. This pain, it is both my enemy and my witness.

The sleeping difficulties, nightmares, visual and auditory memories, intense fear, sadness, profound grief, avoidance of interactions with others from his own country, persistent pain and disability and related functional difficulties – all for him, were the price of change, the human cost of challenging state oppression. The symptoms told a story, one he wished to be heard, not eliminated, alleviated or 'managed'. His suffering was often overwhelming, but he remained adamant: 'I am not sick, I am broken. They broke my body, they did something to my head ... but I am not sick, I am in pain.' Our discussions inevitably returned again and again to the purpose of talking and reaching a shared understanding that what we were engaged in during our 'therapeutic' conversations was perhaps no more than my bearing witness to what he had seen and endured, and that what we were doing in our talk was 'being human, together'.

Yet the health-related literature on torture is saturated with studies and professional accounts 'demonstrating' that torture 'causes' 'psychopathology'. The psychological field of torture is increasingly associated with 'traumatology', or 'victimology', documenting the psychological 'disorders' related to torture, some attempting theoretical explications of their relationship, bio-psychological mechanisms or processes, and considering effective 'treatments'. Thus, in the last 20 years, the discourse of trauma has become the dominant language used to convey the horror of torture, effortlessly conflating torture with trauma. The psychologization of torture is evident in several areas, summarized here.

Torture as biological

Psychology has traditionally resorted to biological explanations for the human capacity for, and 'predisposition' to, aggressive behaviour, as if torture were a wilful expression of individual viciousness, rather than State-sanctioned, systematically designed and administered, purposive violence. For example, gender-based persecution and torture (such as rape) in situations of armed conflict has been explained by emphasizing the biological basis for (men's) violence (to women), locating the problem in individual biological disposition, thereby constructing violence as inevitable, beyond the control of the individual. Torture, viewed as an act of aggression, a drive, is then made (apparently) meaningful without even a cursory glance towards the socio-political context in which it is practised and legitimated.

Torture as situational

Zimbardo's (2008) work offers explanations of torture which do not focus on individual predispositions to aggression, but on the environment – suggesting that under certain conditions, and certain environments, it is understandable that (most) individuals will succumb to situational pressures and engage in aggressive acts, including torture. In this sense torture is almost made meaningful, by implying that the problem is not the individual torturer, but the environment and situational pressures, locating blame in the environment, or its architects (as in the 'war on terror'), potentially absolving individuals of responsibility for atrocities. Ironically, these explanations rely on a familiar dichotomy – who or what is to blame – the individual (their biology or psychology), or the environment? Rather than theorize the relationship between socio-political context and torture in ways, which address the processes by which State responsibility is dissolved, obscured and transformed into individual responsibility, psychological explanations present the individual as responsible for perpetrating torture, yet seemingly as having no agency.

Torture as 'trauma'

With respect to torture, psychology has invested heavily in the trauma discourse. Most forms of violence have consequences in law and, unsurprisingly, both psychology and law collude to privilege objectivity and individualism, relying on notions of 'psychiatric disorder' to provide both 'scientific' explanations of, and 'evidence' for (acts of violence as well as its effects). Several psychiatric diagnoses have emerged in response to the punishment of perpetrators of violence (or its absence). For example, Post Traumatic Stress Disorder (PTSD) emerged in post-Vietnam USA, advocated by anti-war proponents demanding recognition of the injury and suffering sustained by veterans who, it was argued should be seen as ill and in need of psychiatric help, not punishment and judgement as 'baby killers' or 'murderers' (Young, 1995; Summerfield, 1999). Early proponents of 'Battered Women's Syndrome' (BWS) were, similarly, campaigners seeking to establish legal recognition of the 'syndrome' to explain why some women, in long-term abusive and violent relationships, kill their partners (Raitt & Zeedyk, 2000). 'Rape Trauma Syndrome' was allegedly 'discovered' in 1970s, and described as a potentially powerful tool in the prosecutor's armoury (Keogh, 2007) to establish lack of consent. Similarly, efforts by psychologists and psychiatrists to establish whether there is such a phenomenon as 'Torture Syndrome' were arguably driven not by psychological theories but, rather, by efforts to demonstrate the impact of torture, as part of a political struggle by legal, health and other professionals to challenge torture.

Laudable as they may be as efforts to challenge violence, these diagnoses have also been used to not only argue that the impact of violence is severe and can be enduring, but also to defend perpetrators. Diagnosis has conflated the *act* of violence, including torture (understood as 'trauma') with its *effects*, reproducing the dominant discourse of trauma. Some of the difficulties with the trauma discourse, particularly with regards to torture, are discussed below (see also Johnstone, this volume).

Firstly, assumptions are made of linear causal relationships between torture and its effects. Yet, torture is rarely a one-off event, usually being perpetrated repeatedly, over several periods of detention, and in the context of historical and enduring marginalization, persecution, other human rights violations and structural inequalities resulting in poverty, lack of access to education, healthcare, adequate housing and unemployment.

Secondly, in using diagnoses such as 'PTSD', there is an assumption that the impact of torture (ignoring the impact of other social inequalities and injustices) can be reliably captured in a categorization of symptoms, within the individual, and in ways which are universally valid, independent of theory and meaningful (to health professionals) (see Bracken et al., 1997; Summerfield, 1999, 2001; Patel, 2003).

Thirdly, the reliance on diagnosis to direct attention to 'trauma' neglects how trauma discourse relegates and regulates survivors' subjectivities with respect to how they make sense of their own experiences, if and how they seek help, and their expectations and efforts in recovery or in striving for justice. The emphasis is not on resilience, survival and agency, but vulnerability (a 'genetic vulnerability' or 'cultural vulnerability') as a predisposition to stress and psychiatric disorder, while pathologizing stoicism and silence (seen as 'denial', 'dissociation', 'passivity', 'emotional numbness' or 'shame'); problematizing meaning-making (for example, talk of seeing spirits, angels or ancestors, and of hearing the voices of comrades still imprisoned or killed are understood as 'hallucinations' and mistrust of and suspiciousness towards those in authority, health professionals or those from a person's own community is seen as 'paranoia').

Fourthly, the focus on effects of torture often excludes any analysis of the causes and the context in which distress and suffering develops, and related psycho-social-political processes. Thus, psychology invests energy and resources into studying effects, while not asking who did this? How? Why? What are the historical influences (for example subjugation and discrimination)? What are the current influences (e.g., poverty, homelessness, racism, missing family members, hostile immigration system) and context in which such practices continue with impunity? Furthermore, so narrow is our gaze that only 'effects' fitting pre-existing psychological models and psychiatric classification systems are captured – minimizing or ignoring those difficulties which cannot be expressed in terms of concepts we already have to hand. The failure to scrutinize the context of torture also extends to the absence of analysis of the multiplicity of identities of torture survivors, as produced within intersecting axes of power relations – for example, 'why are some people tortured?' is important to theorize. The intersection of gender and ethnicity is evident in the use of systematic rape and torture in armed conflicts (for example in Rwanda and Bosnia) and the intersection of gender, ethnicity and religion (in Kosovo). When we have no explanation for genocide, torture and 'ethnic cleansing', or why women may be complicit in the sexual torture of other women, or the torture of children, relatives, or those previously friends and neighbours, for example, we fail to meaningfully acknowledge our biased models and limited understandings, instead becoming more efficient at demonstrating how torture and other gross human rights violations 'cause' trauma and pathology. Similarly, we fail to name or examine the apparent contradictions in the use of violence, for example, in the 'military humanism' underlying international intervention in the war in Kosovo.

Further, in focussing on effects alone, trauma approaches pathologize distress and encourage the inference that diagnoses (such as PTSD) are themselves indicative of vulnerability, as a personal attribute. Hence, the person is 'vulnerable because they have a diagnosis', not that they were 'vulnerable to torture because of their ethnicity/religious beliefs/ political activity'. Perhaps more importantly they are vulnerable to being pathologized, dehumanized and reduced to a bag of fragmented symptoms, by us. As torture survivors and others note (see Johnstone, this volume; Summerfield, 1999) it is understandable that a person may react severely to extreme events. At what point a survivor's response to torture crosses the threshold into abnormality is essentially arbitrary and a moral question, exposing what health professionals judge to be a proportionate or 'appropriate' response to gross human rights violations. A diagnosis cannot attest to the severity, magnitude, gravity or immorality of torture, nor does its absence indicate that allegations of torture are false, not serious, or that the harm and suffering endured are within 'acceptable limits'. To assert that diagnoses are indicators for professional interventions renders the torture survivor a damaged, helpless person 'in need' of psychological technology to facilitate a return to 'normality'. The grandiosity and absurdity of this assumption is highlighted when we consider the millions of torture survivors globally, who function, notwithstanding immense suffering, debility and distress, without professional intervention – those who after release or escape from detention pursue political activities, employment, education and family life – risking repeated detention and torture, those who flee thousands of miles to seek asylum, but who do not present to health professionals, and those who find support, comfort, courage and solidarity with others in similar situations.

Sixthly, psychology's uncritical focus on distress at the level of the individual psyche has both disguised the impact of torture beyond the individual to their families, and ignored its effect on whole communities in terms of suspiciousness, mistrust, fragmentation and lack of cohesion, economic instability and impact on daily survival. Profound distress and suffering are individualized, as noted above, and the impact on communities quantified in studies, as if to objectively 'prove' the 'prevalence' of psychopathology in communities affected by conflict and torture. The individual's health is understood in Cartesian terms, as a collection of physical and psychological symptoms; and communities as a collection of individuals. Community well-being and survival, meaning-making and collective narratives remain largely untheorized and ignored. Distress is also conceptualized in terms of the individual's failure to cope, with responsibility for and capacity to change located within individuals, as if they should be able to self-transform, independently of their social, material and political context. Where the community's role in recovery and survival is addressed, responsibility for change, adaptation and forgiveness (seen as a means to reconciliation) remains with the very communities that have suffered torture and other violence and injustices.

Finally, trauma approaches inevitably de-politicize torture, ignoring the socio-political and economic contexts that contribute to and sustain torture, as illustrated by the almost exclusive focus on victims and 'their pathology', and the rarity of attention to perpetrators, including the State or non-State actors. The efficiency of psychology in de-politicizing torture is not surprising when we consider how persistently psychology has invested in being a 'science': objective, value-free and worthy of authority and public trust. Psychology has prized 'scientific neutrality' and, in clinical practice, emphasized and reified 'professional neutrality'. However, as Žižek (2005) reminds us, the *political* is the structuring principle in society, such that 'every neutralisation of some partial content as "non-political" is a political gesture par excellence'. In both regards, the stances of 'scientific' and 'professional' neutrality, while understandable responses to our own helplessness and impotence in not being able to adequately theorize or address global injustices and their impact, are nonetheless political gestures effectively condoning oppression, defending, legitimating and colluding with torture and its perpetrators, while locating blame and responsibility for change within the individual torture survivor.

Human rights: An antidote to the psychologization of distress?

If the psychologization of torture is to be rejected, can psychologists do anything to address torture, without psychologizing? Forays into other disciplines can be tempting, searching for alternative models and technologies to address what are, actually, primarily moral (rather than psychological) questions: why do people torture other people? Why do States endorse torture? Why do we look the other way? Should we try to stop torture, and how?

In much of my earlier writing, in arguing against the psychologiza-tion and pathologization of distress related to torture, I have advocated a human-rights-based approach to prevention of torture activities, psychological service development and practice with torture survivors. A human-rights approach is not a therapy, or a method, rather a politi-cal and moral stance that reorients psychological practice. Adopting human rights as a framework seeks to politicize torture, by resorting to apparently 'universal' norms, as codified in international law.

The danger here is of replacing one oppressive discourse with another. In de-medicalizing distress, we may instead psychologize dis-tress. And in trying to avoid psychologizing distress consequent upon social inequality and gross human rights violations, we may fall into to another familiar dualism: individual vs. society. If we uncritically 'legalise' psychological theory and practice (i.e. torture is wrong because it is illegal), we risk enacting *un trompe l'oeil*, failing to recognize that the project engaged in is the (re)moralizing of distress. That torture is wrong is not a fact. The unspoken questions – answered in the negative by so many States – are 'why is torture wrong, for whom and under which circumstances might it be justified (or not), regardless of the distress and suffering it leads to?' While the response in international law is clear in its absolute prohibition of torture, even in emergency situations, this is a moral stance, notwithstanding its codification in law and broad inter-national consensus.

As apparently unhelpful as it may appear to be, the very idea of human rights is a social construction (e.g., Donnelly, 1999; Waters, 1996), despite the widely held view that human rights are 'natural rights' and are universally held by all people equally, existing independently of recognition or implementation by the State and society (Nickel, 1987). Yet, human rights are – of course – a political idea constructed in the West with moral foundations (Henkin, 1989) expressing the political relationship that, ideally, prevails between individuals and the State.

While the human rights approach has been challenged by governments and scholars on grounds of Eurocentricity and from philosophical, political, ideological and feminist perspectives, I argue that socially con-structed, limited and ideologically tainted as they may be, the concept and regime of human rights, like psychology, offer a tool. As Ignatieff (2001) suggests, what is important is what human rights can do for peo-ple, underlining the assumption (questionable, given the very existence of torture) that no one would want to contest a person's right to, and pursuit of, a 'good life' which meets their security, economic and welfare needs. The question posed is, can there be any version of human rights (or psychology) which can be considered emancipatory for all, given their Western liberal roots and their individualistic, Eurocentric and de-politicizing tendencies? I suggest that individuals and communities can and do exercise agency and may be better enabled to seek ways to 'protect themselves against injustice' by using a human rights framework (cf. Ignatieff, 2001: 57) – as evidenced in many emancipatory struggles (e.g. by those fighting for women's rights, minority rights, disability rights) as well as in post-colonial independence struggles.

As psychologists, reaching to human-rights law to address and politicize, rather than psychologize, torture and its impact have considerable appeal. Similarly, lawyers are increasingly reaching to psychologists, psychiatrists, physicians and others in their efforts to facilitate the implementation of international humanitarian and human-rights law, looking to 'scientific evidence', which is assumed to be neutral, definitive and reliable. This is, of course a problematic assumption. With respect to the prohibition of torture, I offer two examples, although limited space precludes a detailed examination of the relevant legal arguments here.

As psychologists, reaching to human rights law to address and politicize, rather than psychologize, torture and its impact has considerable appeal. Similarly, lawyers are increasingly reaching to psychologists, psychiatrists, physicians and others in their efforts to facilitate the implementation of international humanitarian and human rights law, looking to 'scientific evidence', which is assumed to be neutral, definitive and reliable. This is, of course a problematic assumption. With respect to the prohibition of torture, I offer two examples.

In many European states, there has been increasing reliance on, and dismissal of scientific, medical or psychological evidence offered as expert opinion in support of allegations of torture, as part of asylum claims. Central to this practice is the claim that torture can be evidenced, or inferred, to differing degrees, based upon physical scars, signs, impairment and psychological difficulties. In the last 15 years, it would appear the threshold for what constitutes reliable evidence of torture has shifted dramatically, in decisions on asylum claims by the UKBA or immigration judges. With respect to 'psychological evidence' it seems no longer enough to describe in detail the nature of psychological difficulties, experiences and related difficulties in relationships and functioning, if psychiatric diagnoses are not invoked. It is as if a diagnosis offers 'objective' 'verification' of 'damage' beyond 'ordinary' misery, whose cause could be related to torture, though which is often assumed to be a consequence of hardships endured in exile (housing, destitution, strains of asylum process). That is, it seems that a diagnosis is taken to indicate a reasonable likelihood that the person was in fact tortured, and therefore telling the truth, and therefore can be considered a credible witness. Likewise, legal representatives of those tortured increasingly expect that expert witnesses use diagnoses, assuming that the absence of a diagnosis in medico-legal reports may risk the evidence being dismissed or ignored.

Perpetuating a vicious circle, psychologists thus seek to demonstrate, and decision-makers to dismiss, the severity of suffering and its relationship to torture, each assuming that the severity of distress (and experience of torture) can be proved by a diagnosis (or disproved by its absence). Diagnoses are here what they seem, not self-evident objective truths, but rather strategic devices invoked by all parties for a purpose – to decide whether an allegation of torture is reliable, the person a credible witness and a 'genuine' refugee deserving of legal protection and asylum. At stake is the person's safety, and quite possibly their life.

Another example is evidenced in recent debates in international law on gendering torture. Developments in international law have led to a recognition that the failure of a government to prohibit acts of violence against women, or to establish adequate legal protections against such acts, constitutes a failure of State protection, and therefore acts of violence against women can constitute torture when they are of the nature and severity envisaged by the concept of torture in international law, and the State has failed to provide effective protection. Acts of sexual violence in peacetime and conflict can amount to torture, including rape, abduction and sexual slavery, forced marriage, forced impregnation, female genital mutilation (FGM), trafficking and intimate partner violence. Despite advances in the mainstreaming of gender in international human rights law, and in gendering torture, the reliance on dominant psychological discourses which essentialize the notion of harm continues.

Thus uncritical reliance on psychological and medical terminology, including diagnosis, to support the argument that intimate partner violence, FGM and human trafficking can amount to torture, as with 'official' (State perpetrated) torture (in resulting in the same psychological difficulties and psychiatric disorders) (see Novak, 2008) leads to very serious, and potentially counter-productive consequences. In drawing on the dominant trauma discourse, gender oppression is neglected and reproduced, violence de-politicized, 'harm' individualized, psychologized and essentialized, and women pathologized and invalidated.

Further, in the absence of distress meeting the threshold required for 'severe physical or mental pain and suffering', entitlement to protection may be questioned (or reparation measures in law limited, in terms of compensation or healthcare). Meanwhile, longer-term consequences of violence against women in terms of the diminution of their social well-being (ability and opportunities to form and maintain trusting and secure relationships and social networks) and economic well-being (ability and opportunities to ensure economic security) are overlooked.

In this respect the former UN Special Rapporteur on Torture, Manfred Novak's suggestion that medicine and psychology are professions which 'should be looked to more systematically when analysing whether a specific violation may constitute torture or not' (Novak, 2008: 25) should be questioned carefully. In the context of the 'war on terror' the idea that a medico-psychological viewpoint has a compelling explanatory and 'objective' capacity to identify torture as specific actions which cause 'severe' harm and suffering, is one of the reasons why ethical and legal problems persist with respect to the role of psychologists and physicians in specifying what is or is not torture, and especially in the related role of assisting interrogators to determine how far they can go without causing severe pain and suffering, to minimize the risk of accusations of torture (see Granville-Chapman & Patel, 2005; Patel, 2007a, 2007b; Sveaass, 2007; Pope & Gutheil, 2009) In both instances distress is essentialized, thereby diverting our gaze from the moral (and therefore both the particular, and contested) nature of both human-rights, and of psychology. While I have argued that this form of politicizing of psychology is problematic, the question remains, what are we to do?

Alternatives to moonlighting

One alternative to moonlighting in other disciplines may be proactively to seek colleagues across disciplines and to attempt integrative theorizing and practice. Examples of such work include interdisciplinary action or policy-related research or research-exploring State implementation of duties with respect to the prohibition of torture, and implications for policy and health and social care service delivery; or strategic litigation relying on experience and understandings from psychology, medicine and law to challenge policies and practices impacting adversely on the well-being of torture survivors; facilitating torture survivors in seeking justice and reparation and in accessing and negotiating health and social care (individual advocacy); or advocacy at social and/or legal policy levels, nationally and internationally.

Yet, the challenges of integrative and interdisciplinary work are manifold. For example, lack of conceptual clarity about the indivisible and interrelated nature of human rights (civil, political, economic, social and cultural rights), and the multi-dimensionality of well-being and health, is limiting and necessary to address in research, advocacy and practice. Neither health nor human rights research is atheoretical, both offering competing explanations of the same phenomena, or explanations at different levels (political, economic, intrapsychic and interpersonal), which can be paralysing. Partial understandings of other disciplines and their limitations can lead to an uncritical, and crudely pragmatic, use of concepts, theories and 'evidence'. One argument in support of such pragmatism could be that the task of challenging and preventing torture is larger than the bodies and tools we have to hand – and interdisciplinary, inter-agency and international cooperation and collaboration can only contribute to greater resources, broader range of skills and frameworks for under-standing and more tools to utilize.

While synthesis or a robust integration across disciplines may not be possible, one significant difficulty remains – the absence of meth-odologies to address torture which do not have their philosophical foundations in liberalism, with every 'solution' advocated (in law, political science, psychology and medicine) being vulnerable to charges of Eurocentricity and individualism. In the case of psychology we risk deliberately or inadvertently psychologizing human distress and misery located in social, political and material experiences of historical degra-dation, persecution, marginalization, poverty and torture. Worse still, we risk psychologizing both politics and survival.

While psychology has played a malignant role in developing, refining, perpetuating and being complicit in torture (e.g. Patel, 2007a, 2007b; Harper, 2007), and contributed to the psychologizing of torture (Patel, 2003), I would also argue that however limited, partial and flawed psy-chology may be, it does have a role in the prevention of torture (Patel, 2007c), working with individuals, their families and communities as well as at different levels, targeting particular structures, policies and practices – at the local, national, European and international levels – beyond the psychologization of politics and torture.

Beyond psychologization?

Mindful of Albee's (1995: 347) remark that 'soup kitchens, however humane, do not change the numbers of the hungry', some reflections on what it would mean to move beyond the psychologization of torture are offered below.

- Examining our professional codes and ethical frameworks, recognizing their political and philosophical foundations, their individualism and implied individual-society dualism (e.g. individual responsibility versus social responsibility; individual 'good' rather than 'social good'), and their tendency to de-contextualize 'ethical' judgements and practice. For example, recent debates related to the role of psychologists in torture, or 'enhanced interrogation techniques' in the 'war on terror' demonstrate the fluidity of our ethical frameworks, which are evidently amenable to political pressures (see Pope & Gutheil, 2009; Harper, 2007; Kwiatkowski, 2007; Patel, 2007a, 2007b).
- Interrogating our own understandings for their historical and contextual specificity, and exposing the limitations of psychological theories of distress and its relationship to torture, social inequalities and injustices, and making transparent our reductionist tendencies which sanitize complexity. In all theorizing, practice and research, exposing our conceptualization of power, and attending to power, material and discursive. This would also mean challenging misrepresentations and abuses of psychology.
- Transparency about (a) What is being defined as the 'problem'– torture, distress, the absence of a legislative framework for the protection of torture survivors or its effective implementation, social inequalities, impunity, lack of reparation and redress? (b) Theorizing the location of the 'problem' (individual/society? Language, processes or structures? Policy or practice?). And (c) The implications for practice.
- Transparency about how we (a) conceptualize justice (a principle, an act or an outcome? Justice for individual torture survivors or social justice, as defined by whom – torture survivors, practitioners, academics?); and (b) how we theorize the relationship between justice (including notions of equality, fairness, redress and reparation) and well-being.
- Transparency about our conceptualization of change and sources of resistance to change. What needs to change (individuals torture survivors, their families, communities, social policies, laws, State practice etc.), why, what *could* be changed, by whom, with which co-actors/ agencies and how, using which methods or resources?
- Redefining the role of mental-health professionals as (a) having both individual and social responsibility, (b) being political agents, contributing to the collective task of addressing and preventing distress and its determinants, towards individual, social, economic

and political well-being; (c) using a variety of methods and resources (theoretical, practical, therapeutic etc.), being explicit about their limitations and their potential for ideological abuse; (d) collaborating with other disciplines, agencies (NGOs, INGOs, IGOs), networks (professional, interdisciplinary, service user and community networks of torture survivors) in prevention activities; (e) utilizing existing legal mechanisms nationally and internationally, as well as targeting local, national, European and international structures, polices and decision-makers in advocating for change, towards the betterment of social and political conditions related to the safety, security and well-being of torture survivors.

- De-mystifying psychology by exposing attempts to psychologize politics and by exposing the limitations of psychological explanations when applied to social, economic and political phenomena and experiences, such as experiences of torture as an extreme form of State-endorsed, systematic discrimination and violence.
- Recognizing that distress and 'symptoms' tell a story about gross injustice, a story which needs to be heard, witnessed and publicly acknowledged. In that sense, in all our endeavours, therapy, research and advocacy we need to commit ourselves to bearing witness to atrocity and suffering, exposing and challenging injustices.
- Honesty and humility in our activities – acknowledging that in psychologizing or de-psychologizing misery and distress, what we are all doing, however unintentionally, whatever our stated aim, is politicizing distress and therefore, actively moralizing behind the armour of 'health professional' status.

Re-envisioning psychology as a tool

In conclusion, in psychology's efforts to contribute to addressing gross human-rights violations such as torture, we have convinced ourselves that either we are psychologizing, or politicizing distress and torture, without declaring that like all other actors in the field, we are moralizing about humanness and human suffering. On one occasion, one torture survivor, who had waited four years for a decision on his asylum claim without permission to work in the UK, tipped over 30 unopened packets of anti-depressants and painkillers, prescribed by his GP, in front of me, saying:

> Look at this, look, I don't want this, I see this, and it makes me so sad – I never needed anything like this before, I was a healthy man,

now look at me, I am 48 kilos, I have nothing to live for, nothing. The war, it was very hard, I saw terrible things, I was badly tortured, you know. The darkness and the cold in this country makes me so sad, it reminds me of the years in prison ... I don't want these pills, I want my wife, I want to see my country, I want to see sun ... I don't care if I lose my benefits – I want to work, I want to use my arms, my legs, my body, I want to be useful again, to feel like a human being – it is not the life of a human to only sit, wait, sleep, eat ... I am not an animal, not a cockroach, I am a man ... I can do things, even if not like before, I can do something.

Is it always necessary to suggest that something is harmful (hence the temptation to medicalize and psychologize), or that it is illegal, in order to argue that it is *therefore* wrong, and inhumane? What is repugnant about acknowledging that torture is cruel, inhumane and that common sense tells us that it is wrong; that we should never defend it and that when people have been tortured perpetrators should be held accountable; that we should offer kindness, support, warmth and help to those who have been tortured? In this spirit would it be wrong to say that we should use whatever tools we have (psychological or otherwise), if we are committing to social justice and to upholding the dignity and humanity of all?

That is to say, for many torture survivors, medicalizing and psychologizing misery can be functional, a route to safety, security and life. Survival is not just escaping prison and torture, travelling thousands of miles deprived of sanitary facilities, exposed to harsh conditions, numerous dangers, illness and starvation. Surviving can be 'negotiating the system', in whatever way is necessary, to stay safe and to stay alive. Torture survivors are not passive victims or passive recipients of services. In the West, for some, medicalizing or psychologizing their misery may facilitate access to safe housing, possibly asylum, perhaps healthcare. For many, health *is* justice, a symbolic defiance of their torturers and the perpetrating State. Health enables the exercise of choice – to resume political activities, to pursue education, to seek employment, to have a family life, to seek justice and to hold the perpetrating State to account. In short, perhaps de-medicalizing misery is functional for academics and health practitioners with critical leanings, much as medicalizing and psychologizing misery can be functional for some torture survivors – after all, are we not all active agents in seeking survival, and change, in the moment?

This is not to advocate a crude utilitarianism on part of psychologists and others, arguing that 'anything goes' if the means justify the consequences. We need professional ethical frameworks, as well as legal frameworks, which codify moral rules as safeguards, but their essential-izing of ethics and inherent biases must not be hidden, disguised or denied. Critical reflection and judgement must not be rejected, and indeed our imperfect and limited psychological understandings must be exposed for what they are, moral arguments in support of moral positions on well-being, justice and humanity. In the enterprise of de-medicalizing misery, and de-psychologizing torture, perhaps what is necessary is that our moral position is transparent when we do medi-calize or psychologize experience. Psychology, like human-rights law, is after all only a tool, and it is what it is, built on sand, flawed, ideologi-cally driven, but sometimes useful. What is required of us all is honesty in what we do with what we have to hand.

Acknowledgements

Listening to torture survivors who have experienced extreme cruelty and the depth of pain and despair, I have witnessed the most profound beauty and height of the human spirit and endurance – by them I am perpetually moved, and humbled, and to them I am grateful. Thanks to Mark Rapley for the numerous discussions of ideas, his insights and enduring support and encouragement which led to this chapter. Thanks also to the Medical Foundation for the Care of Victims of Torture – the views expressed here are those of the author and do not necessarily reflect those of the Medical Foundation.

19
What Is to Be Done?

Joanna Moncrieff, Jacqui Dillon and Mark Rapley

In the medieval and early modern world, madness was everyone's affair. Local officials administered poor relief to families who required assistance with the care of their afflicted relatives, they gave help to affected individuals themselves, and they made arrangements for other members of the community to care for people who had become mad when domestic or private arrangements did not suffice or broke down (Rushton, 1988). Madness was assumed to be easily recognizable by laypeople, but it was not determined randomly or without care. Where there was a local problem, the parish officers or county magistrates, sometimes assisted by a jury of ordinary people, and taking evidence from relatives, neighbours and the person themselves, assessed people's state of mind, and determined whether or not they should be regarded as mad or insane (Roffe & Roffe, 1995). The often-temporary nature of madness was acknowledged, and arrangements were stopped or reversed when the person regained their senses.

In stark contrast, as tens of thousands of people every year discover, contemporary statutory arrangements place responsibility for the (now frequently lifelong) disenfranchisement of the mad solely into the hands of the psy professions and the police, with what little was left of lay oversight in the form of the magistracy removed via the provisions of the 1959 Mental Health Act.

Madness, misery and distress are experiences that – as far as we can tell – human beings have always faced. Only over the last 200 years, however, have these experiences come to be regarded as the exclusive territory of specialists, and specifically of medical experts, considerably more recently than that (Scull, 1979; Scull, Mackenzie & Hervey, 1996). Of course the triumph of the psy professions has been predicated on establishing as a truth the proposition that knowledge of such matters is beyond the understanding of ordinary people. In his critical history of the psy professions Nikolas Rose notes how recent our current understanding of ourselves, indeed the very idea of 'being normal', is and its inseparability from the exercise of power and surveillance by the state.

> Notable [is] the emergence of *normality* as itself the product of management under the tutelage of experts and the emergence of *risk* as danger *in potentia* to be diagnosed by experts and managed prophylactically in the name of social security.
>
> (Rose, 1996: 117)

Moreover, Rose, following Foucault, points out elsewhere that this now taken-for-granted truth about what it means to be human did not evolve through its own intrinsic merit, but was, like other established 'truths', enthroned by power. That is to say:

> Truth is not only the outcome of construction, but of contestation. There are battles over truth, in which evidence, results, arguments, laboratories, status and much else are deployed as resources in the attempts to win allies and force something into the true. Truth, that is to say, is always enthroned by acts of violence.
>
> (Rose, nd)

In this volume we have attempted to show that the modern conception of madness and misery as diseases, illnesses or disorders that can only be understood within a specialist body of knowledge, fails to do justice to the range and meaning of the experiences these concepts refer to. More seriously, by designating people's distress as illness, we ignore the abuse that individuals may have suffered, and in a wider sense, we obscure the features of modern society that make sanity a precarious state for many people. We enthrone a very particular, and very partisan, 'truth' by wreaking violence on the life experience and subjectivity of those we purport to 'help'. Diagnoses of schizophrenia, depression, or 'reactive attachment disorder' are entirely inadequate descriptions of the problems and difficulties that people experience, and the unfolding life story in which those problems are set. Such labels render people's experiences as meaningless as if they denoted a rash, a boil or a cough (cf. Parry, 2009). Moreover, the experiences we have come to be familiar with under the rubric of 'psychiatric symptoms' may be more of a signal that all is not well, a signal that something needs to change, than a problem itself. But, as we have seen in this collection, this perspective is one that is anathema to currently hegemonic medicalized understandings.

As many of our contributions attest, mental turmoil is *not* meaningless, but a reaction to a world that is experienced as hostile or overwhelming or both. In their interactions with 'expert' mental health professionals, however, these entirely human reactions to a frequently difficult and sometimes arbitrarily cruel world are stripped of meaning and personal significance. It is, by definition, their encounters with psy-professionals, which effect the transformation of despair, withdrawal, disorientation and distress into meaningless 'sickness'. This is indeed firstly *to do* harm. To the contrary, finding a sense of meaning in distressing and confusing experience appears to confer strength to help people overcome or learn to live with their distress, and re-engage in the world in a meaningful way. Foucault wrote of the loss of *significance* of madness, as it was transformed by the Enlightenment into unreason, into something that was simply wrong. Along with this view came the corollary, that madness needs to be corrected. As psychiatric medicine took control of madness, correction became cure (Foucault, 1961). Correcting and curing are profoundly disempowering approaches to misery and madness. They leave little room for people to come to understand their difficulties in ways that make sense to them, and which may allow them to find their own ways of dealing with them.

If, as Audre Lorde contends, 'the master's tools will never dismantle the master's house' then perhaps it is time to discard the tools with which we have constructed the medicalized edifice that is contemporary psychology and psychiatry. That is to say we have, should we wish to employ them, both an entirely adequate vocabulary for distress and misery of all stripes and also, as Spinoza (1677) suggests, simply by virtue of our common humanity a perfectly adequate set of capacities for assisting our fellows in the – essentially moral – human task of perseverance in our being.

So we hope that this volume will help people to appreciate that madness and misery are not other people's problems. Neither are they, of necessity, the exclusive preserve of medicine. They belong to us all. As John Donne (1624) suggests, it is hubris to ask for whom the bell tolls. As citizens we have a bond of common humanity to respect and, as a society, we have a responsibility to understand what drives people mad and to help people to take back what control they can of their lives.

Notes

1 Carving Nature at its Joints? DSM and the Medicalization of Everyday Life

1. See http://www.facebook.com/pages/DSM-5-Diagnostic-and-Statistical-Manual-of-Mental-Disorders/260197062886.
2. We are perplexed as to quite how the *type of care* a child has received from others can be considered a 'diagnostic criterion' for a 'mental disorder' supposedly affecting the individual diagnosed. Can we imagine, say, 'happy family relationships' – 'philogenic care' perhaps – seriously being proposed as a 'diagnostic criterion' for a genuine childhood medical condition like measles, mumps or chickenpox?
3. *Am I doing it right?* is the (designedly?) guilt-inducing strapline on advertisements for a 'helpful' UK government 'parenting advice service' – see http://www.babylifecheck.co.uk/.

2 Dualisms and the Myth of Mental Illness

1. It is important to point out that, according to Schaler (2004), Szasz rejects the label 'anti-psychiatrist'.
2. The Vienna Circle was a group of philosophers whose work was important to the development of logical positivism, a central feature of which was the principle of verifiability. This concerns the idea that the meaning of individual sentences is specified by the steps that are taken to determine their truth or falsity. For this reason logical positivism is also sometimes referred to as linguistic empiricism. Logical positivists saw no real distinction between philosophy and the philosophy of science (hence positivism). Members of the Vienna Circle included Moritz Schlick (whose work Szasz cites), Rudolph Carnap and Otto Neurath.
3. Historicism has a number of meanings, but the sense that Szasz is referring to here concerns the view that social history is determined, and progresses out of necessity according to a set of rules. It is closely related to, but not the same as holism, the view that society is greater than the sum of the individuals that constitute society, and that in turn, society shapes and influences their destinies. Both historicism and holism feature prominently in Marxism, a political philosophy that Szasz clearly abhors.
4. He also points out that Charcot was an immensely powerful figure. He was very well connected with aristocratic acquaintances. However, Szasz refers to contemporary reports of inconsistencies in Charcot's views about hysteria. He interprets these observations to indicate that Charcot was either confused about the contribution of emotional factors, or preferred not to admit to believing that they were significant when he was seen in social gatherings where he was reported to have said that hysteria was a neurological disorder.

5. He presumably makes this point in part to account for the reported inconsistencies in Charcot's attitude towards the 'psychosocial'.
6. Szasz is referring here to his appeal, based in the philosophy of the Vienna Circle, for clarity in the use of language.
7. Susan Sontag (1979) has described in detail the metaphoric significance of TB and cancer, and more recently, AIDS (1989).
8. Again, we agree with Szasz as far as the influence of culture on phenomenology in psychiatry is concerned, but we disagree strongly with the way in which he polarizes the debate and imposes over-simplistic binary distinctions by writing the body out of psychiatry, and culture out of medicine.
9. Or at least the early phenomenology of Husserl for, as Matthews (2002) points out, later ideas about phenomenology appear to have moved away from a strictly scientific approach, under the influence of his most prominent student, Martin Heidegger.
10. Those interested in following this in greater detail are referred to Bracken and Thomas (2005), particularly pages 113–16.
11. The fundamental principles here map directly on to contemporary models of mind such as cognitivism, where we might think of 'schema' as being equivalent to representations.
12. It is also worth noting here that logical positivism is rooted in the Cartesian tradition. It assumes that careful reflection on our use of language, and also an appeal to the Universal principles of formal logic, means we can be certain about the truth status of particular instances of language use.
13. Although there are similarities between the two philosophers (Merleau-Ponty borrows the expression being-in-the-world from Heidegger), Merleau-Ponty diverges from Heidegger in that the latter sets out a general ontology, or theory of Being. In contrast, Merleau-Ponty's objective was more modest than Heidegger's, simply to draw attention to our understanding of ourselves through the physical, social and historical facts of human existence. One relevant outcome of this is that we can achieve a clearer role of the significance and importance of science in our lives. This emerges, for example, in Merleau-Ponty's preoccupation with psychological and neurological theories of human experience.
14. Matthews (2002) points out that in the original translation of *Phenomenology of Perception* the French word *désaveu* was incorrectly rendered as a 'rejection' (of science), when a better word is *foreswearing* as it appears in the later translations (see Merleau-Ponty, 1962: viii). This indicates that Merleau-Ponty was not hostile to science, but wanted to place it in what he considered to be an appropriate relationship to human experience.
15. Merleau-Ponty's position on how we are to understand perception is radically different. He argues that if we set scientific and empirical accounts of perception to one side, and try to see the world not as science would have us see it, but as we actually experience it, then we will see that the concept of 'sensation' is misleading, and bears very little relationship to anything in our experience. Matthews (2002: 50) points out that this is because Cartesianism forces sensations into an uneasy position somewhere between the subjective and objective domains. They must be objective in the sense that they are related in a causal path to objects in the external world. At the same time they must be a part of my subjective experience

if indeed they are to be a part of myself. Thus confusion arises through dualism, which attempts to fuse the subjectivity of personal experience with the empirical or scientific perspective that sensations are also part of the objective world.

16. Merleau-Ponty considers in detail the phantom limb experiences of amputees, who not infrequently experience the limb in the position it was at the instant of trauma. This suggests that the experience is in some way linked to the personal history of the individual who experiences it. He argues that such an experience cannot be adequately accounted for by psychology or neurology alone. A phantom limb can also reappear as memories are recalled to an amputee, but a phantom limb is not itself a memory. The subject may experience it in the present, but with no awareness of its origins in the past. Langer points out that memory and the emotions are not to be regarded here as intellectual operations (i.e. part of the *cogitatio*), but as preobjective ways of relating to the world. Although phantom limb experiences can be accounted for in physiological or psychological terms, the separating out of the 'psychological' from the 'physiological' that we encounter with Cartesianism makes it impossible to reconnect the two in our attempts to understand the particularity of the experience in an individual.

17. We are not arguing here that our consciousness is the same thing as our brain, as materialist philosophers would argue.

18. He argues that Descartes' division of human being into the body (*res extensa*) and mind (*res cogitans*) places our awareness of our bodies in a paradoxical situation. Is it a part of the self, or an object in the physical world? It occupies a similarly anomalous situation to sensation, as we saw earlier. He argues instead for a new way of thinking about the relationship between self and matter, so that my body is no longer just another object in the world, but it becomes instead a visible expression of myself, or my ego. In this sense, because it is through the body that I engage in projects and activities that are meaningful for me, the body itself is laden with meaning and significance.

19. The Holy People are a central feature of the Navajo creation myth.

20. Peyote ingestion can result in severe vomiting, and this is usually interpreted in rituals as a punishment by the Holy People for wrong thinking and speaking.

21. The difficulty here, of course is that we are all tied in any case to the cultural systems that shape how we present our distress, and who we present it to. In the US system of health care there is no equivalent to the British general practitioner or family doctor. Those who can afford health care go directly to the specialist of their choice. Szasz's analysis appears to be blind to the effect that culture has on disease, illness, and how we present for help.

5   The Social Context of Paranoia

1. This perspective is, of course, beautifully illustrated in R. D. Laing's (1960) case study of '*The Ghost of the Weed Garden*'.

6 From Bad Character to BPD: The Medicalization of 'Personality Disorder'

1. The idea of PD also protects the psy professions from their failure to have any convincing explanations for bizarre and socially unacceptable conduct. For an analysis of the way in which PD apparently explains the inexplicable, silences 'lay' voices, and preserves psy's sole authority to speak of these matters, see Rapley, McCarthy & McHoul (2003).
2. It is unclear whether 'striving to achieve (unpalatable) long-term strategic goals' – to be a highly effective mafia boss, to profitably exploit child labourers, or to 'ethnically cleanse' one's country, for example – would be considered as 'abnormal' under this formulation.

10 Discourses of Acceptance and Resistance: Speaking out about Psychiatry

1. This is not to say that these categories are mutually exclusive, people can and do explain and describe their situations drawing on the social and the biological to construct how they make sense of their situation. What I am drawing attention to is the incommensurability of biological explanations (that are reductionist) and social explanations (which may be much more contingent). These different regimes of truth offer different means of making sense of mental health.

12 'I'm Just, You Know, Joe Bloggs': The Management of Parental Responsibility for First-episode Psychosis

1. Importantly, Masson proposes that Freud's 'assault on truth' was driven by the fact that the seduction theory explicitly held parents directly responsible for the generation of his patients' distress. This, Masson points out, was not conducive to the building of a successful private practice dependent upon fee-paying parents.
2. As Read et al. (2004b) note this is to seriously misread Laing who emphasized that families are influenced by the imperfect societies in which they are located, and that parents are themselves the product of their own family backgrounds.
3. See Rapley (2011) and McHoul & Rapley (2005) for a detailed explication of the epistemological and methodological position we adopt.
4. The material in this chapter is drawn from the first author's unpublished DClinPsy thesis at the University of East London. All interviews, which were informal and semi-structured, were organized around an exploration of an initial question 'What has been happening for your daughter / son to be referred to an EIP team?'.
5. Parents may also elect to save their money and order (free of charge) the Royal College of Psychiatrists' factsheet entitled *'Good Parenting'*, which provides answers to such profound and pertinent questions as 'why is parenting

important?', 'what helps?' and 'how can it go wrong?' (Royal College of Psychiatrists, 2004: 1–2).

6. The relationship between culturally prevalent notions of parental culpability and legal reasoning was exemplified recently when Lord Justice Wall recited Philip Larkin's 'This Be The Verse' in court to warn parents in a divorce case that they risked adversely affecting their son (Pidd, 2009). We note that Larkin (1974) also clearly makes a crucial distinction, as we suggest here, between parental 'responsibility' and parental 'intent'.

13   The Myth of the Antidepressant: An Historical Analysis

1. Which of course they do. And also cause, among other things, the irreversible and disabling neurological condition *Tardive Dyskinesia*.

16   Toxic Psychology

1. Rose (1998) provides a helpful discussion of the psy professions, indeed the 'psy-complex': that constellation of professional groups the names of which are prefixed by psy- or psycho- (e.g. psychiatry, psychology, psychoanalysis psychiatric nursing) and which are concerned with the disciplining of the individual subject.

2. Wolfensberer's concept of 'deathmaking' refers to those human service practices which (deliberately, or more often, unconsciously) cause physical or spiritual harm, including causing or hastening death, to their recipients. Examples of deathmaking practices include the causing of self-evidently toxic conditions like Neuroleptic Malignant Syndrome and neuroleptic-induced brain disorders such as Tardive Dyskinesia, but also service practices which expose people to abuse and/or neglect. It is perhaps of note that the DSM 5 (see www.DSM5.org) lists neuroleptic-induced brain disorders not as the iatrogenic assaults that they are, but rather as 'mental disorders' in their own right.

17   Psychotherapy: Illusion with No Future?

1. This predicament was neatly summed up in the chorus of the pop singer Lily Allen's 2008 hit *The Fear*.

Bibliography

Abramson, L. Y., Seligman, M. E. P. & Teasdale, J. D. (1978). 'Learned Helplessness in Humans: Critique and Reformulation', *Journal of Abnormal Psychology*, 87, 49–74.

Adams, W. L. (2008). 'The Listening Cure', *Time Magazine*, 21 February.

Albee, G. (1995). 'Ann and Me', *Journal of Primary Prevention*, 15, 4, 331–47.

Als-Nielsen, B., Chen, W., Gluud, C. & Kjaergard, L. L. (2003). 'Association of Funding and Conclusions in Randomized Drug Trials', *Journal of the American Medical Association*, 290, 921–8.

Alwin, N., Blackburn, R., Davidson, K., Hilton, M., Logan, C. & Shine, J. (2006). *'Understanding Personality Disorder: A Professional Practice Board Report by the British Psychological Society* (Leicester: British Psychological Society).

American Psychiatric Association (1952). *Diagnostic and Statistical Manual of Mental Disorders*, 1st edn (Washington, DC: Author).

American Psychiatric Association (1980). *Diagnostic and Statistical Manual of Mental Disorders*, 3rd edn (Washington, DC: Author).

American Psychiatric Association (1994). *The Diagnostic and Statistical Manual of Mental Disorders*, 4th edn (Washington, DC: Author).

American Psychiatric Association (2000). *Diagnostic and Statistical Manual of Mental Disorders*, 4th edn, Text Revision (Washington, DC: Author).

American Psychiatric Association (2003). *Statement on Diagnosis and Treatment of Mental Disorders*. Release no 03–39, 25 September (Washington, DC: Author).

Amnesty International (2010). *Amnesty International Report 2010: The State of the World's Human Rights* (London: Author).

Andrews, G. (2001). 'Should Depression be Managed as a Chronic Disease?', *British Medical Journal*, 322, 419–22.

Andrews, B. & Hunter, E. (1997). 'Shame, Early Abuse and Course of Depression in a Clinical Sample', *Cognition and Emotion*, 11, 373–81.

Angermeyer, M. C., Holzinger, A. & Matschinger, H. (2010). 'Mental Health Literacy and Attitude Towards People with Mental Illness: A Trend Analysis Based on Population Surveys in the Eastern Part of Germany', *European Psychiatry*, 24, 4, 225–32.

Armstrong, D. (1983). *Political Anatomy of the Body: Medical Knowledge in Britain in the Twentieth Century* (Cambridge: Cambridge University Press).

Ayd, F. J., Jr (1961a). 'A Critique of Antidepressants', *Diseases of the Nervous System*, 22, 5, (Pt 2) 32–6.

Ayd, F. J., Jr (1961b). *Recognising the Depressed Patient* (New York: Grune & Stratton).

Azam, A. (1876). 'Le dédoublement de la personnalité, suite de L'histoire de Felida X', *Revue Scientifique*, IIe serie, 265–9.

Baker, P. (1989). *Hearing Voices* (Manchester: Hearing Voices Network).

Balbernie R. (2001). 'Circuits and Circumstances: The Neurobiological Consequences of Early Relationship Experiences and How They Shape Later Behaviour', *Journal of Child Psychotherapy*, 27, 3, 237–55.

Baldessarini, R., Ghaemi, S. N. & Viguera, A. C. (2002). 'Tolerance in Antidepressant Treatment', *Psychotherapy and Psychosomatics*, 71, 177–9.

Barber, B. R. (2007). *Consumed: How Markets Corrupt Children, Infantilise Adults and Swallow Citizens Whole* (New York: Norton).

Barbui, C., Furukawa, T. A. & Cipriani, A. (2008). 'Effectiveness of Paroxetine in the Treatment of Acute Major Depression in Adults: A Systematic Re-examination of Published and Unpublished Data from Randomized Trials', *Canadian Medical Association Journal*, 178, 3, 296–305.

Barnes, C., Mercer, G. & Shakespeare, T. (2000). *Exploring Disability: A Sociological Introduction* (Cambridge: Polity Press).

Barrett, R. J. (1988). 'Clinical Writing and the Documentary Construction of Schizophrenia', *Culture, Medicine & Psychiatry*, 12, 265–99.

Barthes, R. (1957). *Mythologies* (Paris: Editions du Seuil).

Barzun, J. (1965). *Race: A Study of Superstition* (New York: Harper and Row).

Basch, M. F. (1981). 'Self-object Disorders and Psychoanalytic Theory: A Historical Perspective', *Journal of the American Psychoanalytic Association*, 29, 337–51.

Beach, W. A. & Metzger, T. R. (1997). 'Claiming Insufficient Knowledge', *Human Communication Research*, 23, 562–88.

Bebbington, P. E. & Kuipers, L. (1994). 'The Predictive Utility of Expressed Emotion in Schizophrenia: An Aggregate Analysis', *Psychological Medicine*, 24, 707–18.

Bebbington, P., Bhugra, D., Brugha, T., Singleton, N., Farrell, M., Jenkins, R., Lewis, G. & Meltzer, H. (2004). 'Psychosis, Victimization and Childhood Disadvantage: Evidence from the Second British National Survey on Psychiatric Morbidity', *British Journal of Psychiatry*, 185, 220–6.

Bell, V., Halligan, P. W. & Ellis, H. D. (2006). Diagnosing Delusions: 'A Review of Inter-rater Reliability', *Schizophrenia Research*, 86, 76–9.

Bentall, R. P. (1990). *Reconstructing Schizophrenia* (London: Routledge).

Bentall, R. P. (1992). 'A Proposal to Classify Happiness as a Psychiatric Disorder', *Journal of Medical Ethics*, 18, 94–8.

Bentall R. P. (2003). *Madness Explained: Psychosis and Human Nature* (London: Penguin).

Bentall, R. P. (2006). 'The Environment and Psychosis: Rethinking the Evidence', in W. Larkins & A. Morrison (eds) *Trauma and Psychosis: New Directions for Theory and Therapy* (London: Routledge).

Berrios, G. E. (1991). 'Delusions as "Wrong Beliefs": A Conceptual History', *British Journal of Psychiatry*, 159 (suppl. 14), 6–13.

Bijl, R. V., Ravelli, A. & Van Zessen. G. (1998). Prevalence of Psychotic Disorder in the General Population: Results from the Netherlands Mental Health Survey and Incidence Study', *Social Psychiatry Epidemiology*, 33, 587–96.

Blackman, L. (2007). 'Psychiatric Culture and Bodies of Resistance', *Body and Society*, 13, 2, 1–23.

Blanchard, J. J. & Brown, S. B. (1998). 'Structured Diagnostic Interview Schedules', in C. R. Reynolds (ed.) *Assessment*, Series eds: A. S. Bellack & M. Hersen, *Comprehensive Clinical Psychology*, vol. 4 (Amsterdam: Elsevier).

Blashfield, R. K. & McElroy, R. A. (1987). 'The 1985 Journal Literature on Personality Disorders', *Comprehensive Psychiatry*, 28, 536–46.

Bleuler, E. & Brill, A. A. (1924). *Textbook of Psychiatry* (Oxford: Macmillan).

Blier, P. & Trimblay, P. (2006). 'Physiologic Mechanisms Underlying the Antidepressant Discontinuation Syndrome', *Journal of Clinical Psychiatry*, 67 (Supplement 4), 8–13.

Board, B. J. & Fritzon, K. (2005). 'Disordered Personalities at Work', *Psychology, Crime & Law*, 11, 1, 17–32.

Bond, C. H. (1915). 'The Position of Psychiatry and the Role of the General Hospitals in its Improvement', *Journal of Mental Science*, 61, 1–17.

Boseley, S. (2003). 'Seroxat Maker Abandons "No Addiction" Claim', *The Guardian*, 3 May.

Bourru, H. & Burot, P. (1888). *Variations de la Personnalité* (Paris: Baillière).

Boydell, J., van Os, J., McKenzie, K., Allardyce, J., Goel, R., McGreadie, R. G. & Murray, R. M. (2001). 'Incidence of Schizophrenia in Ethnic Minorities in London: Ecological Study into Interactions with Environment', *British Medical Journal*, 323, 1336–8.

Boyle, M. (nd). *Untitled* available from: http://www.caslcampaign.com/campaign_scientific_arguments.php?article=21. Accessed 11 April 2010.

Boyle, M. (1997). *Rethinking Abortion: Psychology, Gender, Power and the Law* (London: Routledge).

Boyle, M. (2002a). *Schizophrenia: A Scientific Delusion?* 2nd edn (London: Routledge).

Boyle, M. (2002b). It's All Done with Smoke and Mirrors: Or, How to Create the Illusion of a Schizophrenic Brain Disease', *Clinical Psychology*, 12, 9–16.

Boyle, M. (2006). 'Developing Real Alternatives to Medical Models', *Ethical Human Psychology and Psychiatry*, 8, 191–200.

Boyle, M. (2006). *From 'Schizophrenia' to 'Psychosis': Paradigm Shift or More of the Same?* Paper presented at BPS Division of Clinical Psychology Annual Conference, London, December.

Boyle, M. H. & Jadad, A. R. (1999). 'Lessons from Large Trials: The MTA Study as a Model for Evaluating the Treatment of Childhood Psychiatric Disorder', *Canadian Journal of Psychiatry*, 44, 991–8.

Bracken, P. & Thomas, P. (2001). 'Postpsychiatry: A New Direction for Mental Health', *British Medical Journal*, 322, 724–7.

Bracken, P. & Thomas, P. (2005). *Postpsychiatry: Mental Health in a Postmodern World* (Oxford: Oxford University Press).

Bracken, P. & Thomas, P. (2008). 'Cognitive Therapy, Cartesianism and the Moral Order', in R. House & D. Loewenthal (eds) *Against and For CBT: Towards a Constructive Dialogue?* (Ross-on-Wye: PCCS Books).

Bracken, P. & Thomas, P. (2010). 'From Szasz to Foucault: On the Role of Critical Psychiatry', *Philosophy, Psychiatry and Psychology*, 17, 3, 219–28.

Bracken, P., Giller, J. & Summerfield, D. (1997). 'Rethinking Mental Health Work with Survivors of Wartime Violence and Refugees', *Journal of Refugee Studies*, 10, 4, 431–42.

Breggin, P. R. (1998). 'Electroshock: Scientific, Ethical, and Political Issues', *International Journal of Risk & Safety in Medicine*, 11, 3, 5–40.

Breggin, P. (1991). *Toxic Psychiatry* (New York: St. Martin's Press).

Breggin, P. (2000). 'The NIMH Multimodal Study of Treatment for Attention Deficit Hyperactivity Disorder: A Critical Analysis', *International Journal of Risk and Safety in Medicine*, 13, 1, 15–22.

Breggin, P. & Cohen, D. (2007). *Your Drug May Be Your Problem* (New York: Perseus Books).

British Medical Association and Pharmaceutical Society of Great Britain (1963). *British National Formulary* (London: Authors).

Brown, J. F. & Menninger, K. A. (1940). *Psychodynamics of Abnormal Behavior* (New York: McGraw-Hill).

Brown, G. W., Monck, E. M., Carstairs, G. M. & Wing, J. K. (1962). 'Influence of Family Life on the Course of Schizophrenic Illness', *British Journal of Preventative Social Medicine*, 16, 2, 55–68.

Browne, K. & Herbert, M. (1997). *Preventing Family Violence* (Chichester: Wiley).

Bullmore, E., Fletcher, P. & Jones, P. B. (2009). 'Why Psychiatry Can't Afford to Be Neurophobic', *British Journal of Psychiatry*, 194, 4, 293–5.

Bullimore, P. (2010). 'The Paranoia Group', *Asylum: The Magazine for Democratic Psychiatry*, 17, 1, 26.

Bullimore, P. Dillon, J. Hammersley, P. McLaughlin, T. & Romme, M. (2007). 'Bad Science', *Open Mind*, January.

Burkitt, I. (1999). *Bodies of Thought: Embodiment, Identity and Modernity* (London: Sage).

Burton, M. (2004). 'Liberating Psychology in Latin America', *The Psychologist*, 17, 10, 584–7.

Busfield, J. (2006). 'Pills, Power, People: Sociological Understandings of the Pharmaceutical Industry', *Sociology*, 40, 2, 297–314.

Calder, J. (2005). 'Histories of Child Abuse', *Journal of Critical Psychology, Counselling and Psychotherapy*, 5, 3, 111–23.

California State Senate (1956). *California 1955/56 Senate Interim Committee on the Treatment of Mental Illness: First Partial Report* (Sacramento CA: Author).

Callcott, P. & Turkington, D. (2006). 'CBT for Traumatic Psychosis', in W. Larkin & A. P. Morrison (eds) *Trauma and Psychosis: New Directions for Theory and Therapy* (London: Routledge).

Campbell, M. & Morrison A. P. (2007). 'The Relationship Between Bullying, Psychotic Like Experiences and Appraisals in 14–16 Year Olds', *Behaviour Research and Therapy*, 45, 7, 1579–91.

Carey, B. (2010). 'Revising Book on Disorders of the Mind', *New York Times*, 10 February.

Carothers, J. C. (1953). *The African Mind in Health and Disease: A Study in Ethnopsychiatry*. WHO Monograph Series No. 17 (Geneva: WHO).

Cartwright, S. A. (1851). 'Report on the Diseases and Physical Peculiarities of the Negro Race', *New Orleans Medical and Surgical Journal*, vol. 7, May, 691–715.

Casey, P. R. & Tyrer, P. (1990). 'Personality Disorder and Psychiatric Illness in General Practice', *British Journal of Psychiatry*, 156, 2, 261–5.

Castel, R. (1991). 'From Dangerousness to Risk', in G. Burchell, C. Gordon & P. Miller (eds) *The Foucault Effect: Studies in Governmentality* (London: Harvester Wheatsheaf).

Castillo, H. (2000). 'You Don't Know What It's Like', *Mental Health Care*, 4, 2, 53–8.

Cauwels, J. (1992). *Imbroglio: Rising to the Challenges of Borderline Personality Disorder* (New York: W. W. Norton).

Chalmers, A. F. (1990). *Science and its Fabrication* (Milton Keynes: Open University Press).

Chan, A. -W. & Altman, D. G. (2005). Identifying Outcome Reporting Bias in Randomised Trials on PubMed: Review of Publications and Survey of Authors', *British Medical Journal*, 330, 7494, 753–6.

Charney, D. S., Heninger, G. R., Sternberg, D. E. & Landis, H. (1982). 'Abrupt Discontinuation of Tricyclic Antidepressant: Evidence for Noradrenergic Hyperactivity',. *British Journal of Psychiatry*, 141, 377–86.

Clark, M. (1981). 'The Rejection of Psychological Approaches to Mental Disorder in Late Nineteenth Century British Psychiatry', in Scull, A. (ed.) *Madhouses, Mad-doctors and Madmen* (London: Althone Press).

Cloninger, C. R. & Svrakic, D. M. (2008). 'Personality Disorders', in S. H. Fatemi, P. J. Clayton & N. F. R. W. Sartorius (eds) *The Medical Basis of Psychiatry*, 3rd edn (New Jersey: Humana Press).

Coleman, R. (1999). 'Hearing Voices and Political Oppression', in C. Newnes, G. Holmes & C. Dunn, (eds) *This is Madness: A Critical Look at Psychiatry and the Future of Mental Health Services* (Ross-on-Wye: PCCS Books).

Connel, R. W. (2000). *The Men and the Boys* (Berkeley: University of California Press).

Connel, R. W. (2002). *Gender* (Cambridge: Polity Press).

Crane, G. E. (1956). 'Further Studies on Iproniazid Phosphate, Isonicotinil-isopropyl-hydrazine Phosphate Marsilid', *Journal of Nervous and Mental Disease*, 124, 3, 322–31.

Crane, G. E. (1957). 'Iproniazid (marsilid) Phosphate, a Therapeutic Agent for Mental Disorders and Debilitating Diseases', *Psychiatric Research Reports of the American Psychiatric Association*, 135, 8, 142–52.

Crittenden, P. M. (2006). 'A Dynamic-maturational Model of Attachment', *Australian and New Zealand Journal of Family Therapy*, 27, 2, 105–15.

Cromby, J. & Harper, D. (2009). 'Paranoia: A Social Account', *Theory & Psychology*, 19, 3, 335–61.

Cromby, J., Diamond, B., Kelly, P., Moloney, P., Priest P. & Smail D. (eds) (2006). 'Critical and Community Psychology', Special issue of *Clinical Psychology Forum*, 163, June.

Crossley, N. (1999). 'Fish, Field, Habitus and Madness: The First Wave Mental Health Users Movement in Great Britain', *British Journal of Sociology*, 50, 4, 647–70.

Crowe, M. (2004). 'Never Good Enough – Part 1: Shame or Borderline Personality Disorder?', *Journal of Psychiatric and Mental Health Nursing*, 11, 3, 327–34.

Csordas, T. (1994). 'Introduction: The Body as Representation and Being-in-the-World', in T. Csordas (ed.) *Embodiment and Experience: The Existential Ground of Culture and Self* (Cambridge: Cambridge University Press).

Csordas, T. (1994a). 'Words from the Holy People: A Case Study in Cultural Phenomenology',. in T. Csordas (ed.) *Embodiment and Experience: The Existential Ground of Culture and Self* (Cambridge: Cambridge University Press).

Dally, P. J. & Rohde, P. (1961). 'Comparison of Antidepressant Drugs in Depressive Illnesses', *The Lancet*, 1, 277, 7167, 18–20.

Danzinger, K. (1985). 'The Methodological Imperative in Psychology', *Philosophy of the Social Sciences*, 15, 1, 1–13.

David, A. S. (1999). 'On the Impossibility of Defining Delusion', *Philosophy, Psychiatry & Psychology*, 6, 1, 17–20.

de Mijolla, A. (ed.). *International Dictionary of Psychoanalysis* (Farmington Hills, MI: Thomson Gale).

de Rivera, J. & Sarbin, T. (eds) (1998). *Believed-in Imaginings: The Narrative Construction of Reality* (Washington, DC: American Psychological Association).

Delay, J. & Buisson, J. F. (1958). 'Psychic Action of Isoniazid in the Treatment of Depressive States', *Journal of Clinical and Experimental Psychopathology*, 19, 2 (suppl. 1), 51–5.

Deonna, J. A. & Teroni, F. (2008). 'Differentiating Shame from Guilt', *Consciousness and Cognition*, 17, 4, 1063–400.

Deniker, P. & Lemperiere, T. (1964). 'Drug Treatment of Depression', in E. B. Davies, (ed.). *Depression: Proceedings of the Symposium Held at Cambridge 22nd to 26th September, 1959* (Cambridge: Cambridge University Press).

Department of Health (1989). *Working for Patients* (London: HMSO).

Department of Health (2000). *The Mental Health Policy Implementation Guide* (London: HMSO).

Department of Health (2003). *Expert Briefing: Summer 2003 - Early Intervention for People with Psychosis* (London: HMSO).

Department of Health (2005). *Delivering Race Equality in Mental Health Care: An Action Plan for Reform Inside and Outside Services and the Government's Response to the Independent Inquiry into the Death of David Bennett* (London: HMSO).

Department of Health (2007). *Prescription Cost Analysis: England 2006* (London: Department of Health). Available from:http://www.ic.nhs.uk/ webfiles/publications/pca2006/PCA_2006.pdf accessed 13 July 2010.

Department of Health (2010). *Prescription Cost Analysis, 2009.* (London, HMSO). Available from: http://www.ic.nhs.uk/statistics-and-data-collections/primary-care/ prescriptions/prescription-cost-analysis-england--2009. Accessed 13 July 2010.

Descartes, R. (1968). *Discourse on Method and the Meditations* E. E. Sutcliffe, ed. (London: Penguin).

Dillon, J. & May, R. (2002). Reclaiming Experience, *Clinical Psychology*, vol. 17, 25–7.

Dillon, J. (2006). 'Collective Voices', *Open Mind*, 142, 16–18.

Dilthey, W. (1976). *Selected Writings* (Cambridge: Cambridge University Press).

Disability Rights Commission (2006). *Equal Treatment – Closing the Gap: The Disability Rights Commission Formal Investigation into Physical Health Inequalities Experienced by People with Learning Disabilities and/or Mental Health Problems* (London: Author).

Doanne, J. A., West, K. L., Goldstein, M. J., Rodnick, E. H. & Jones, J. E. (1981). 'Parental Communication Deviance and Affective Style', *Archives of General Psychiatry*, 38, 6, 679–715.

Dobson, K. S., Hollon, S. D., Dimidjian, S., Schmaling, K. B., Kohlenberg, R. J., Gallop, R. J., Rizvi, S. L., Gollan, J. K., Dunner, D. L. & Jacobson, N. S. (2008). 'Randomized Trial of Behavioural Activation, Cognitive Therapy, and Antidepressant Medication in the Prevention of Relapse and Recurrence in Major Depression', *Journal of Consulting and Clinical Psychology*, 76, 3, 468–77.

Dolan, B. & Coid, J. (1993). *Psychopathic and Antisocial Personality Disorders: Treatment and Research Issues* (London: Gaskell).

Dolan, Y. M. (2000). *Beyond Survival: Living Well is the Best Revenge*, 2nd edn, Revised (London: BT Press).

Donne, J. (1624/1839). 'Meditation 17, Devotions upon Emergent Occasions', in *The Works of John Donne, Vol III*, H. Alford (ed.) (London: John W. Parker).

Donnelly, J. (1999). 'The Social Construction of International Human Rights', in T. Dunne & N. Wheeler (eds) *Human Rights in Global Politics* (Cambridge: Cambridge University Press).

Double, D. B. (ed.) (2006). *Critical Psychiatry: The Limits of Madness* (Basingstoke: Palgrave Macmillan).

Down, J. L. M. (1866/1987). 'Observations on an Ethnic Classification of Idiots', *Lectures and Reports from the London Hospital for 1866*, reprinted in C. Thompson (ed.) *The Origins of Modern Psychiatry* (Chichester: Wiley).

Downs, J. (2005a). *Starting and Supporting Hearing Voices Groups* (Manchester: Hearing Voices Network).

Downs, J. (ed.) (2005b). *Coping with Voices and Visions* (Manchester: Hearing Voices Network).

Dowson, J. & Grounds, A. (1995). *Personality Disorders: Recognition and Clinical Management* (Cambridge: Cambridge University Press).

Dreyfus, H. (1991). *Being-in-the-World: A Commentary on Heidegger's Being and Time, Division 1* (Cambridge, MA: MIT Press).

Dryden, C. (1999). *Being Married, Doing Gender: A Critical Analysis of Gender Relationships in Marriage* (London: Routledge).

DSM5.org (2010). *313.89 Reactive Attachment Disorder of Infancy or Early Childhood.* Available from: http://www.dsm5.org/ProposedRevisions/Pages/proposedrevision.aspx?rid=120. Accessed 10 March 2010.

Drugs and Therapeutics Bulletin (1999). 'Withdrawing Patients from Antidepressants', *Drugs and Therapeutics Bulletin*, 37, 7, 49–52.

Dunne, T. & Wheeler, N. (eds) *Human Rights in Global Politics* (Cambridge: Cambridge University Press).

Edginton, J. (Director) (1995). *Horizon: Hearing Voices*. An Otmoor and Mental Health Media Production for BBC Television.

Eekelaar, J. (1993). 'Are Parents Morally Obliged to Care for Their Children?', in J. Eekelaar & P. Sarcevic (eds) *Parenthood in Modern Society: Legal and Social Issues for the Twenty-first Century* (Dordrecht: Martinus Nijhoff).

Ellett, L., Lopes, B. & Chadwick, P. (2003). 'Paranoia in a Nonclinical Population of College Students', *Journal of Nervous and Mental Disease*, 191, 7, 425–30.

Elliott, D., Bjeelajac, P., Fallot, R., Markoff, L. & Glover Reed, B. (2005). 'Trauma-informed or Trauma-denied: Principles and Implementation of Trauma-informed Services for Women', *Journal of Community Psychology*, 33, 4, 461–77.

Emerson, J., Pankratz, L., Joos, S. & Smith, S. (1994). 'Personality Disorders in Problematic Medical Patients', *Psychosomatics: Journal of Consultation Liaison Psychiatry*, 35, 5, 469–73.

Engels, F. (1845/1969). *The Condition of the Working Class in England* (London: Panther).

Epstein, W. (1995). *The Illusion of Psychotherapy* (New Brunswick & London: Transaction Publishers).

Epstein, W. (2006). *Psychotherapy as Religion* (Reno & Las Vegas: University of Nevada Press).

Escher, S. (1993). 'Talking about Voices', in M. Romme & S. Escher (eds) *Accepting Voices* (London: Mind).

Essed, P. (1990). *Everyday Racism*, 2nd edn, trans. Cynthia Jaffé (Alameda, CA: Hunter House), originally published in Dutch as *Alledaags Racisme* (Baarn, Netherlands: Ambo b. v.)

Even, C., Siobud-Dorocant, E. & Dardennes, R. M. (2000). 'Critical Approach to Antidepressant Trials: Blindness Protection is Necessary, Feasible and Measurable', *British Journal of Psychiatry*, 177: 1, 47–51.

Falloon, I. R. H, (2000). 'Problem-solving as a Core Strategy in the Prevention of Schizophrenia and Other Mental Disorders', *Australian and New Zealand Journal of Psychiatry*, 34 (SUPPL.): 185–90.

Fava, G. A. (2003). 'Can Long-term Treatment with Antidepressant Drugs Worsen the Course of Depression?', *Journal of Clinical Psychatry*, 64, 2, 122–33.

Feeley, M. & Simon, J. (1992). 'The New Penology: Notes on the Emerging Strategy of Corrections and Its Implications', *Criminology*, 30, 4, 449–74.

Feighner, J. P., Robins, E., Guze, S. B., Woodruff, R. A., Winokur, G. & Munoz, R. (1972). 'Diagnostic Criteria for Use in Psychiatric Research', *Archives of General Psychiatry*, 26, 1, 57–63.

Fernando, S. (1997). 'Peeling Labels', *Open Mind*, 87, 16–17.

Fernando, S. (2003). *Cultural Diversity, Mental Health and Psychiatry: The Struggle Against Racism* (Hove & New York: Brunner-Routledge).

Fernando, S. (2007). 'From "Whole Systems Change" to No Change', *Openmind*, 143, 25.

Fernando, S. (2010). *Mental Health, Race and Culture*, 2nd Edn (Basingstoke: Palgrave Macmillan).

Ferriter, M. & Huband, N. (2003). 'Experiences of Parents with a Son or Daughter Suffering from Schizophrenia', *Journal of Psychiatric and Mental Health Nursing*, 10, 5, 552–60.

Fonagy, P. & Bateman, A. (2006). 'Progress in the Treatment of Borderline Personality Disorder', *British Journal of Psychiatry*, 188, 1, 1–3.

Fonagy, P. & Target, M. (1995). 'Dissociation and Trauma', *Current Opinion in Psychiatry*, 8, 8, 161–6.

Foress Bennett, J. (1997). 'Credibility, Plausibility and Autobiographical Oral Narrative: Some Suggestions from the Analysis of a Rape Survivor's Testimony', in A. Levett, A. Kottler, E. Burman & I. Parker (eds) *Culture, Power & Difference: Discourse Analysis in South Africa* (London: Zed Books).

Fowler, D., Freeman, D., Steele, C., Hardy, A., Smith, B., Hackman, C., Kuipers, E., Garety, P. & Bebbington, P. (2006). 'The Catastrophic Interaction Hypothesis', in W. Larkin and A. P. Morrison (eds) *Trauma and Psychosis: New Directions for Theory and Therapy* (Hove: Routledge).

Freeman, D. (2007). 'Suspicious Minds: The Psychology of Persecutory Delusions', *Clinical Psychology Review*, 27, 4, 425–57.

Freeman, D. & Freeman, J. (2008). *Paranoia: The Twenty-first Century Fear* (Oxford: Oxford University Press).

Freeman, D. & Garety, P. A. (2000). 'Comments on the Content of Persecutory Delusions: Does the Definition Need Clarification?', *British Journal of Clinical Psychology*, 39, 4, 407–14.

Freud, S. (1973). *Introductory Lectures on Psychoanalysis, Vol. I* (Harmondsworth: Penguin).

Freud, S. (1974). *Studies on Hysteria* (Harmondsworth: Penguin).

Freud, S. (1985). *Civilization, Society and Religion* (Harmondsworth: Penguin).

Freud, S. (1986). *Historical and Expository Works on Psychoanalysis* (Harmondsworth: Penguin).

Fromm-Reichmann, F. (1948). 'Notes on Development of Treatment of Schizophrenics by Psychoanalytic Psychotherapy', *Psychiatry*, 11, 3, 263.

Forster, R. & Gabe, J. (2008). 'Voice or Choice? Patient and Public Involvement in the National Health Service in England under New Labour', *International Journal of Health Services*, 38, 2, 333–56.

Foucault, M. (1961). *Folie et déraison: Histoire de la folie à l'âge classique* (Paris: Plon).

Foucault, M. (1963). *Naissance de la clinique* (Paris: Presses Universitaires de France).

Foucault, M. (1973). *The Birth of the Clinic: An Archaeology of Medical Perception*, trans. A. M. Sheridan Smith (London: Tavistock).

Foucault, M. (1982). 'The Subject and Power', in H. Dreyfus and P. Rabinow', 2nd edn *Michel Foucault: Beyond Structuralism and Hermeneutics* (Chicago: Chicago University Press).

Foucault, M. (2003). *Abnormal: Lectures at the Collège de France 1974–1975* (London: Verso).

Fowler, K. A., O'Donohue, W. & Lilienfeld, S. O. (2007). 'Personality Disorders in Perspective', in K. A. Fowler, W. O'Donohue and S. O. Lilienfeld (eds) *Personality Disorders: Towards the DSM-V* (Thousand Oaks: Sage).

Friedli, L. (2009). *Mental Health, Resilience and Inequalities* (Copenhagen: WHO).

Garfinkel, H. (1956a). 'Conditions of Successful Degradation Ceremonies', *American Journal of Sociology*, 61, 5, 420–4.

Garfinkel, H. (1956b). 'Some Sociological Concepts and Methods for Psychiatrists', *Psychiatric Research Reports*, 6, October, 181–98.

Georgaca, E. (2000). 'Reality and Discourse: A Critical Analysis of the Category of "delusions"', *British Journal of Medical Psychology*, 73, 2, 227–42.

Georgaca, E. (2004). 'Factualization and Plausibility in "Delusional" Discourse', *Philosophy, Psychiatry & Psychology*, 11, 1, 13–23.

Gergen, K. (1997). *Realities and Relationships: Soundings in Social Construction* (Harvard: Harvard University Press).

Gergen, K. J. & Gergen, M. M. (1988). 'Narrative and Self as Relationship', in L. Berkowitz (ed.) *Advances in Experimental Social Psychology, Vol. 21. Social Psychology Studies of the Self: Perspectives and Programs* (San Diego: Academic Press).

Gilbert, P., Pehl, J. & Allan, S. (1994). The Phenomenology of Shame and Guilt: An Empirical Investigation', *British Journal of Medical Psychology*, 67, 1, 23–36.

Gilbert, P. & McGuire, M. (1998). 'Shame, Social Roles and Status: The Psychobiological Continuum from Monkey to Human', in P. Gilbert & B. Andrews (eds) *Shame: Interpersonal Behavior, Psychopathology and Culture* (New York: Oxford University Press).

Goffman, E. (1961). *Asylums: Essays on the Social Situation of Mental Patients and Other Inmates* (New York: Anchor Books).

Goldberg, D. M. (2000). 'Predictions for Psychiatry', *The Journal of the Royal Society of Medicine*, vol. 93, no. 12, December, 649–51.

Goldberg, D. T. (1993). *Racist Culture: Philosophy and the Politics of Meaning* (Oxford: Blackwell).

Goldie, N. (1977). 'The Division of Labour among the Mental Health Professions in M. Stacey, M. Reid, C. Heath & R. Dingwall (eds) *Health and the Division of Labour* (London: Croom Helm).

Goldman, D. (1966). 'Critical Contrasts in Psychopharmacology', in M. Rinkel (ed.) *Biological Treatment of Mental Illness* (New York: L. C. Page).

Goldstein, M. J. (1987). 'The UCLA High-risk Project', *Schizophrenia Bulletin*, 13, 3, 505–14.

Grant, B. F., Hasin, D. S., Stinson, F. S., Dawson, D. A., Chou, S. P., Ruan, W. J. & Pickering, R. P. (2004). 'Prevalence, Correlates, and Disability of Personality Disorders in the United States: Results from the National Epidemiologic Survey on Alcohol and Related Conditions', *Journal of Clinical Psychiatry*, 65, 7, 948–58.

Granville-Chapman, C. & Patel, N. (2005). 'Channel 4's Guantanamo Guidebook: Making a Point or Unethical and Irresponsible?', *British Medical Journal Online*, 9 March.

Grilo, C. M., Sainslow, C. A., Fehon, D. C., Lipschitz, D. S., Martino, S. & McGlashan, T. H. (1999). 'Correlates of Suicide Risk in Adolescent Inpatients Who Report a History of Childhood Sexual Abuse', *Comprehensive Psychiatry*, 40, 6, 422–8.

Gunderson, J. G. & Zanarini, M. C. (1987). 'Current Overview of the Borderline Diagnosis', *Journal of Clinical Psychiatry*, (Suppl.), 48, 5–11.

Gurian, M. (1999). *The Good Son* (New York: Tarcher-Putnam).

Gurian, M. (2001). *Boys and Girls Think Differently!* (San Francisco: Jossey-Bass).

Hacking, I. (1995). *Rewriting the Soul: Multiple Personality and the Sciences of Memory* (Princeton NJ: Princeton University Press).

Haddad, P., Lejoyeux, M. & Young, A. (1998). 'Antidepressant Discontinuation Reactions', Editorial, *British Medical Journal*, 316, 7138, 1105–6.

Hall, G. S. (1904). *Adolescence: Its Psychology and its Relations to Physiology, Anthropology, Sociology, Sex, Crime, Religion and Education, vol. 2* (New York: D. Appleton).

Hall, S. (1997). *Representation: Cultural Representations and Signifying Practices* (London: Sage).

Hall, S. (1992). 'New Ethnicities', in J. Donald and A. Ratansi (eds) *'Race', Culture and Difference* (London: Sage).

Hall, W. (2007). *Harm-Reduction Guide to Coming Off Psychiatric Drugs*. Available from: http://theicarusproject.net/alternative-treatments/harm-reduction-guide-to-coming-off-psychiatric-drugs. Accessed 11 April 2010.

Hallam, R. S. & O'Connor, K. P. (2002). 'A Dialogical Approach to Obsessions', *Psychology and Psychotherapy: Theory Research and Practice*, 75, 3, 333–48.

Hammersley, P., Read, J., Woodall, S. & Dillon. J. (2008). 'Childhood Trauma and Psychosis: The Genie is Out of the Bottle', *Journal of Psychological Trauma*, 6, 2/3, 7–20.

Hammersley, P., Langshaw, B., Bullimore, P., Dillon, J., Romme, M. & Escher, S. (2008). 'Schizophrenia at the Tipping Point', *Mental Health Practice*, 12, 1, 14–19.

Hanish, C. (1970). 'The Personal Is Political', in S. Firestone & A. Koedt (eds) Notes from the Second Year: Women's Liberation (New York: Radical Feminism).

Hansen, S., McHoul, A. & Rapley, M. (2003). *Beyond Help: A Consumer's Guide to Psychology* (Ross-on-Wye, PCCS Books).

Hare, E. H., McCance, C. & McCormick, W. O. (1964). 'Imipramine and "Drinamyl" in Depressive Illness: A Comparative Trial', *British Medical Journal*, 1, 5386, 818–20.

Harper, D. J. (1994). 'The Professional Construction of "Paranoia" and the Discursive Use of Diagnostic Criteria', *British Journal of Medical Psychology*, 67, 2, 131–43.

Harper, D. J. (1996). 'Deconstructing "Paranoia": Towards a Discursive Understanding of Apparently Unwarranted Suspicion', *Theory & Psychology*, 6, 3, 423–48.

Harper, D. J. (1999). *Deconstructing Paranoia: An Analysis of the Discourses Associated with the Concept of Paranoid Delusion*. Unpublished Ph.D. thesis, Manchester Metropolitan University.

Harper, D. J. (2004). 'Delusions and Discourse: Moving Beyond the Constraints of the Modernist Paradigm', *Philosophy, Psychiatry & Psychology*, 11, 1, 55–64.

Harper, D. (2007). 'The Complicity of Psychologists in the Security State', in R. Roberts (ed.) *Just War: Iraq and Psychology* (Ross-on-Wye: PCCS Books).

Harper, D. J. (2008). 'The Politics of Paranoia: Paranoid Positioning and Conspiratorial Narratives in the Surveillance Society', *Surveillance & Society*, 5, 1, 1–32.

Harris, G. & Carey, B. (2008). 'Researchers Fail to Reveal Full Drug Pay', *Sunday New York Times*, 8 June. Available from: http://www.mindfreedom.org/kb/psych-drug-corp/ny-times-biederman-harvard/grassley-v-harvard/ Accessed 9 October 2008.

Haslam, J. (1798). *Observations on Insanity* (London: Rivington).

Haslam, J. (1817). *Considerations on the Moral Management of Insane Persons.* (London: Hunter).

Healthcare Commission (2008). *The Pathway to Recovery: A Review of NHS Acute In-patient Mental Health Services* (London: Author).

Healy, D. (1997). *The Antidepressant Era* (New York: Harvard University Press).

Healy, D. (2002). *The Creation of Psychopharmacology* (Cambridge, MA: Harvard University Press).

Hearn, K. (2004). *Here Kiddie, Kiddie.* Available from: http://alternet.org/drugreporter/20594. Accessed 13 April 2010.

Heise, D. R. (1988). Delusions and the Construction of Reality', in T. F. Oltmanns & B. A. Maher (eds) *Delusional Beliefs* (New York: Wiley).

Henderson, D. & Gillespie, R. D. (1927/1944). *Henderson and Gillespie's Textbook of Psychiatry* (Oxford: Oxford University Press).

Henkin, L. (1989). 'The Universality of the Concept of Human Rights', *Annals*, AAPSS, vol. 506, November, 10–16.

Herman, J. L. (1992). *Trauma and Recovery: From Domestic Abuse to Political Theory* (London: Pandora).

Herrnstein, R. J. & Murray, C. (1994). *The Bell Curve: Intelligence and Class Structure in American life* (New York: Free Press).

Hester, M., Pearson, C. & Harwin, N. (2000). *Making an Impact: Children and Domestic Violence – A Reader* (London: Jessica Kingsley).

Hilpern, K. (2007a). 'How I Beat the Voices in My Head', *The Independent*, 6 March.

Hilpern, K. (2007b). 'Muddy Thinking', *The Guardian*, 9 October.

Hobsbawm, E. (1994). *The Age of Extremes: The Short Twentieth Century 1914–1991* (Harmondsworth: Michael Joseph/Penguin).

Hodge, J. R. (1955). 'The Passive-dependent Versus the Passive-aggressive Personality', *United States Armed Forces Medical Journal*, 6, 1, 84–90.

Holland, S. (1991). 'From Private Symptom to Public Action', *Feminism & Psychology*, 1, 1, 58–62.

Hollon, S. D., DeRubeis, R. J., Shelton, R. C. & Weiss, B. (2002). 'The Emperor's New Drugs: Effect Size and Moderation Effects', *Prevention and Treatment*, 5, Article 27, available from: http://www.journals.apa.org/prevention/volume5/pre0050027c.html.

Holmes, O. W. (1871). Valedictory Address, Delivered to the Graduating Class of the Bellevue Hospital College, 2 March 1871. *New York Medical Journal*, 13, 420–40.

Holmes, G., Hudson, M. & May, R. (2008). 'Coping with Coming Off', *Open Mind*, 150, 12–14.

Holt, E. (1996). 'Reporting on Talk: The Use of Direct Reported Speech in Conversation', *Research on Language and Social Interaction*, 29, 3, 219–45.

Holzinger, A., Kilian, R., Lindenbach, I., Petscheleit, A. & Angermeyer, M. C. (2003). 'Patients' and Their Relatives' Causal Explanations of Schizophrenia', *Social Psychiatry and Psychiatric Epidemiology*, 38, 3, 155–62.

Home Office (1999). *The Stephen Lawrence Inquiry: Report of an Inquiry by Sir William Macpherson of Cluny* (London: HMSO).

Home Office (2003). *Respect and Responsibility – Taking a Stand against Anti-social Behaviour*. White Paper. Cmnd. 5778. (London: HMSO).

Home Affairs Select Committee (2000). *First Report: Managing Dangerous People with Severe Personality Disorder* (London: HMSO).

Hornstein, G. A. (2009a). 'Who Owns the Mind?', *Open Mind*, 157, 6–8.

Hornstein, G. A. (2009b). *Agnes's Jacket: A Psychologist's Search for the Meanings of Madness* (New York: Rodale Press).

House, R. & Loewenthal, D. (eds) (2008). *Against and For CBT: Towards a Constructive Dialogue?* (Ross-on-Wye: PCCS Books).

Howarth, D. (2000). *Discourse* (Buckingham: Open University Press).

Huppert, F. A. (2009). 'A New Approach to Reducing Disorder and Improving Well-being', *Perspectives on Psychological Science*, 4, 1, 108–11.

Husband, C. (1982). '"Race", the Continuity of a Concept', in C. Husband (ed.) *Race in Britain: Continuity and Change* (London: Hutchinson).

Hyman, S. (2000). 'The NIMH Perspective: Next Steps in Schizophrenia Research', *Biological Psychiatry*, 47, 1, 1–7.

Imel, Z. E., Malterer, M. B., McKay, K. M. & Wampold, B. E. (2008). A Meta-analysis of Psychotherapy and Medication in Unipolar Depression and Dysthymia', *Journal of Affective Disorders*, 110, 3, 197–206.

Ingelby, D. (1982). 'The Social Construction of Mental Illness', in P. Wright & A. Treacher (eds) *The Problem of Medical Knowledge: Examining the Social Construction of Medicine* (Edinburgh: Edinburgh University Press).

Ignatieff, M. (2001). *Human Rights as Politics and Idolatry* (Princeton: Princeton University Press).

Ivanovic, M., Vuletic, Z. & Bebbington, P. (1994). 'Expressed Emotion in the Families of Patients with Schizophrenia and its Influence on the Course of Illness', *Social Psychiatry and Psychiatric Epidemiology*, 29, 2, 61–5.

Jacobs, D. H. (1995). 'Psychiatric Drugging: Forty Years of Pseudoscience, Self Interest and Indifference to Harm', *Journal of Mind and Behaviour*, 16, 4, 421–70.

Jacobs, D. H. (2009). 'Is a Correct Psychiatric Diagnosis Possible? Major Depressive Disorder as a Case in Point', *Ethical Human Psychology and Psychiatry: An International Journal of Critical Inquiry*, 11, 2, 83–96.

Jacobs, D. H. & Cohen, D. (2010). 'Does "Psychological Dysfunction" Mean Anything? A Critical Essay on Pathology Versus Agency', *The Journal of Humanistic Psychology*, 50, 3, 312–34.

Jacobsen, E. (1964). 'The Theoretical Basis of the Chemotherapy of Depression', in Davies, E. B. (ed.) *Depression: Proceedings of the Symposium Held at Cambridge 22nd to 26th September 1959* (Cambridge: Cambridge University Press).

Jadad, A. R., Boyle, M., Cunningham, C., Kim, M. & Schachar, R. (1999). *Treatment of Attention-Deficit/Hyperactivity Disorder – Evidence Report: Technology Assessment 11* (Rockville, MD: Agency for Health Care Policy and Research).

James, A. (2001). *Raising our Voices: An Account of the Hearing Voices Movement* (Gloucester: Handsell Publishing).

James, A. (2003). 'Voices of Reason', *The Guardian*, 10 December. Available from: http://society.guardian.co.uk/societyguardian/story/0,7843,1103141,00.html. Accessed 8 February 2010.

James, O. (2005). 'Think Again', *The Guardian*, 22 October.

James, W. (1890). *The Principles of Psychology, 2 vols* (New York: Henry Holt).

Janet, P. (1907). *The Major Symptoms of Hysteria* (London: Macmillan).

Janssen, I., Hanssen, M. A., Bak, M., Bijl, R. V., de Graaf, R., Vollebergh, W. & van Os, J. (2003). 'Discrimination and Delusional Ideation', *British Journal of Psychiatry*, 182, 1, 71–6.

Janssen, I., Krabbendum, L., Bak, M., Hanssen, M., Vollebergh, W., de Graaf, R. & van Os, J. (2004). 'Childhood Abuse as a Risk Factor for Psychotic Experiences', *Acta Psychiatrica Scandinavica*, 109, 1, 38–45.

Jensen, P. S., Arnold, L. E., Swanson, J. M., Vitiello, B., Abikoff, H. B., Greenhill, L. L., Hechtman, L., Hinshaw, S. P., Pelham, W. E., Wells, K. C., Conners, C. K., Elliott, G. R., Epstein, J. N., Hoza, B., March, J. S., Molina, B. S., Newcorn, J. H., Severe, J. B., Wigal, T., Gibbons, R. D. & Hur, K. (2007). '3-year Follow-up of the NIMH MTA Study', *Journal of the American Academy of Child and Adolescent Psychiatry*, 46, 8, 989–1002.

Jefferson, G. (2004) '"At First I Thought": A Normalizing Device for Extraordinary Events', in G. H. Lerner (ed.) *Conversation Analysis: Studies from the First Generation* (Philadelphia: John Benjamins).

Jessner, L. & Ryan,V. G. (1943). *Shock Treatment in Psychiatry* (London: Heineman).

Johns, L. C., Cannon, M., Singleton, N., Murray, R. M., Farrell, M., Brugha, T., Bebbington, P., Jenkins, R. & Meltzer, H. (2004). 'Prevalence and Correlates of Self-reported Psychotic Symptoms in the British Population', *British Journal of Psychiatry*, 185, 298–305.

Johnstone, L. (1999). 'Do Families Cause "Schizophrenia"? Revisiting a Taboo Subject', *Changes*, 17, 2, 77–90.

Johnstone, L. (1993). 'Family Management in "Schizophrenia": Its Assumptions and Contradictions', *Journal of Mental Health*, 2, 3, 255–69.

Johnstone, L. (2000). *Users and Abusers of Psychiatry: A Critical Look at Psychiatric Practice* (London: Routledge).

Johnstone, L. (2007). 'Can Trauma Cause "Psychosis"?' Revisiting (Another) Taboo Subject', *Journal of Critical Psychology, Counselling and Psychotherapy*, 7, 4, 211–20.

Jorm, A. F. (2000). 'Mental Health Literacy', *British Journal of Psychiatry*, 177, 5, 396–401.

Joyce, P. R. & Paykel, E. S. (1989). 'Predictors of Drug Response in Depression', *Archives of General Psychiatry*, 46, 1, 89–99.

Jukes, A. E. (1999). *Men Who Batter Women* (London: Routledge).

Jung, C. G. (1930). 'Your Negroid and Indian Behaviour', *Forum*, 83, 4, 193–9.

Jüni, P., Altman, D. G. & Egger, M. (2001). 'Assessing the Quality of Controlled Clinical Trials', *British Medical Journal*, 323, 7303, 42–6.

Kaldor, M. (2003). *Global Civil Society: An Answer to War* (Cambridge: Polity Press).

Karlowski, T. R., Chalners, T. C., Frenkel, L. D., Kapikian A. Z., Lewis, T. L. & Lynch, J. M. (1975). 'Ascorbic Acid for the Common Cold', *Journal of the American Medical Association*, 231, 10, 1038–42.

Karlsen, S. & Nazroo, J. Y. (2002). 'Relation Between Racial Discrimination, Social Class and Health among Ethnic Minority Groups', *American Journal of Public Health*, 92, 4, 624–31.

Kavanagh, D. J. (1992). 'Recent Developments in Expressed Emotion and Schizophrenia', *British Journal of Psychiatry*, 162: 5, 601–20.

Keogh, A. (2007). 'Rape Trauma Syndrome – Time to Open the Floodgates?', *Journal of Legal and Forensic Medicine*, 15, 4, 221–4.

Kemper, T. D. (1987). A Manichean Approach to the Social Construction of Emotions', *Cognition and Emotion*, 1, 4, 353–65.

Kilcommons, A. M. & Morrison, A. P. (2005). 'Relationships between Trauma and Psychosis: An Exploration of Cognitive and Dissociative Factors', *Acta Psychiatrica Scandinavica*, 112, 5, 351–9.

Kimmel, M. (2004). *The Gendered Society* (New York: Oxford University Press).

Kindlon, D. & Thompson, M. (2000). *Raising Cain: Protecting the Emotional Life of Boys* (New York: Ballantine Books).

King, S. (2000). 'Is Expressed Emotion Cause or Effect in the Mothers of Schizophrenic Young Adults?', *Schizophrenia Research*, 45, 1–2, 65–78.

King, M., Coker, E., Leavey, A., Hoare, A. & Johnson-Sabine, D. (1994). 'Incidence of Psychotic Illness in London: Comparison of Ethnic Groups', *British Medical Journal*, 309, 6962, 1115–9.

King, N., Finlay, L., Ashworth, P., Smith, J. A., Langdridge, D. & Butt, T. (2008). '"Can't Really Trust That, so What Can I Trust?": A Polyvocal, Qualitative Analysis of the Psychology of Mistrust', *Qualitative Research in Psychology*, 5, 2, 80–102.

King, S., Griffin, S., Hodges, Z., Weatherly, H., Asseburg, C., Richardson, G., Golder, S., Taylor, E., Drummond, M. & Riemsma, R. (2006). 'A Systematic Review and Economic Model of the Effectiveness and Cost-effectiveness of Methylphenidate, Dexamfetamine and Atomoxetine for the Treatment of Attention Deficit Hyperactivity Disorder in Children and Adolescents', *Health Technology Assessments*, 10, 23, 1–146.

Kirsch, I. (1985). 'Response Expectancy as a Determinant of Experience and Behavior', *American Psychologist*, 40, 11, 1189–202.

Kirsch, I. (ed.) (1999). *How Expectancies Shape Experience* (Washington, DC: American Psychological Association).

Kirsch, I. (2010). *The Emperor's New Drugs: Exploding the Antidepressant Myth* (New York: Basic Books).

Kirsch, I. & Sapirstein, G. (1998). 'Listening to Prozac but Hearing Placebo: A Meta-analysis of Antidepressant Medication', *Prevention and Treatment*, 1 (Article 0002a). Available from: http://www.journals.apa.org/prevention/volume1/pre0010002a.html.

Kirsch, I., Moore, T. J., Scoboria, A. & Nicholls, S. S. (2002). The Emperor's New Drugs: An Analysis of Antidepressant Medication Data Submitted to the US Food and Drug Administration', *Prevention and Treatment*, 5, article 23. Available from: http://www.namiscc.org/Research/2002/DrugEfficacy.htm. Accessed 5 April 2010.

Kirsch, I., Deacon, B. J., Huedo-Medina, T. B., Scoboria, A., Moore, T. J. & Johnson, B. T. (2008). 'Initial Severity and Antidepressant Benefits: A Meta-analysis of Data Submitted to the Food and Drug Administration'. *PLoS Medicine*, 5(2). Available from: http://medicine.plosjournals.org/perlserv/?request=get-document&doi=10.1371/journal.pmed.0050045.

Kirsch, M. (2007). 'Voices in Your Head? You May Not Be Crazy', *The Times*, 23 January.

Klassen, A., Miller, A., Raina, P., Lee, S. K., & Olsen, L. (1999). Attention-deficit Hyperactivity Disorder in Children and Youth: A Quantitative Systematic

Review of the Efficacy of Different Management Strategies', *Canadian Journal of Psychiatry*, 44, 10, 1007–16.

Klein, R. (2001). *The New Politics of the National Health Service*, 4th edn (Harlow: Prentice Hall).

Klerman, G. L. (1978) 'The Evolution of a Scientific Nosology', in Shershow, J. C. (ed.) *Schizophrenia: Science and practice* (Cambridge, MA: Harvard University Press).

Klerman, G. L. (1990). 'The Psychiatric Patient's Right to Effective Treatment: Implications of Osheroff vs. Chestnut Lodge', *American Journal of Psychiatry*, 147, 4, 409–18.

Klerman, G. L., Dimascio, A., Weissman, M., Prusoff, B. & Paykel, E. S. (1974). Treatment of Depression by Drugs and Psychotherapy', *American Journal of Psychiatry*, 131, 2, 186–91.

Knight, T. (2009). *Beyond Belief: Alternative Ways of Working With Delusions, Obsessions and Unusual Experiences* (Berlin: Peter Lehmann Publishing). Available from: http://www.peter-lehmann-publishing.com/beyond-belief.htm. Accessed 15 January 2010.

Kraepelin, E. (1893/1919). *Psychiatrie: Ein lehrbuch fur studierende und ärtze*, 4th edn (Edinburgh: Livingstone).

Kraepelin, E. (1904). *Clinical Psychiatry*, trans. A. R. Diefendorf (New York: Macmillan).

Kraepelin, E. (1913). *Manic Depressive Insanity and Paranoia*, translation of *Lehrbuch der Psychiatrie*, *Vols 3 and 4*, 8th edn (trans. R. M. Barclay) (Edinburgh: Livingstone).

Kraepelin, E. (1921). *Manic-Depressive Insanity and Paranoia*, trans. and edited R. M. Barclay & G. M. Robertson (Edinburgh: Livingstone).

Krafft-Ebbing, R. von (1905). *Textbook of Insanity Based on Clinical Observation for Practitioners and Students in Medicine* (Philadelphia: F. A. Davis).

Kuhn, R. (1957). 'Treatment of Depressive States with an Iminodibenzyl Derivative (G 22355)', *Schweizer Medicalicsher Wochenschrift*, 87, 35/36, 1135–40.

Kuhn, R. (1958). 'The Treatment of Depressive States with G 22355 (Imipramine Hydrochloride)', *American Journal of Psychiatry*, 115, 5, 459–64.

Kuhn, T. S. (1970). *The Structure of Scientific Revolutions*, 2nd edn (Chicago: University of Chicago Press).

Kuipers, L., Birchwood, M. & McCreadie, R. G. (1992). 'Psychosocial Family Intervention in Schizophrenia: A Review of Empirical Studies', *British Journal of Psychiatry*, 160, 2, 272–5.

Kwiatkowski, R. (2007). 'Science and Ethics Underlie Our Actions', *Science and Public Affairs*, 10 March.

Lacasse, J. R. & Leo, J. (2005). 'Serotonin and Depression: A Disconnect between the Advertisements and the Scientific Literature', *PLoS Medicine*, 2: e392. doi:10.1371/journal.pmed.0020392.

Laing, R. D. (1960). *The Divided Self* (London: Tavistock).

Laing, R. D. (1969). *The Politics of the Family* (New York: Pantheon).

Laing, R. D. & Esterson, A. (1964). *Sanity, Madness and the Family*, 2nd edn (London: Tavistock).

Lancet (2008). 'Children and Psychiatric Drugs: Disillusion and Opportunity', *The Lancet*, (Editorial), 372, 9645, 1194.

Land, J. (2006). 'Schizophrenia Label "Should Be Abolished"', *Press Association*, October.

Lane, C. (2007). *Shyness: How Normal Behavior Became a Sickness* (New York: Vail-Ballou).

Langer, M. (1989). *Merleau-Ponty's Phenomenology of Perception: A Guide and Commentary* (London: Macmillan).

Largactil advertisement (1964). *British Medical Journal*, 5 September.

Larkin, P. (1974). *High Windows* (New York: Farrar, Straus and Giroux).

Larkin, W. & Morrison, A. P. (2006). *Trauma and Psychosis: New Directions for Theory and Therapy* (London: Routledge).

Laurance, J. (2010). 'Sex Addiction Sells – for the Drug Industry: Latest Psychiatrist's Bible is Criticised for Pathologising People's Everyday Habits', *The Independent*, 12 February.

Layard, R. (2006). *The Depression Report: A New Deal for Depression and Anxiety Disorders*. The Centre for Economic Performance's Mental Health Policy Group, June. Available from: http://cep.lse.ac.uk/_new/staff/person.asp?id=970. Accessed 10 March 2010.

Leber (1998). Unpublished Document.

Leeming, D. & Boyle, M. (2004). 'Shame as a Social Phenomenon: A Critical Analysis of the Concept of Dispositional Shame', *Psychology and Psychotherapy: Theory, Research and Practice*, 77, 3, 375–96.

Leff, J. (1973). 'Culture and the Differentiation of Emotional States', *British Journal of Psychiatry*, 123, 574, 299–306.

Leff, J. (1981). *Psychiatry Around the Globe: A Transcultural View* (New York: Marcel Dekker).

Lehmann, H. E., Cahn, C. H. & DeVerteuil, R. L. (1958). 'The Treatment of Depressive Conditions with Imipramine (G 22355)', *Canadian Psychiatric Association Journal*, 3, 4, 155–64.

Lehmann, H. E. & Kline, N. S. (1983). 'Clinical Discoveries with Antidepressant Drugs', in M. J. Parnham & J. Bruinvels (eds), *Discoveries in Pharmacology, Vol. 1* (London: Elsevier).

Leighton, A. H. & Hughes, J. M. (1961). 'Culture as Causative of Mental Disorder', *Millbank Memorial Fund Quarterly*, 39, 3, 446–70.

Lemma, A. (2003). *Introduction to the Practice of Psychoanalytic Psychotherapy* (Chichester: Wiley).

Leudar, I. & Thomas, P. (2000). *Voices of Reason, Voices of Insanity: Studies of Verbal Hallucinations* (London: Routledge).

Lewis, M. (1993). 'Self-conscious Emotions: Embarrassment, Pride, Shame and Guilt', in M. Lewis & J. M. Haviland (eds) *Handbook of Emotions* (New York: Guilford Press).

Lewontin, R. C., Rose, S. & Kamin, L. (1984). *Not In Our Genes: Biology, Ideology and Human Nature* (Penguin: Harmondsworth).

Lidz, R. W. & Lidz, T. (1949). 'The Family Environment of Schizophrenic Patients'. *American Journal of Psychiatry*, 106, 5, 332–45.

Link, B. G., Dohrenwend, B. P. & Skodol, A. E. (1986). 'Socio/Economic Status and Schizophrenia: Noisome Occupational Characteristics as a Risk Factor', *American Sociological Review*, 51: 2, 242–58.

Linnet, P. (2004). 'A Matter of Semantics', *Asylum*, 12, 2, 10–14.

Littlewood, R. (2002). *Pathologies of the West: An Anthropology of Mental Illness in Europe and America* (London: Continuum).

Livesley, W. J. (ed.) (2001). *Handbook of Personality Disorders: Theory, Research, and Treatment* (New York: Guilford Press).

Livesley, W. J., Schroeder, M. L., Jackson, D. N. & Lang, K. L. (1994). 'Categorical Distinctions in the Study of Personality Disorder: Implications for Classification', *Journal of Abnormal Psychology*, 103, 1, 6–17.

Lorde, A. (1984). The Master's Tools Will Never Dismantle the Master's House', in A. Lorde (ed.) *Sister Outsider: Essays and Speeches* (New York: The Crossing Press).

Loomer, H. P., Saunders, J. C., & Kline, N. S. (1957). A Clinical and Pharmacodynamic Evaluation of Iproniazid as a Psychic Energizer. *Psychiatric Research Reports of the American Psychiatric Association*, 13, 8, 129–41.

LSE, The Centre for Economic Performances Mental Health Policy Group (2006). *The Depression Report: A New Deal for Depression and Anxiety Disorders* (London: Author).

McCabe, R., Leudar, I. & Antaki, C. (2004). 'Do People with Schizophrenia Display Theory of Mind Deficits in Clinical Interactions?', *Psychological Medicine*, 34, 3, 401–12.

McCabe, R., Heath, C., Burns, T. & Priebe, S. (2002). 'Engagement of Patients with Psychosis in the Consultation: Conversation Analytic Study', *British Medical Journal*, 325, 7373, 1148–51.

McCracken, J. T., McGough, J., Shah, B., Cronin, P. & Hong, D. (2002). 'Risperidone in Children with Autism and Serious Behavioral Problems', *New England Journal of Medicine*, 347, 5, 314–21.

McCrone, P., Dhanasiri, S., Patel, A., Knapp, M. & Lawton-Smith, S. (2008). *Paying the Price: The Cost of Mental Health Care in England to 2026* (London: King Edward's Hospital Fund for London).

McDonagh, M. S. & Peterson, K. (2005). *Drug Class Review on Pharmacologic Treatments for ADHD* (Portland: Oregon Health and Science University).

McGlashan & Johannssen (1996). 'Early Detection and Intervention with Schizophrenia: Rationale', *Schizophrenia Bulletin*, 22: 2, 201–22.

McGorry, P. D. (2000). 'The Nature of Schizophrenia: Signposts to Prevention', *Australian and New Zealand Journal of Psychiatry*, 34 (SUPPL.): 14–21.

McGorry, P. D., Edwards, J., Mihalopoulos, C., Harrigan, S. M. & Jackson, H. J. (1996). 'EPPIC: An Evolving System of Early Detection and Optimal Management', *Schizophrenia Bulletin*, 22, 2, 305–26.

McHoul, A. (2008). *What Are We Doing When We Analyse Conversation?* Keynote Address, 6th Australasian Symposium on Conversation Analysis and Membership Categorisation Analysis, Brisbane, November 5th–7th. Available from http://aiemca.net/?page_id=229. Accessed 14 January 2010.

McHoul, A. & Rapley, M. (2005). 'A Case of ADHD Diagnosis: Sir Karl and Francis B Slug It Out on the Consulting Room Floor', *Discourse and Society*, 16, 3, 419–49.

McNab, C., Haslam, N. & Burnett, P. (2007). 'Expressed Emotion, Attributions, Utility Beliefs, and Distress in Parents of Young People with First Episode Psychosis', *Psychiatry Research*, 151, 1–2, 97–106.

Magnavita, J. (2003). *Handbook of Personality Disorders: Theory and Practice* (New York: Wiley).

Maher, B. A. (1992). 'Delusions: Contemporary Etiological Hypotheses', *Psychiatric Annals*, 22, 260–8.

Malson, H. & Burns, M. (2009). *Critical Feminist Approaches to Eating Disorders* (Hove: Routledge).

Mann, J. (1999). *The Elusive Magic Bullet: The Search for the Perfect Drug* (New York: Oxford University Press).

Mann, A. M. & MacPherson, A. S. (1959). 'Clinical Experience with Imipramine (G22355) in the Treatment of Depression', *Canadian Psychiatric Association Journal*, 4, 1, 38–47.

Masson, J. M. (1984). *The Assault on Truth: Freud's Suppression of the Seduction Theory* (New York: Farrar, Straus and Giroux).

Masson, J. M. (ed.) (1985). *The Complete Letters of Sigmund Freud to Wilhelm Fliess 1887–1904* (Letter of 21/09/1899) (Cambridge, MA: Harvard).

Masson, J. M. (1988). *Against Therapy* (London: Harper Collins).

Matthews, E. (2002). *The Philosophy of Merleau-Ponty* (Chesham: Acumen).

Maudsley, H. (1874). *Responsibilities in Mental Disease*, 2nd edn (London: Kegan Paul).

Maudsley, H. (1884). *Body and Will* (New York: Appleton).

May, R., Angel, E. & Ellenberger, H. (eds) (1958). *Existence: A New Dimension in Psychiatry and Psychology* (New York: Basic Books).

May, R. (1958a) 'The Origins and Significance of the Existential Movement in Psychology', in R. May, E. Angel, & H. Ellenberger (eds) *Existence: A New Dimension in Psychiatry and Psychology* (New York: Basic Books).

May, R. (2007). 'Working Outside the Diagnostic Frame', *The Psychologist*, 20, 5, 300–1.

Mayer-Gross, W., Slater, E., & Roth, M. (1954/1960). *Clinical Psychiatry* (London: Cassell).

Medawar, C. & Hardon, A. (2004). *Medicines out of Control? Anti-depressants and the Conspiracy of Goodwill* (Amsterdam: Aksant Academic).

Mendeleev, D. I. (1901). *Principles of Chemistry* (New York: Collier).

Menninger, K, with Mayman, M. & Pruyser, P. (1963). *The Vital Balance* (New York: Viking Press).

Merleau-Ponty, M. (1962). *Phenomenology of Perception*, trans. C. Smith (London: Routledge & Kegan Paul).

Middleton, N., Gunnell, D., Whitley, E., Dorling, D. & Frankel, S. (2001). 'Secular Trends in Antidepressant Prescribing in the UK', *Journal of Public Health Medicine*, 23, 4, 263–7.

Miller, A. (2005). *The Body Never Lies: The Lingering Effects of cruel Parenting* (New York: Norton & Company).

Miller, T. (2008). 'Panic between the Lips: Attention Deficit Hyperactivity Disorder and Ritalin®', in C. Krinsky (ed.) *Moral Panics Over Contemporary Children and Youth* (London: Ashgate).

Millon, T. (2004). *Matters of the Mind: Exploring the Story of Mental Illness from Ancient Times to the New Millennium* (Hoboken, NJ: John Wiley).

Millon, T. (ed.) (1983). *Theories of Personality and Psychopathology* (New York: Holt, Rinehart, and Winston).

Millon, T. (1981). *Disorders of Personality* (New York: Wiley).

Millon, T. (1969). *Modern Psychopathology: A Biosocial Approach to Maladaptive Learning and Functioning* (Philadelphia: Saunders).

Millon, T., Meagher, S. E. & Grossman, S. D. (2001) in W. J. Livesley, (ed.) *Handbook of Personality Disorders: Theory, Research, and Treatment* (New York: Guilford Press).

Mirowsky, J. & Ross, C. E. (1983). 'Paranoia and the Structure of Powerlessness', *American Sociological Review*, 48, 2, 228–39.

Moerman, D. (2002). *Meaning, Medicine and the 'Placebo' Effect* (Cambridge: Cambridge University Press).

Moerman, D. E. (2002). '"The Loaves and the Fishes": A Comment on The Emperor's New Drugs: An Analysis of Antidepressant Medication Data Submitted to the US Food and Drug Administration', *Prevention and Treatment*, 5, Article 29. Available from: http://www.journals.apa.org/prevention/volume5/pre0050029c.html.

Moffitt, T. E. & Caspi, A. (1998). 'Annotation: Implications of Violence between Intimate Partners for Child Psychologists and Psychiatrists', *Journal of Child Psychology and Psychiatry*, 39, 2, 137–44.

Mold, A. (2010). 'Patient Groups and the Construction of the Patient-consumer in Britain: An Historical Overview', *Journal of Social Policy*, published online by Cambridge University Press 13 April 2010.

Moncrieff, J. (1999). 'An Investigation into the Precedents of Modern Drug Treatment in Psychiatry', *History of Psychiatry*, 10, 40, (Pt 4), 475–90.

Moncrieff, J. (2006). 'Psychiatric Drug Promotion and the Politics of Neoliberalism', *British Journal of Psychiatry*, 188, 4, 301–2.

Moncrieff, J. (2007). 'Co-opting Psychiatry: The Alliance between Academic Psychiatry and the Pharmaceutical Industry', *Epidemiologia e Psichiatria Sociale* 16, 3, 192–6.

Moncrieff, J. (2008a). *The Myth of the Chemical Cure* (Basingstoke: Palgrave Macmillan).

Moncrieff J. (2008b). 'Neoliberalism and Biopsychiatry: A Marriage of Convenience', in C. Cohen & S. Timimi (eds) *Liberatory Psychiatry* (Cambridge: Cambridge University Press).

Moncrieff, J. & Cohen, D. (2005). 'Rethinking Models of Psychotropic Drug Action', *Psychotherapy and Psychosomatics*, 74, 3, 145–53.

Moncrieff, J. & Cohen, D. (2006). 'Do Antidepressants Cure or Create Abnormal Brain States?', *PLoS Medicine*, 3, 7. Available from: http://www.plosmedicine.org/article/info%3Adoi%2F10.1371%2Fjournal.pmed.0030240. Accessed 5 April 2010.

Moncrieff, J. & Crawford, M. J. (2001). 'British Psychiatry in the 20th Century – Observations from a Psychiatric Journal', *Social Science and Medicine*, 53, 3, 349–56.

Moncrieff, J., Hopker, S. & Thomas, P. (2005). 'Psychiatry and the Pharmaceutical Industry: Who Pays the Piper?', *Psychiatric Bulletin*, 29, 3, 84–5.

Moncrieff, J. & Timimi, S. (2010). 'Is ADHD a Valid Diagnosis in Adults? No', *British Medical Journal*, vol. 340, c547.

Moor, J. H & Tucker, G. J. (1979). 'Delusions: Analysis and Criteria', *Comprehensive Psychiatry*, 20, 4, 388–93.

Moore, D. W. (2005). *Three in Four Americans Believe in Paranormal: Little Change from Similar Results in 2001*. Available from: http://www.gallup.com/poll/16915/Three-Four-Americans-Believe-Paranormal.aspx. Accessed 13 January 2010.

Moore, M., Yuen, H. M., Dunn, N., Mullee, M. A., Maskell, J. & Kendrick, T. (2009). 'Explaining the Rise in Antidepressant Prescribing: A Descriptive Study Using the General Practice Research Database', *British Medical Journal*, 339, b3999.

Morel, B. -A. (1852) *Traite des Mentales* (Paris: Masson).

Morey, L. C. (1988). 'The Categorical Representation of Personality Disorder: A Cluster Analysis of DSM-III-R Personality Features', *Journal of Abnormal Psychology*, 97, 3, 314–21.

Morgan, M. (1998). 'Qualitative Research: Science or Pseudo-science?', *The Psychologist*, 11 (October): 481–3.

Morgan, S. & Taylor, E. (2007). Antipsychotic Drugs in Children with Autism', *British Medical Journal*, 334, 7603, 1069–70.

Morgan, C., Dazzan, P., Morgan, K., Jones, P., Harrison, G., Leff, J., Murray, R., & Fearon, P. (2006). 'First Episode Psychosis and Ethnicity: Initial Findings from the AESOP Study', *World Psychiatry*, 1, 1, 40–6.

Morris, J. B. & Beck, A. T. (1974). 'The Efficacy of Antidepressant Drugs: A Review of Research (1958–1972)', *Archives of General Psychiatry*, 30, 5, 667–74.

Morrison, A. P. (1989). *Shame: The Underside of Narcissism* (Hillsdale NJ: Analytic Press).

Morrison, A. P. (2001). 'The Interpretation of Intrusions in Psychosis: An Integrative Cognitive Approach to Hallucinations and Delusions', *Behavioural and Cognitive Psychotherapy*, 29, 3, 257–76.

Morrison, A. P., Read, J. & Turkington, D. (2005), 'Trauma and Psychosis: Theoretical and Clinical Implications', (Editorial) *Acta Psychiatrica Scandinavica*, 112, 5, 327–9.

Morrison, T. (1990). *Playing in the Dark: Whiteness and the Literary Imaginination* (London: Picador, Pan Macmillan).

Moskowitz, A. & Corstens, D. (2008). 'Auditory Hallucinations: Psychotic Symptom or Dissociative Experience?', *Journal of Psychological Trauma*, 6, 2/3, 35–63.

Moskowitz, A., Schafer, I. & Dorahy, M. J. (eds) (2008). *Psychosis, Trauma and Dissociation: Emerging Perspectives on Severe Psychopathology* (Chichester: Wiley).

Moss, B. F. J., Thigpen, C. H. & Robinson, W. P. (1953). 'Report on the Use of Succinyl Choline Dichloride (a Curare-like Drug) in Electroconvulsive Therapy', *American Journal of Psychiatry*, 109, 12, 895–8.

Moynihan, R., Heath, I. & Henry, D. (2002). 'Selling Sickness: The Pharmaceutical Industry and Disease Mongering', *British Medical Journal*, 324, 1–2, 886–91.

MTA Cooperative Group. (1999). 'A 14-month Randomised Clinical Trial of Treatment Strategies for Attention-Deficit/ Hyperactivity Disorder', *Archives of General Psychiatry*, 56, 12, 1073–86.

Mueser, K. T., Rosenberg, S. D., Goodman, L. A. & Trumbetta, S. L. (2002). 'Trauma, PTSD and the Course of Severe Mental Illness: An Interactive Model', *Schizophrenia Research*. 53, 1–2, 123–43.

Muntaner, C., Tien, A. Y., Eaton, W. W. & Garrison, R. (1991). 'Occupational Characteristics and the Occurrence of Psychotic Disorder', *Social Psychiatry and Psychiatric Epidemiology*, 26: 6, 273–80.

Mytas, N. (2009). 'Clinical and Neurological Differentiation in ADHD', *ADHD in Practice*, 1, 6, 22–3.

Nagel, T. (1986). *The View from Nowhere* (Oxford: Oxford University Press).

Nardil advertisement (1960). *American Journal of Psychiatry*, March, XII.

Nardil advertisement (1961). *British Medical Journal*, 14 January.

National Institute for Clinical Excellence (2004). *Depression: Management of Depression in Primary and Secondary Care: Clinical Practice Guideline Number 23* (London: Author).

Newman J. & Clarke J. (2009). *Publics, Politics and Power: Changing the Public of Public Services* (London: Sage).

Newnes, C. (2001). 'Speaking Out', *Ethical Human Sciences and Services*, 3, 1, 135–42.

Newnes, C. (1991). 'ECT, the DCP and ME', *Clinical Psychology Forum*, 36, 20–4.

Newton, S. (2004). *The Global Economy 1944–2000* (London: Arnold).

Niamid Advertisement (1962). *British Medical Journal*, 27th January.

Nickel, J. (1987). 'The Contemporary Idea of Human Rights', in J. Nickel (ed.), *Making Sense of Human Rights: Philosophical Reflections on the Universal Declaration of Human Rights* (Los Angeles: University of California Press).

NIMH(E) (2003). *Personality Disorder: No Longer a Diagnosis of Exclusion* (London: Department of Health).

NIMH(E) (2004). *Breaking the Cycle of Rejection* (London: Department of Health).

NIMH(E) (2009). History of EI development in UK. Available from www.iris-initiative.org.uk/about-us/history-of-ei-development-in-uk.html. Accessed 1 April 2009.

NIMH Psychopharmacology Service Center Collaborative Study Group (1964). 'Phenothiazine Treatment in Acute Schizophrenia', *Archives of General Psychiatry*, 10: 246–61.

Norfolk, Suffolk and Cambridgeshire Strategic Health Authority (2003). *Independent Inquiry into theDeath of David Bennett* (Cambridge: Author).

Novak, M. (2008). *Report of UN Special Rapporteur on Torture and Other Cruel, Inhuman or Degrading Treatment or Punishment* A/HRC/7/3. (Geneva: United Nations).

Olafson, E. (1987). *Heidegger and the Philosophy of Mind* (New Haven CT: Yale University Press).

Oltmanns, T. F. (1988). 'Approaches to the Definition and Study of Delusions', in T. F. Oltmanns & B. A. Maher (eds) *Delusional Beliefs* (New York: Wiley).

Omi, M. & Winant, H. (1994) *Racial Formation in the United States, From the 1960s to the 1990s* (New York and London: Routledge).

Online Etymology Dictionary (2010). *Paranoia*. Available from: http://www.etymonline.com/index.php?search=paranoia&searchmode=none. Accessed: 10 March 2010.

Ornitz, E. M. (1973). 'Childhood Autism: A Review of the Clinical and Experimental Literature', *California Medicine*, 118, 4, 21–47.

Os, J. van (2004). 'Does the Urban Environment Cause Psychosis?', *British Journal of Psychiatry*, 184, 4, 287–8.

Os, J. van (2009). 'A Salience Dysregulation Syndrome', *British Journal of Psychiatry*, 194, 2, 101–3.

Osofsky, J. (1999). 'The Impact of Violence on Children', *The Future of Children: Domestic Violence and Children*, 9, 3, 33–49.

Oxtoby, A., Jones, A. & Robinson, M. (1989). 'Is Your "Double-blind" Design Truly Double-blind?' *British Journal of Psychiatry*, 155, 5, 700–1.

Overall, J. E., Hollister, L. E., Meyer, F., Kimbell, I., Jr. & Shelton, J. (1964). 'Imipramine and Thioridazine in Depressed and Schizophrenic Patients: Are There Specific Antidepressant Drugs?', *Journal of the American Medical Association*, 189, 8, 605–8.

Parry, P. (2009). 'Cough Disorder: An Allegory on DSM-IV', *Medical Journal of Australia*, 191, 11/12, 674–6.

Parstellin advertisement (1962). *British Medical Journal*, 10 February.

Patel, N. (2003). 'Clinical Psychology: Reinforcing Inequalities or Facilitating Empowerment?', *International Journal of Human Rights*, 7, 1, 16–39.

Patel, N. (2007a). 'Torture, Psychology and the "War on Terror"', in R. Roberts (ed.) *Just War: Iraq and Psychology* (Ross-on-Wye: PCCS Books).

Patel, N. (2007b). 'The BPS Should do More: Science and Ethics, the Case of Psychology', *Science and Public Affairs*, 11 March. Patel, N. (2007c). 'The Prevention of Torture: A Role for Clinical Psychologists?', *Journal of Critical Psychology, Counselling and Psychotherapy*, 7, 4, 229–46.

Paterson, A. S. (1963). *Electrical and Drug Treatments in Psychiatry* (London: Elsevier).

Paul, A. M. (2004). *The Cult of Personality Testing* (New York: Free Press).

Pellegrino, E. D. (1979). 'The Socio-cultural Impact of Twentieth Century Therapeutics', in M. J. Vogel & C. E. Rosenberg (eds) *The Therapeutic Revolution*. (Philadelphia, PA: University of Pennsylvania Press).

Perry, J. C. & Klerman, G. L. (1978). 'The Borderline Patient: A Comprehensive Analysis of Four Sets of Diagnostic Criteria', *Archives of General Psychiatry*, 35, 2, 141–50.

Peters, E. R., Joseph, S. A. & Garety, P. (1999a). 'Measurement of Delusional Ideation in the Normal Population: Introducing the PDI (Peters et al. Delusions Inventory)', *Schizophrenia Bulletin*, 25, 3, 553–76.

Peters, E., Day, S., McKenna, J. & Orbach, G. (1999b). 'Delusional Ideation in Religious and Psychotic Populations', *British Journal of Clinical Psychology*, 38, 1, 83–96.

Peters, E. R. (2001). 'Are Delusions on a Continuum? The Case of Religious and Delusional Beliefs', in I. Clarke (ed.) (2001) *Psychosis and Spirituality: Exploring the New Frontier* (London: Whurr).

Peters, E., Joseph, S., Day, S. & Garety, P. (2004). 'Measuring Delusional Ideation: The 21-Item Peters et al. Delusions Inventory (PDI)', *Schizophrenia Bulletin*, 30, 4, 1005–22.

Petrie, A. A. W. (1945). 'Psychiatric Developments: The Presidential Address Delivered at the One Hundred and Third Annual Meeting of The Association on Wednesday, 29th November, 1944', *British Journal of Psychiatry*, 91, 384, 267–80.

Philipp, M., Kohnen, R. & Hiller, K. O. (1999). 'Hypericum Extract Versus Imipramine or Placebo in Patients with Moderate Depression: Randomised Multicentre Study of Treatment for Eight Weeks', *British Medical Journal*, 319, 7224, 1534–9.

Pick, D. (1989). *Faces of Degeneration: A European Disorder, c. 1848–c. 1918.* (Cambridge: Cambridge University Press).

Pidd, H. (2009). 'They Quote you Larkin, Your Appeal Court Judges', *The Guardian*, 30 April. Available from: http://www.guardian.co.uk/uk/2009/apr/30/divorce-judge-philip-larkin. Accessed 16 March 2010.

Pilgrim, D. (2001). 'Disordered Personalities and Disordered Concepts', *Journal of Mental Health*, 10, 3, 253–65.

Pilgrim, D. (2007). 'The Survival of Psychiatric Diagnosis', *Social Science & Medicine*, 65, 3, 536–47.

Pilgrim, D. & Bentall, R. P. (1999). 'The Medicalisation of Misery: A Critical Realist Approach to the Concept of Depression', *Journal of Mental Health*, 8, 3, 261–74.

Pilgrim, D. & Rogers, A. (2005). 'Editorial: Social Psychiatry and Sociology', *Journal of Mental Health*, 14, 4, 317–20.

Pinfold, V. (2005). 'Letter to the Editor as Spokesperson for Rethink', *The Guardian*, 4 November.

Pollack, W. (1998). *Real Boys* (New York: Henry Holt).

Pope, K. & Gutheil, T. (2009). 'The Interrogation of Detainees: How Doctors' and Psychologists' Ethical Policies Differ', *British Medical Journal*, 338, 61653, 1178–80.

Popper, K. (1963). *Conjectures and Refutations: The Growth of Scientific Knowledge* (London: Routledge and Keegan Paul).

Porter, A. M. W. (1970). 'Depressive Illness in a General Practice: A Demographic Study and a Controlled Trial of Imipramine', *British Medical Journal*, 1, 5699, i, 773–8.

Porter, R. (1997). *The Greatest Benefit to Mankind: A Medical History of Humanity from Antiquity to the Present* (London: Harper Collins).

Powell, F. (2007). *The Politics of Civil Society: Neoliberalism or Social Left?* (Bristol: Policy Press).

Prien, R., Caffery, E. & Kett, C. (1974). 'Factors Associated With Treatment Success in Lithium Carbonate Prophylaxis: Report of the Veterans Administration and National Institute of Mental Health Collaborative Study Group', *Archives of General Psychiatry*, 31, 189–92.

Priest, R. G., Vize, C., Roberts, A., Roberts, M. & Tylee, A. (1996). 'Lay People's Attitudes to Treatment of Depression: Results of Opinion Poll for Defeat Depression Campaign Just before Its Launch', *British Medical Journal*, 313, 7601, 858–9.

Rabkin, J. G., Markowitz, J. S., Stewart, J., McGrath, P., Harrison, W., Quitkin, F. M. & Klein, D. F. (1986). 'How Blind is Blind? Assessment of Patient and Doctor Medication Guesses in a Placebo-controlled Trial of Imipramine and Phenelzine', *Psychiatry Research*, 19, 1, 75–86.

Raitt, F. E. & Zeedyk, M. S. (2000). *The Implicit Relation of Psychology and Law: Women and Syndrome Evidence* (London: Routledge).

Rapley, M. (2011). 'Ethnomethodology/Conversation Analysis', in D. Harper & A. R. Thompson (eds) *Qualitative Research Methods in Mental Health & Psychotherapy: A Guide for Students & Practitioners* (Basingstoke: Palgrave Macmillan).

Rapley, M., McCarthy, D. & McHoul, A. (2003). 'Mentality or Morality? Membership Categories, Multiple Meanings and Mass Murder', *British Journal of Social Psychology*, 42, 3, 427–44.

Rapley, M. & McHoul, A. (2004). 'Paying Attention', *Meanjin*, 63, 4, 60–7.

Rasmussen, N. (2006). 'Making the First Antidepressant: Amphetamine in American Medicine 1929–1950', *Journal of the History of Medicine and Allied Sciences*, 61, 3, 288–23.

Raune, D., Kuipers, E. & Bebbington, P. E. (2004). 'Expressed Emotion at First-episode Psychosis: Investigating a Carer Appraisal Model', *British Journal of Psychiatry*, 184, 4, 321–6.

Read, J. (1997). 'Child Abuse and Psychosis: A Literature Review and Implications for Professional Practice', *Professional Psychology: Research and Practice*, 28, 5, 448–56.

Read, J. (2002). *Abuse 'Triggers' Schizophrenia*. Available from: www.namiscc.org/newsletters/January02/AbuseAndSchizophrenia.htm. Accessed 31 March 2010.

Read, J. (2005). 'The Bio-bio-bio Model of Madness', *The Psychologist*, 18, 10, 596–7.

Read, J., Agar, K., Argyle, N. & Aderhold, V. (2003). 'Sexual and Physical Abuse During Childhood and Adulthood as Predictors of Hallucinations, Delusions and Thought Disorder', *Psychology and Psychotherapy: Theory, Research and Practice*, 76, 1, 1–22.

Read, J., Goodman, L., Morrison, A. P., Ross, C. A. & Aderhold, V. (2004a). 'Childhood Trauma, Loss and Stress', in J. Read, L. R. Mosher & R. P. Bentall (eds) *Models of Madness: Psychological, Social and Biological Approaches to Schizophrenia* (Hove: Routledge).

Read, J. & Gumley, A. (2008). 'Can Attachment Theory Help Explain the Relationship between Childhood Adversity and Psychosis?', *Attachment*, 2, 1, 1–35.

Read, J. & Hammersley, P. (2006). 'Can Very Bad Childhoods Drive Us Crazy? Science, Ideology and Taboo', in J. Johanssen, B. Martindale & J. Cullberg (eds) *Evolving Psychosis* (London: Routledge).

Read, J. & Haslam, N. (2004). 'Public Opinion: Bad Things Happen and Can Drive You Crazy', in J. Read., L. Mosher, & R. P. Bentall, (eds) *Models of Madness* (Hove: Brunner-Routledge).

Read, J. & Ross, C. A. (2003). 'Psychological Trauma and Psychosis: Another Reason Why People Diagnosed Schizophrenic Must Be Offered Psychological Therapies', *Journal of the American Academy of Psychoanalytic and Dynamic Psychiatry*, 31, 1, 247–68.

Read, J., Rudegeair, T. & Farrelly, S. (2006). 'Relationship between Child Abuse and Psychosis', in W. Larkin and A. P. Morrison (eds) *Trauma and Psychosis: New Directions for Theory and Therapy* (London: Routledge).

Read, J., Seymour, F. & Mosher, L. R. (2004b). 'Unhappy Families', in J. Read, L. R. Mosher & R. P. Bentall (eds) *Models of Madness: Psychological, Social and Biological Approaches to Schizophrenia* (Hove: Routledge).

Read, J., van Os, J., Morrison, A. P. & Ross, C. A. (2005). 'Childhood Trauma, Psychosis and Schizophrenia: A Literature Review with Theoretical and Practical Implications', *Acta Psychiatrica Scandinavica*, 112, 5, 330–50.

Reich, W. (1928). 'Character Analysis', *Internationale Zeitschrift für Psychoanalyse*, 14, 180–96.

Reiser, D. E. & Levenson, H. (1984). 'Abuses of the Borderline Diagnosis: A Clinical Problem with Teaching Opportunities', *American Journal of Psychiatry*, 141, 12, 1528–32.

Rhodes, J. E. & Jakes, S. (2000). 'Correspondence between Delusions and Personal Goals: A Qualitative Analysis', *British Journal of Medical Psychology*, 73, 2, 211–25.

Ribot, T. (1885). *Les Maladies de la Personnalité* (Paris: Alcan).

Rimke, H. & Hunt, A. (2002). 'From Sinners to Degenerates: The Medicalization of Morality in the c19th', *History of the Human Sciences*, 15, 1, 59–88.

Ritalin advertisement (1964). *British Medical Journal*, 24 October.

Roberts, G. (1991). 'Delusional Belief Systems and Meaning in Life: A Preferred Reality?', *British Journal of Psychiatry*, 159 (suppl. 14), 19–28.

Roffe D. & Roffe, C. (1995). 'Madness and Care in the Community: A Medieval Perspective', *British Medical Journal*, 311, 7021, 1708–12.

Rogers, A. & Pilgrim, D. (1997). The Contribution of Lay Knowledge to the Understanding and Promotion of Mental Health', *Journal of Mental Health*, 6, 23–36.

Rogers, A. & Pilgrim, D. (2003). *Mental Health and Inequality* (Basingstoke: Palgrave Macmillan).

Rogers, A. and Pilgrim, D. (2010) *A Sociology of Mental Health and Illness*, 4th edn (Maidenhead: Open University Press).

Romme, M. (2000). *Redefining Hearing Voices*. Available from: http://www. psychminded.co.uk/critical/marius.htm. Accessed 11 April 2010.

Romme, M. & Escher, S. (1989a). 'Hearing Voices', *Schizophrenia Bulletin*, 15, 2, 209–16.

Romme, M. & Escher, S. (1989b). 'Effects of Mutual Contacts from People with Auditory Hallucinations', *Perspectief*, 3, 37–43.

Romme, M. & Escher, S. (1990). 'Heard but Not Seen', *Open Mind*, 49, 16–18.

Romme, M. & Escher, S. (1993). *Accepting Voices* (London: MIND).

Romme, M. & Escher, S. (2000). *Making Sense of Voices* (London: MIND).

Romme, M., Escher, A., Dillon, J., Corstens, D. & Morris, M. (2009). *Living with Voices* (Ross-on-Wye: PCCS Books).

Ronson, J. (2001). *Them: Adventures with Extremists* (London: Picador).

Rose, N. (nd). *Power and Subjectivity: Critical History and Psychology*. Available from: http://www.academyanalyticarts.org/rose1.htm. Accessed 14 July 2010.

Rose, N. (1990). *Governing the Soul: The Shaping of the Private Self* (London: Routledge).

Rose, N. (1998). *Governing the Soul: The Shaping of the Private Self* (Cambridge: Cambridge University Press).

Rose, N. (1996a). *Inventing Our Selves: Psychology, Power and Personhood* (Cambridge: Cambridge University Press).

Rose, N. (1996b). 'Psychiatry as a Political Science: Advanced Liberalism and the Administration of Risk', *History of the Human Sciences*, 9, 2, 1–23.

Rose, N. (1996c). 'Power and Subjectivity: Critical History and Psychology', in C. F. Graumann & K. J. Gergen, (eds) *Historical Dimensions of Psychological Discourse* (Cambridge: Cambridge University Press).

Rose, N. (2003). 'Neurochemical Selves', *Society*, 41, 1, 46–59.

Rose, N. (2004). 'Becoming Neurochemical Selves', in N. Stehr (ed.) *Biotechnology, Commerce and Civil Society* (New Brunswick, NJ: Transaction Publishers).

Rose, S., Lewontin, R. C. & Kamin, L. J. (1984). *Not In Our Genes: Biology, Ideology and Human Nature* (New York: Pantheon).

Rosenberg, C. E. (1977). 'The Therapeutic Revolution: Medicine, Meaning and Social Change in 19th Century America', *Perspectives in Biological Medicine*, 20, 4, 485–506.

Rosenberg, C. E. (1986). 'Disease and Social Order in America: Perceptions and Expectations', *Milbank Quarterly*, 64 (suppl. 1), 34–55.

Rosenhan, D. L. (1973). 'On Being Sane in Insane Places', *Science*, 179, 70, 250–8.

Ross, C., Anderson, G. & Clark, P. (1994). 'Childhood Abuse and Positive Symptoms of Schizophrenia', *Hospital and Community Psychiatry*, 45, 5, 489–91.

Ross, C. E., Mirowsky, J. & Pribesh, S. (2001). 'Powerlessness and the Amplification of Threat: Neighbourhood Disadvantage, Disorder and Mistrust', *American Sociological Review*, 66, 4, 568–91.

Royal College of Psychiatrists (2004). 'Good Parenting: Factsheet for Parents and Teachers', *Mental Health and Growing Up Factsheet 2* (London: Author).

Rushton P. (1988). 'Lunatics and Idiots: Mental Disability, the Community, and the Poor Law in North-east England, 1600—1800', *Medical History*, 32, 1, 34–50.

Russell, M. A. H. (1976). 'What is Dependence?', in G. Edwards, et al. (eds) *Drugs and Drug Dependence* (Westmead: Saxon House).

Ryle, G. (1948). *The Concept of Mind* (London: Hutchinson).

Sacks, H. (1992). *Lectures on Conversation* 2 vols. Edited by G. Jefferson with introductions by E. A. Schegloff (Oxford: Basil Blackwell).

Sadler, W. S. (1953). *Practice of Psychiatry* (London: Henry Kimpton).

Sampson, E. E. (1981). 'Cognitive Psychology as Ideology', *American Psychologist*, 36, 7, 730–43.

SANE (2002). In 'Abuse "Triggers Schizophrenia" Claim NZ Psychologists', available from: http://www.psychminded.co.uk/news/news2002/0102/abuse. htm. Accessed 09 August 2011.

Sarbin, T. R. (1990). 'Metaphors of Unwanted Conduct: A Historical Sketch', in D. W. Leary (ed.) *Metaphors in the History of Psychology* (New York: Cambridge University Press).

Sarbin, T. R. & Mancuso, J. C. (1970). 'Failure of a Moral Enterprise: Attitudes of the Public Toward Mental Illness', *Journal of Consulting and Clinical Psychology*, 35, 2, 159–73.

Sarbin, T. R. & Mancuso, J. C. (1980). *Schizophrenia: Medical Diagnosis or Moral Verdict?* (New York: Pergamon).

Sargant, W. & Slater, E. (1944). *An Introduction to Physical Methods of Treatment in Psychiatry* (Edinburgh: Churchill Livingstone).

Sartre, J.-P. (1944/1989). *No Exit and Three Other Plays*, trans. S. Gilbert: No Exit/ Huis Clos, pp. 1–46 (New York: Vintage).

Saroten advertisement (1962a). *British Medical Journal*, 13 January.

Saroten advertisement (1962b). *British Medical Journal*, 7 July.

Schachter, H., Pham, B., King, J., Langford, S. & Moher, D. (2001). 'How Efficacious and Safe is Short-acting Methylphenidate for the Treatment of Attention-Deficit Disorder in Children and Adolescents? A Meta-analysis', *Canadian Medical Association Journal*, 165, 11, 1475–88.

Schaler, J. (2004). 'Introduction', in J. Schaler, (ed.) *Szasz under Fire: The Psychiatric Abolitionist Faces his Critics* (Chicago: Open Court).

Sharfstein, S. (2006). 'New Task Force Will Address Early Childhood Violence', *Psychiatric News*, 41, 3, 3.

Schatzberg, A. F., Haddad, P., Kaplan, E. M., Lejoyeux, M., Rosenbaum, J. F., Young, A. H. & Zajecka, J. (1997). 'Serotonin Reuptake Inhibitor Discontinuation Syndrome: A Hypothetical Definition. Discontinuation Consensus Panel', *Journal of Clinical Psychiatry*, 58 (suppl. 7), 5–10.

Scheff, T. (1984). *Being Mentally Ill: A Sociological Theory* 2nd edn (New York: Aldine).

Schneider K. (1923/1958). *Psychopathic Personalities* (Vienna: Deuticke). Trans. M. W. Hamilton (London: Cassell).

Schütz, A. (1962). *Collected Papers, Vol. I: The Problem of Social Reality* (The Hague: Martinus Nijhoff).

Scull, A. (1979). *Museums of Madness: The Social Organization of Insanity in Nineteenth Century England* (London: Allen Lane).

Scull, A., Mackenzie, C. & Hervey, N. (1996). *Masters of Bedlam: The Transformation of the Mad-doctoring Trade* (Princeton NJ: Princeton University Press).

Seddon, T. (2008). 'Dangerous Liaisons: Personality Disorder and the Politics of Risk', *Punishment Society*, 10, 3, 301–17.

Seidenberg, R. & Decrow, K. (1983). *Women Who Marry Houses: Panic and Protest in Agoraphobia* (London: McGraw Hill).

Senior, P. R. & Bhopal, R. (1994). 'Ethnicity as a Variable in Epidemiological Research', *British Medical Journal*, 309, 6950, 327–30.

Seu, I. B. (1998). 'Shameful Women: Accounts of Withdrawal and Silence', in K. Henwood, C. Griffin, & A. Phoenix (eds) *Standpoints and Differences: Essays in the Practice of Feminist Psychology* (London: Sage).

Shapiro, A. K. & Shapiro, E. (1997). *The Powerful Placebo: From Ancient Priest to Modern Physician* (Baltimore: Johns Hopkins University Press).

Sharfstein, S. S. (2005). 'Big Pharma and American Psychiatry: The Good, the Bad, and the Ugly', *Psychiatric News*, 40, 16, 19 August.

Shaw, G. B. (1908/1987). *The Doctor's Dilemma* (Harmondsworth: Penguin).

Shaw, C. & Proctor, G. (2005). 'Women at the Margins: A Critique of the Diagnosis of Borderline Personality Disorder', *Feminism & Psychology*, 15, 4, 483–90.

Shea, S., Turgay, A., Carroll, A., Schulz, M. & Orlik, M. (2004). 'Risperidone in the Treatment of Disruptive Behavioral Symptoms in Children with Autistic and Other Pervasive Developmental Disorders', *Pediatrics*, 114, 5, 634–41.

Shepherd, M. (1994). 'Neurolepsis and the Psychopharmacological Revolution: Myth and Reality', *History of Psychiatry*, 5, 17 (Pt 1), 89–96.

Shorter, E. (1997). *A History of Psychiatry: From the Era of the Asylum to the Age of Prozac* (New York: Wiley).

Skodol, A. E., Gunderson, J. G., Pfohl, B., Widiger, T. A., Livesley, W. J. & Siever, L. J. (2002). 'The Borderline Diagnosis 1: Psychopathology, Comorbidity, and Personality Structure', *Biological Psychiatry*, 51, 12, 936–50.

Smail, D. (2005). *Power, Interest and Psychology: Elements of a Social Materialist Understanding of Distress* (Ross-on-Wye: PCCS Books).

Smail, D. (2001). *The Nature of Unhappiness* (London: Constable and Robinson).

Smiley, T. (2001). *Clinical Psychology and Religion: A Survey of the Attitudes and Practices of Clinical Psychologists in South East England* (Unpublished Psych. D thesis: University of Surrey).

Smith, D. B. (2007). 'Can You Live With the Voices in Your Head?', *New York Times*, 25 March.

Social Surveys/Gallup Poll Ltd (1994). 'Lying', *Gallup Political and Economic Index*, 404, 24.

Social Surveys/Gallup Poll Ltd. (1995). 'Paranormal Behaviour', *Gallup Political Index*, 415, 24.

Social Surveys/Gallup Poll Ltd. (1997). 'Trust in People', *Gallup Political Index*, 437, 26.

Sommers, C. H. (2000). *The War Against Boys* (New York: Simon and Schuster).

Sontag, S. (1979). *Illness as Metaphor* (London: Allen Lane).

Sontag, S. (1989). *AIDS and Its Metaphors* (London: Allen Lane).

Special Hospitals Service Authority (SHSA) (1993). *Report of the Committee of Inquiry into the Death in Broadmoor Hospital of Orville Blackwood and a Review of the Deaths of Two Other Afro-Caribbean Patients: 'Big, Black and Dangerous?'* Chairman Professor H. Prins (London: Author).

Speed, E. (2002). Irish Mental Health Social Movements: A Consideration of Movement Habitus', *Irish Journal of Sociology*. 11, 1, 61–80.

Speed, E. (2006). 'Patients, Consumers and Survivors: A Case Study of Mental Health Service User Discourses', *Social Science & Medicine*, 62, 1, 28–38.

Speed, E. (2007). 'Discourses of Consumption or Consumed by Discourse? A Consideration of What "Consumer" Means to the Service User', *Journal of Mental Health*, 16, 3, 307–18.

Speed, E. (2010). Applying Soft Bureaucracy to Rhetorics of Choice: UK NHS 1983–2007 in S. Clegg, M. Harris and H. Höpfl (eds) *Managing Modernity: The End of Bureaucracy?* (Oxford: Oxford University Press).

Speed, E. (forthcoming). 'Applying Soft Bureaucracy to Rhetorics of Choice: UK NHS 1983–2007', in S. Clegg, M. Harris and H. Höpfl (forthcoming) (eds) *Managing Modernity: Beyond Bureaucracy?* (Oxford: Oxford University Press).

Spencer, E., Birchwood, M. & McGovern D. (2001). 'Management of First-episode Psychosis', *Advances in Psychiatric Treatment*, 7, 2, 133–42.

Spinoza, B. de (1677/1996). *Ethics* trans. E. Curley. (London: Penguin).

Spitzer, E. (2004). Major Pharmaceutical Firm Concealed Drug Information: GlaxoSmithKline misled doctors about the safety of drug used to treat depression in children. *Press Release: Office of the New York State Attorney General, 2 June 2004*. Available from: http://www.oag.state.ny.us/press/2004/jun/jun2b_04.html.

Spitzer, M. (1995). 'Conceptual Developments in the Neurosciences Relevant to Psychiatry', *Current Opinion in Psychiatry*, 8, 5, 317–29.

Spitzer, R. L. (1975). 'On Pseudoscience in Science, Logic in Remission, and Psychiatric Diagnosis: A Critique of Rosenhan's "On Being Sane inInsane Places"'. *Journal of Abnormal Psychology*, 84, 5, 442–52.

Stagnitti, M. (2005). *Antidepressant Use in the US Civilian Non-Institutionalised Population, 2002*. Statistical Brief #77 (Rockville, MD: Medical Expenditure Panel, Agency for Healthcare Research and Quality).

Stastny, P. & Lehmann, P. (eds). (2007). *Alternatives Beyond Psychiatry* (Shrewsbury: Lehmann Publications).

Stewart, M., Brown, J. B., Weston, W. W., McWhinney, I. R., McWilliam, C. L. & Freeman, T. R. (2003). *Patient-centred Medicine: Transforming the Clinical Method* 2nd edn (Abingdon: Radcliffe Medical Press).

Stone, A. A. (1990). 'Law, Science, and Psychiatric Malpractice: A Response to Klerman's Indictment of Psychoanalytic Psychiatry', *American Journal of Psychiatry*, 147, 4, 419–27.

Stoppard, J. M. (2000). *Understanding Depression: Feminist Social Constructionist Approaches* (London: Routledge).

Such, E. & Walker, R. (2005). 'Young Citizens or Policy Objects? Children in the "Rights and Responsibilities" Debate', *Journal of Social Policy*, 34, 39–57.

Summerfield, D. (1999). 'A Critique of Seven Assumptions Behind Psychological Trauma Programmes in War-affected Areas', *Social Science & Medicine*, 48, 10, 1449–62.

Summerfield, D. (2001). 'The Invention of Post Traumatic Stress Disorder and the Social Usefulness of a Psychiatric Category', *British Medical Journal*, 322, 7278, 95–8.

Sveaass, N. (2007). 'Destroying Minds: Psychological Pain the Crime of Torture', *New York City Law Review*, 11, 1, 303.

Svrakic, D., Lecic-Tosevski, D. & Divac-Jovanovic, M. (2009). DSM Axis II: Personality Disorders or Adaptation Disorders? *Current Opinion in Psychiatry*, vol. 29, 111–17.

Swazey, J. (1974). *Chlorpromazine in Psychiatry* (Cambridge, MA: MIT Press).

Szasz, T. (1960). 'The Myth of Mental Illness', *American Psychologist*, 15, 2, 113–8.

Szasz, T. (1961/1974). *The Myth of Mental Illness: Foundations of a Theory of Personal Conduct* Revised edition (New York: Harper Collins).

Szasz, T. (1976). 'Schizophrenia: The Sacred Symbol of Psychiatry', *British Journal of Psychiatry*, 129, 4, 308–16.

Szasz, T. (2007). *The Medicalization of Everyday Life* (New York: Syracuse University Press).

Szwed, J. F. (1998). *Space is the Place: The Lives and Times of Sun Ra* (Cambridge, MA: Da Capo Press).

Teasdale, J. D. (1985). 'Psychological Treatments for Depression: How Do They Work?', *Behaviour Research & Therapy*, 23, 2, 157–65.

Teroni, F. & Deonna, J. A. (2008). 'Differentiating Shame from Guilt', *Consciousness and Cognition*, 17, 3, 725–40.

Tew, J. (ed.) (2005). *Social Perspectives in Mental Health: Developing Social Models to Understand and Work with Mental Distress* (London: Jessica Kingsley).

The Chambers Dictionary (2003). (Edinburgh: Chambers Harrap).

The National Institute of Mental Health Psychopharmacology Service Center Collaborative Study Group (1964). 'Phenothiazine Treatment in Acute Schizophrenia', *Archives of General Psychiatry*, 10, 3, 246–58.

Thomas, P. & May, R. (2005). *Basic Information About Medication* (Manchester: Hearing Voices Network).

Thomas, A. & Sillen, S. (1972) *Racism and Psychiatry* (New York: Brunner-Mazel).

Thomson, R. (1982). 'Side Effects and Placebo Amplification', *British Journal of Psychiatry*, 140, 1, 64–8.

Thornicroft, G. (2006). *Shunned: Discrimination against People with Mental Illness* (Oxford: Oxford University Press).

Tienari, P. (1991). 'Interaction between Genetic Vulnerability and Family Environment: The Finnish Adoption Study of Schizophrenia', *Acta Psychiatrica Scandinavica*, 84, 5, 460–5.

Tienari, P., Wynne, L. C., Moring, I. L., Naarala, M., Sori, A., Wahlberg, K. E., Saarento, O., Seitamaa, M., Kaleva, M. & Läksy, K. (1994). 'The Finnish Adoptive Study of Schizophrenia: Implications for Family Research', *British Journal of Psychiatry*, 164 (SUPPL. 23), 20–6.

Tilly, C. (2004). *Social Movements, 1768–2004* (Boulder, CO: Paradigm).

Timimi, S. (2002). *Pathological Child Psychiatry and the Medicalization of Childhood* (London: Brunner-Routledge).

Timimi, S. (2004). Rethinking Childhood Depression', *British Medical Journal*, 329, 7479, 1394–6.

Timimi, S. (2005). *Naughty Boys: Anti-social Behaviour, ADHD, and the Role of Culture* (Basingstoke: Palgrave Macmillan).

Timimi, S. (2006). 'Childhood Depression?', in S. Timimi & B. Maitra (eds) *Critical Voices in Child and Adolescent Mental Health* (London: Free Association Books).

Timimi, S. (2007). *Misunderstanding ADHD: The Complete Guide for Parents to Alternatives to Drugs* (Milton Keynes: Author).

Timimi, S. (2008). 'Child Psychiatry and Its Relationship to the Pharmaceutical Industry: Theoretical and Practical Issues', *Advances in Psychiatric Treatment*, 14, 1, 3–9.

Timimi, S. & Leo, J. (eds) (2009). *Rethinking ADHD: From Brain to Culture* (Basingstoke: Palgrave Macmillan).

Timimi, S. & Maitra, B. (eds) (2006). *Critical Voices in Child and Adolescent Mental Health* (London: Free Association Books).

Timimi, S. & Radcliffe, N. (2005). 'The Rise and Rise of ADHD', in C. Newnes and N. Radcliffe (eds) *Making and Breaking Children's Lives* (Ross on Wye: PCCS Books).

Tofranil advertisement (1961). *British Medical Journal*, 14 January.

Townsend, A., Hunt, K. & Wyke, S. (2003). 'Managing Multiple Morbidity in Mid-life: A Qualitative Study of Attitudes to Drug Use', *British Medical Journal*, 327, 7419, 837–40.

Tryptizol advertisement (1964). *British Medical Journal*, 12 September.

Uslaner, E. (2002). *The Moral Foundations of Trust* (Cambridge: Cambridge University Press).

Ussher, J. (1991). *Women's Madness: Misogyny or Mental Illness?* (Hemel Hempstead: Harvester Wheatsheaf).

van der Kolk, B. (2005). 'Child Abuse & Victimization', *Psychiatric Annals*, 35, 5, 374–8.

van Os, J., Hanssen, M., Bijl, R. V. & Ravelli, A. (2000). 'Strauss (1969) Revisited: A Psychosis Continuum in the General Population?', *Schizophrenia Research*, 45, 1–2, 11–20.

van Os, J. (2004). Does the Urban Environment Cause Psychosis? *British Journal of Psychiatry*, 184: 287–8.

Vetere, A. & Cooper, J. (2005). 'Working Systemically with Family Violence: Risk, Responsibility and Collaboration', *Journal of Family Therapy*, 23, 4, 378–96.

Visser, H. M. & Van der Mast, R. C. (2005). 'Bipolar Disorder, Antidepressants and Induction of Hypomania or Mania: A Systematic Review', *World Journal of Biological Psychiatry*, 6, 4, 231–41.

Wahl, O. (1987). 'Public Versus Professional Conceptions of Schizophrenia', *Journal of Community Psychology*, 15, 2, 285–91.

Wallcraft, J. & Michaelson, J. (2001). 'Developing a Survivor Discourse to Replace the 'Psychopathology' of Breakdown and Crisis', in C. Newnes, G. Holmes & C. Dunn (eds) *This is Madness Too: Critical Perspectives on Mental Health Services* (Ross-on-Wye: PCCS Books).

Warner, R. (2000). *The Environment of Schizophrenia: Innovations in Practice, Policy, and Communications* (London: Brunner-Routledge).

Waters, M. (1996). 'Human Rights and the Universalisation of Interests: Towards a Social Constructionist Approach', *Sociology*, 30, 3, 593–600.

Wedel, J. (1995). 'US Aid to Central and Eastern Europe 1990–1994: An Analysis of Aid Models and Responses', in J. Hardt & R. Kaufman (eds). *East-Central European Economies in Transition* (Washington, DC: US Government Printing Press).

Weeks, D. & James, J. (1997). *Eccentrics* (London: Phoenix).

Whitaker, R. (2002). *Mad in America* (Cambridge, MA: Perseus).

Whitaker, R. (2004). 'The Case against Anti-psychotic Drugs: A 50–year History of Doing More Harm Than Good', *Medical Hypotheses*, 62, 1, 5–13.

Whitaker, R. (2010). *Anatomy of an Epidemic: Magic bullets, Psychiatric Drugs, and the Rise of Mental Illness in America* (New York: Crown).

Whitfield, C. L., Dubeb, S. R., Felittic, V. J. & Anda, R. F. (2005). 'Adverse Childhood Experiences and Hallucinations', *Child Abuse and Neglect*, 29, 7, 797–810.

Widiger, T. A., Frances, A. J., Harris, M., Jacobsberg, L., Fyer, M. & Manning, D. (1991). 'Comorbidity among Axis II Disorders', in J. Oldham (ed.) *Personality Disorder: New Perspectives on Diagnostic Validity* (Washington, DC: American Psychiatric Press).

Wilkinson, R. & Pickett, K. (2009). *The Spirit Level: Why More Equal Societies Almost Always Do Better* (London: Penguin).

Willig, C. (1997). 'The Limitations of Trust in Intimate Relationships: Constructions of Trust and Sexual Risk Taking', *British Journal of Social Psychology*, 36, 2, 211–21.

Wilson, M. (1993). 'DSM-III and the Transformation of American Psychiatry: A History', *American Journal of Psychiatry*, 150, 3, 399–410.

Wirth-Cauchon, J. (2001). *Women and Borderline Personality Disorder: Symptoms and Stories* (New Brunswick: Rutgers University Press).

Wittgenstein, L. (1975). *On Certainty*, G. E. M. Anscombe & G. H. von Wright, eds trans. D. Paul & G. E. M. Anscombe (Oxford: Basil Blackwell).

Wolfensberger, W. (1987). *The New Genocide of Handicapped and Afflicted People* (New York: University of Syracuse).

Young, A. (1995). *The Harmony of Illusions: Inventing Post-traumatic Stress Disorder* (New Jersey: Princetown University Press).

Young, A. & Haddad, P. (2000). 'Discontinuation Symptoms and Psychotropic Drugs', *Lancet*, 355, 9210, 1184.

Zimbardo, P. (2008). *The Lucifer Effect: Understanding How Good People Turn Evil* (New York: Random House).

Zimmerman, M. (1994). 'Diagnosing Personality Disorders', *Archives of General Psychiatry*, 51, 3, 225–49.

Žižek, S. (2005). 'The Obscenity of Human Rights: Violence as Symptom', available from: http://libcom.org/library/the-obscenity-of-human-rights-violence-as-symptom. Accessed 17 September 2010.

Zubin, J. & Spring, B. (1977). 'Vulnerability – A New View of Schizophrenia', *Journal of Abnormal Psychology*, 86, 2, 103–26.

Index

Page numbers followed by **n** indicate notes. **n** is followed by chapter number, period and note number.